Information Technology

for the

Health Professions

Third Edition

Lillian Burke

Barbara Weill

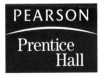

PEARSON

Prentice Hall

Upper Saddle River, New Jersey

Library of Congress Cataloging-in-Publication Data

Burke, Lillian.
    Information technology for the health professions /
Lillian Burke, Barbara Weill.—3rd ed.
        p. ; cm.
    Includes bibliographical references and index.
    ISBN-13: 978-0-13-159933-8 (alk. paper)
    ISBN-10:   0-13-159933-X (alk. paper)
    1. Medical informatics.   I. Weill, Barbara.
II. Title.
    [DNLM: 1. Medical Informatics.
2. Information Systems. W 26.5 B959i 2008]
    R858.B856 2008
    610.285—dc22   2008002675

Notice: The authors and publisher of this volume have taken care that the information and technical recommendation contained herein are based on research and expert consultation, and are accurate and compatible with the standards generally accepted at the time of publication, Nevertheless, as new information becomes available, changes in clinical and technical practices become necessary. The reader is advised to carefully consult manufacturers' instructions and information material for all supplies and equipment before use, and to consult with a healthcare professional as necessary. This advice is especially important when using new supplies or equipment for clinical purposes. The authors and publisher disclaim all responsibility for any liability, loss, injury, or damage incurred as a consequence, directly or indirectly, of the use and application of any of the contents of this volume.

Publisher: Julie Levin Alexander
Executive Editor: Mark Cohen
Associate Editor: Melissa Kerian
Assistant Editor: Nicole Ragonese
Managing Editor for Production: Patrick Walsh
Production Liaison: Christina Zingone
Production Editor: Edith Bicknell, TexTech International
Manufacturing Manager: Ilene Sanford
Manufacturing Buyer: Pat Brown
Design Director: Jayne Conte
Cover Designer: Bruce Kenselaar
Director of Marketing: Karen Allman
Senior Marketing Manager: Harper Coles
Marketing Specialist: Michael Sirinides

Marketing Assistant: Lauren Castellano
Director, Image Resource Center: Melinda Patelli
Manager, Rights and Permissions: Zina Arabia
Manager, Visual Research: Beth Brenzel
Manager, Cover Visual Research & Permissions:
    Karen Sanatar
Image Permission Coordinator: Fran Toepfer
Composition/Full-Service Management: TexTech
    International/Edith Bicknell
Cover Illustration: Campbell Laird/SIS/
    Getty Images, Inc.
Printer/Binder: Edwards Bros.
Cover Printer: Phoenix Color, Hagerstown, MD

Credits and acknowledgments borrowed from other sources and reproduced, with permission, in this textbook appear on appropriate page within text.

Pearson Education Ltd., *London*
Pearson Education Australia Pty, Limited, *Sydney*
Pearson Education Singapore, Pte. Ltd.
Pearson Education North Asia Ltd., *Hong Kong*
Pearson Education, Canada, Inc., *Toronto*
Pearson Educación de Mexico, S.A. de C.V.
Pearson Education—Japan, *Tokyo*
Pearson Education Malaysia, Pte. Ltd.
Pearson Education, Upper Saddle River, New Jersey

10 9 8 7 6 5 4 3 2
ISBN-13: 978-0-13-159933-8
ISBN-10:   0-13-159933-X

To our families, for their inspiration, understanding, patience, faith in us, and love.

Molly and Harry, Richard, Andrea and Daniel

—L.B.

Hazel and Rob, Mike, Buffy and Jon, Joanne and Melissa and Sarah

—B.W.

Contents

CHAPTER 4 *Telemedicine*   57

CHAPTER 5 *Information Technology in Public Health*   85

CHAPTER 6 *Information Technology in Radiology*   111

CHAPTER 7 *Information Technology in Surgery—the Cutting Edge*   **133**

CHAPTER 8 *Information Technology in Pharmacy*   159

CHAPTER 9 *Information Technology in Dentistry*   187

CHAPTER 10 *Informational Resources: Computer-Assisted Instruction, Expert Systems, Health Information Online* **211**

CHAPTER 11 *Information Technology in Rehabilitative Therapies: Computerized Medical Devices, Assistive Technology, and Prosthetic Devices* **241**

Preface to the Third Edition

The third edition of *Information Technology for the Health Professions* has been expanded and updated with new information. Some of the chapters have been reorganized. Two new chapters of current interest have been added: Medical Informatics: The Health Information Technology Decade (Chapter 2) and Information Technology in Public Health (Chapter 5).

Chapter 1 is a very short introduction to computers and computer literacy. Classes with any computer background may omit this chapter. The new Chapter 2 extensively deals with medical informatics, the electronic health record, and the Health Information Technology decade (2004–2014). We are in the midst of a federally declared decade that will supposedly end with the universal use of computer systems in health care. These systems would be dependable, secure, and fully interoperable by 2014. A shortened Chapter 3 deals with issues of administration, accounting, and insurance in a health care environment. An expanded Chapter 4 deals with the continual development of telemedicine.

A new Chapter 5 examines the role of computers in public health. With new diseases challenging health care systems worldwide and previously conquered diseases reemerging, public health is a particularly relevant topic. Healthcare-associated infections lead to almost 100,000 deaths per year in the United States. Computers are intimately involved in public health because even to know whether an epidemic exists, counting and statistics are necessary. The issues involved in global warming are also mentioned here.

Chapter 6 deals with radiology, stressing the expansion of interventional radiology. Chapter 7, on surgery, has added sections on NASA Extreme Environment Mission Operation (NEEMO), a NASA project that attempts distance surgery in extreme environments. The Operating Room of the Future integrates on a "wall of knowledge" all the information needed for an operation; the wall includes current images, lists of personnel, and any other relevant information in real time. Chapter 8 on pharmacy includes information on new developments in biotechnology. A caution on the Food and Drug Administration (FDA) is also included, given information about FDA funding and PDUFA (Prescription Drug User Fee Act). Information from the FDA should be checked in the same way as information from any other source. The use of stem cells, with their potential for rehabilitative medicine, is mentioned. Chapter 9 examines the use of computer technology in dentistry. Chapter 10 looks at information resources made available by computers and networks. A section on the expanding use of computers in psychiatry has been added.

Computerized devices, adaptive technology, and functional electrical stimulation (FES) technology are examined in Chapter 11, which also includes a new section on computers in rehabilitative therapies. Chapter 12 is on the security and privacy of information, with emphasis on medical information. New information on the Health Insurance Portability and Accountability Act (HIPAA) has been added; the current lack of enforcement may make the law irrelevant. New threats to privacy, including the REAL ID Act, are examined. The effect of the interaction of HIPAA and the USA PATRIOT Act (Uniting and Strengthening America by Providing Appropriate Tools Required to Intercept and Obstruct Terrorism Act of 2001) on the privacy of medical records is not yet known.

A note on point of view: Over the past few years, politics and science have clashed over myriad issues including stem cell research and global warming. The debates over whether global warming is taking place and whether human action contributes to it, is not a debate within the scientific community. In each debate, we take the consensus of the scientific community as our point of view.

Lillian Burke
Barbara Weill

Reviewers

Reviewers of the Third Edition

Richard Boan, PhD
Professor, Allied Health
  Sciences
Midlands Technical College
West Columbia, South Carolina

Joseph Burke, BS, MS
Instructor, Information
  Technology
Sanford-Brown College
Fenton, Missouri

Pamela Greenstone, RHIA
Adjunct Instructor, Allied
  Health and Public Safety
Cincinnati State Technical and
  Community College
Cincinnati, Ohio

Heather Merkley, M.Ed., RHIA
Assistant Professor, Health
Weber State University
Ogden, Utah

Nancy Powell, RHIT, BS
Director/Instructor, Health
  Information Technology
South Plains College
Lubbock, Texas

Nick Thireos
Director, Medical Informatics
Rochester Institute of
  Technology
Rochester, New York

Reviewers of Previous Editions

Patt Elison-Bowers
Associate Professor, Health
  Studies
Boise State University
Boise, Idaho

Deedee McClain Smith, CDA,
  RDH, MS
Director, Dental Health
  Professions Program
York Technical College
Rock Hill, South Carolina

Diane Premeau
Director, Health Information
  Programs
Chabot College
Hayward, California

Theresa Lyn Schlabach,
  OTR/L, BCP, MA
Instructor, Occupational
  Therapy
St. Ambrose University
Davenport, Iowa

Patricia Shaw, MEd, RHIA
Associate Professor, Health
  Administrative Services
Weber State University
Ogden, Utah

R. Bruce Steinbach, RRT
Director, Respiratory Therapy
Pitt Community College
Greenville, North Carolina

Philip Vuchetich
Creighton University
Omaha, Nebraska

Deborah Weaver, RN, PhD
Associate Professor, Nursing
Valdosta State University
Valdosta, Georgia

James A. Yanci, MS, MT(ASCP),
  CLS(NCA)
Adjunct Faculty
Youngstown State University
Youngstown, Ohio

CHAPTER 1

Introduction to Information Technology—Hardware, Software, and Telecommunications

CHAPTER OUTLINE

- **Learning Objectives**
- **Information Technology and Computer Literacy**
- **Hardware and Software**
  - *Hardware*
    - Input Devices
    - Processing Hardware and Memory
    - Output Devices
    - Secondary Storage Devices
  - *Software*
    - System Software
    - Application Software
- **An Overview of Networking, Connectivity, and Telecommunications**
- **Uses of Telecommunications and Networking**
- **The Expansion of Wireless Technology: Cell Phones, Global Positioning Systems, Wi-Fi, and Personal Digital Assistants (PDAs)**
- **The Internet and the World Wide Web**
  - *Intranets/Extranets*
  - *Internet Services*
- **In the News**
- **Chapter Summary**
- **Key Terms**
- **Review Exercises**
- **Notes**
- **Additional Resources**
- **Related Web Sites**

LEARNING OBJECTIVES

Upon completion of this chapter, you will be able to

- Define information technology, computer, and computer literacy and understand their significance in today's society.
- Describe the classification of computers into supercomputers, mainframes, microcomputers, minicomputers, personal digital assistants (PDAs), and embedded computers.
- Differentiate between hardware and software and discuss the different hardware components of a computer.
- Describe the difference between system and application software, know what an operating system is, and know what various application programs are used for what tasks.
- Discuss the significance of connectivity and networking.
- Discuss the recent expansion of the uses of wireless technologies including cell phones, Global Positioning System (GPS) technology, and PDAs with Internet access.
- List the components necessary for telecommunications to take place.
- State the uses of telecommunications and networking.

INFORMATION TECHNOLOGY AND COMPUTER LITERACY

The term **information technology (IT)** includes not only the use of computers but also communications networks and computer literacy—knowledge of how to use computer technology. As in other fields, the basic tasks of gathering, allocating, controlling, and retrieving information are the same. The push to use IT in all aspects of health care, from the electronic health record (EHR) to integrated hospital information technology (HIT) systems, makes it crucial for health care professionals to be familiar with basic computer concepts. In this chapter, we will focus on computer literacy, computers, and networks. Currently, computer literacy involves several aspects. A computer-literate person knows how to make use of a computer in his or her field to make tasks easier and to complete them more efficiently, has a knowledge of terminology, and understands in a broad, general fashion what a computer is and what its capabilities are. **Computer literacy** involves knowledge of the Internet and the World Wide Web and the ability to take advantage of their resources and to critically judge the information.

A **computer** is an electronic device that accepts data (raw facts) as input, processes, or alters them in some way and produces useful information as output. A computer manipulates data by following step-by-step instructions called a **program**. The program, the data, and the information are temporarily stored in memory while processing is going on, and then permanently stored on secondary storage media for future use. Computers are accurate, fast, and reliable.

HARDWARE AND SOFTWARE

To understand the myriad uses of IT in health care, you need to familiarize yourself with computer terminology, hardware, and software applications. Every computer performs similar functions. Specific hardware is associated with each function.

Input devices take data that humans understand and digitize those data, that is, translate them into binary forms of ones and zeroes, ons and offs that the computer processes; a **processing unit** manipulates data; output devices produce information that people understand; memory and **secondary storage devices** hold information, data, and programs (Figure 1.1 ■).

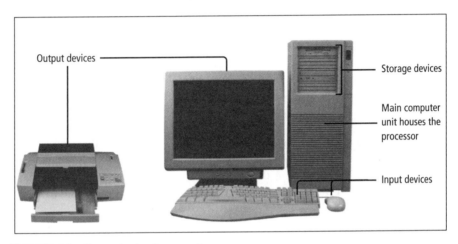

Output devices

Storage devices

Main computer unit houses the processor

Input devices

■ **FIGURE 1.1**   Computer hardware system.

Although all computers perform similar functions, they are not the same. There are several categories based on size, speed, and processing power: supercomputers are the largest and most powerful. Supercomputers are used for scientific purposes, such as weather forecasting and drug design. Supercomputers take complex mathematical data and create simulations of epidemics, pandemics, and other disasters. Mainframes are less powerful and are used in business for input/output intensive purposes, such as generating paychecks or processing medical insurance claims. Minicomputers are scaled-down mainframes; they are multiuser computers that are used by small businesses. Microcomputers (personal computers) are powerful enough for an individual's needs in word processing, spreadsheets, and database management. Small handheld computers called **personal digital assistants (PDAs)** originally could hold only a notepad, a calendar, and an address book. Today, sophisticated PDAs are used throughout the health care system. Physicians can write prescriptions on PDAs, consult online databases, and capture patient information and download it to a hospital computer. PDAs also hold reference manuals and are used in public health to gather information and help track diseases and epidemics. The **embedded computer** is a single-purpose computer on a chip of silicon, which is embedded in anything from appliances to humans. An embedded computer may help run your car, microwave, pacemaker, or watch. A chip embedded in a human being can dispense medication, among other things.

Hardware

The physical components of a computer are called **hardware**. Pieces of hardware may be categorized according to the functions each performs: input, process, output, and storage. As you recall, inside the computer, all data are represented by the **binary digits (bits)** 1 (one) and 0 (zero). To translate data into 1s and 0s is to **digitize**.

Input Devices

Input devices function to take data that people understand and translate those data into a form that the computer can process. Input devices may be divided into two categories: **keyboards** and direct-entry devices.

Direct-entry devices include pointing devices, scanning devices, smart and optical cards, speech and vision input, touch screens, sensors, and human-biology input devices.

The pointing device with which you are most familiar is the **mouse**, which you can use to position the insertion point on the screen, or make a choice from a menu. Other pointing devices are variations of the mouse. Light pens, digitizing tablets, and pen-based systems allow you to use a pen or stylus to enter data. The marks you make or letters you write are digitized.

Most **scanning devices** digitize data by shining a light on an image and measuring the reflection. Bar-code scanners read the universal product codes; optical mark recognition devices can recognize a mark on paper; optical character recognition devices can recognize letters. Special scanning equipment called magnetic ink character recognition (MICR) is used by banks to read the numbers at the bottoms of checks. You are familiar with fax machines, which scan images, digitize them, and send them over telecommunication lines. Some scanning devices, called image scanners, scan and digitize whole pages of text and graphics. One scanning device of particular interest to those with impaired eyesight is the Kurzweil scanner—hardware and software—which scans printed text and reads it aloud to the user.

Radio frequency identification (RFID) tags (input devices) are now used to identify anything from the family dog to the sponge the surgeon left in your body, by sending out radio waves. One medical insurance company is conducting a two-year trial with chronically ill patients who will have an RFID the size of a grain of rice implanted. The RFID will contain their medical histories. It transmits 30 feet without the person's knowledge.[1] In 2006, one U.S. company implanted chips in two of its employees "as a way of controlling access to a room where it holds security video footage for government agencies and police."[2]

Several different kinds of cards are used as input devices: your automated teller machine (ATM) card or charge card contains a small amount of data in the magnetic stripe. A smart card can hold more data and contains a microprocessor. Smart cards have been used as debit cards. Several states now use smart cards as driver's licenses. The card includes a biometric identifier and may include other personal information as well. Privacy advocates fear that there is so much information on the cards that they can become a target for identity thieves. An optical card holds about two thousand pages. The optical card may be used to hold your entire medical history, including test results and X-rays. If you are hospitalized in an emergency, the card—small enough to carry in your wallet—would make this information immediately available.

Vision input systems are currently being developed and refined. A computer uses a camera to digitize images and stores them. The computer "sees" by having the camera take a picture of an object. The digitized image of this object is then compared to images in storage. This technology can be used in adaptive devices, such as in glasses that help Alzheimer's patients. The glasses include a database of names and faces; a camera sees a face, and if it "recognizes" the face, it gives the wearer the name of the subject.

Speech input systems allow you to talk to your computer, and the computer processes the words as data and commands. A speech-recognition system contains a dictionary of digital patterns of words. You say a word and the speech-recognition system digitizes the word and compares the word to the words in its dictionary. If it recognizes the word, the command is executed. There are speech dictation packages tailored to specific professions. A system geared toward medicine would include an extensive vocabulary of digitized medical terms and would allow the creation of patient records and medical reports. This system can be used as an input device by physicians who, in turn, can dictate notes, even while, for example, operating. Speech recognition is also especially beneficial as an enabling technology, allowing those who do not have the use of their hands to use computers. In English, many phrases and words sound the same, for example, hyphenate and -8 (hyphen eight). Speech-recognition software allows mistakes such as these to be corrected by talking. The newest speech-recognition software does not need training and gets "smarter" as you use it. It looks at context to get homophones (to, too, two) correct.[3]

Of particular interest to health professionals are input devices called **sensors.** A sensor is a device that collects data directly from the environment and sends those data to a computer. Sensors are used to collect patient information for clinical monitoring systems, including physiological, arrhythmia, pulmonary, and obstetrical/neonatal systems. In critical care units, monitoring systems make nurses aware of any change in a patient's condition immediately. They detect the smallest change in temperature, blood pressure, respiration, or any other physiological measurement.

The newest kinds of input devices are called human-biology input devices. They allow you to use your body as an input device. They include biometrics, which are being used in security systems to protect data from unauthorized access. **Biometrics** identify people by their body parts. Biometrics include fingerprints, hand prints, face recognition, and iris scans. Once thought to be almost 100 percent accurate, biometric identification systems are now recognized as far from perfect.

Line-of-sight input allows the user to look at a keyboard displayed on a screen and indicate the character selected by looking at it. Implanted chips have allowed locked-in stroke patients (a syndrome caused by stroke where a person cannot respond, although he or she knows what is going on) to communicate with a computer by focusing brain waves (brain wave input); this is experimental; research is continuing.[4]

Processing Hardware and Memory

Once data are digitized, they are processed. Processing hardware is the brain of the computer. Located on the **main circuit board** (or **motherboard**), the **processor** or **system unit** contains the **central processing unit (CPU)** and **memory**. The CPU has two parts: the **arithmetic-logic unit**, which performs arithmetic operations and logical operations of comparing; and the **control unit**, which directs the operation of the computer in accordance with the program's instructions.

The CPU works closely with memory. The instructions of the program being executed must be in memory for processing to take place. Memory is also located on chips on the main circuit board. The part of memory where current work is temporarily stored during processing is called **random-access memory (RAM)**. It is temporary and volatile. The other part of memory is called **read-only memory (ROM)** or **firmware**; it contains basic start-up instructions, which are burned into a chip at the factory; you cannot change the contents of ROM.

Many computers have **open architecture** that allows you to add devices. The system board contains **expansion slots**, into which you can plug expansion boards for additional hardware. The board has sockets on the outside, called **ports**. You can plug a cable from your new device into the port. The significance of open architecture is the fact that it enables you to add any hardware and software interfaces to your existing computer system. This means you can not only expand the memory of your computer but also add devices that make your computer more amenable to uses in medicine. **Expansion boards** also allow the use of virtual reality simulators, which help in teaching certain procedures.

Output Devices

Once data are processed, **output devices** translate the language of bits into a form humans can understand. Output devices are divided into two basic categories: those that produce **hard copy**, including **printers** and **plotters**; and those that produce **soft (digital) copy**, including **monitors** (the most commonly used output device). Soft copy is also produced by speakers that produce speech, sound, or music.

Secondary Storage Devices

The memory we have discussed so far is temporary or volatile. To save your work permanently, you need secondary storage devices. **Magnetic disk** and magnetic tape and **optical disks** are used as secondary storage media. Magnetic media (disk, diskette, tape, and high-capacity Zip disks) store data and programs as magnetic spots or electromagnetic charges. High-capacity optical disks (**compact disks [CDs]** or **digital video disks [DVDs]**) store data as pits and lands burned into a plastic disk. **Solid-state memory devices** include flash memory cards used in notebooks, memory sticks, and very compact key chain devices; these devices have no moving parts, are very small, and have a high capacity. USB flash drives have a huge capacity for information.

Software

Software refers to the programs—the step-by-step instructions that tell the hardware what to do. Without software, hardware is useless. Software falls into two general categories: system software and application software.

System Software

System software consists of programs that let the computer manage its resources. The most important piece of system software is the operating system. The **operating system** is a group of programs that manage and organize resources of the computer. It controls the hardware, manages basic input and output operations, keeps track of your files saved on disk and in memory, and directs communication between the CPU and other pieces of hardware. It coordinates how other programs work with the hardware and with each other. Operating systems also provide the **user interface**—that is, the way the user communicates with the computer. For example, Windows provides a **graphical user interface**, pictures or icons that you click on with a mouse. When the computer is turned on, the operating system is **booted** or loaded into the computer's RAM. No other program can work until the operating system is booted.

Application Software

Application software allows you to apply computer technology to a task you need done. There are application packages for many needs.

   Word-processing software allows you to enter text for a paper, report, letter, or memo. Once the text is entered, you can format it, that is, make it look the way you want it to look. You can change the size, style, and face of the type. In addition, margins and justification can be set to any specifications. Style checkers can help you with spelling and grammar. Word-processing software also includes thesauri, headers and footers, index generators, and outlining features.

   Electronic spreadsheets allow you to process numerical data. Organized into rows and columns intersecting to form cells, spreadsheets make doing arithmetic almost fun. You enter the values you want processed and the formula that tells the software how to process them and the answer appears. If you made a mistake entering a value, just change it and the answer is **automatically recalculated**. Spreadsheet software also allows you to create graphs easily—just by indicating what cells you want graphed. Electronic health records (EHRs) can use spreadsheets to graph a series of a patient's blood values over time.

Database management software permits you to manage large quantities of data in an organized fashion. Information in a database is organized in tables. The database management software makes it easy to enter data, edit data, sort or organize data, search for data that meets a particular criterion, and retrieve data. Once the structure of the table is defined and the data entered, that data can be used for a variety of purposes without being retyped. Eye-pleasing, businesslike reports can easily be generated by simply defining their structure.

There are also specialized software packages used in specific fields such as medicine. For example, there are specialized accounting programs used in medical offices. Microsoft is considering developing a new software package for the health care industry.[5]

Communications software includes Web browsers, such as Internet Explorer. These programs allow you to connect your computer to other computers in a network.

AN OVERVIEW OF NETWORKING, CONNECTIVITY, AND TELECOMMUNICATIONS

Telecommunications form the third component of IT. The implications of telecommunications for the medical world will be more fully explored in Chapter 4. Although you can enjoy the wonders of the Internet and surf the World Wide Web with very little technical knowledge, this section introduces you to some of the complexities behind networking, connectivity, telecommunications, and the Internet and gives you a foundation for appreciating the impact of these developments on health care.

Standing alone, your computer has access only to the data and information stored on its hard drive and on the disks you insert in its disk drives. If you can connect your personal computer to a network, however, you have access to the data and information on that network as well. The fact that computers can be connected is referred to as **connectivity**. Connectivity greatly enhances the power of your computer, bringing immense stores of information to your fingertips and making it possible for you to interact with people around the world. Connectivity is the prerequisite for developing the field of telemedicine. Computers and other hardware devices that are connected form what is called a **network**. Networks come in all sizes, from small **local area networks (LANs)**, which span one room, to **wide area networks (WANs)**, which may span a state, nation, or even the globe, like the Internet and World Wide Web. Networks can be private or connected through telephone lines, making them **telecommunications networks**. Given the right mix of hardware and software, computers are connected globally.

When computers are connected, the data and information that travel between them must follow some path. There are several communications channels—either wired or wireless. Communications can be high bandwidth (broadband or high speed) or low bandwidth (slow). Most hospitals use broadband connections such as dedicated T1–T3 lines. A slow dial-up connection, however, may be used for sending e-mail and small attachments.

Bluetooth technology is used to create small personal area networks. **Bluetooth** is a wireless technology that can connect digital devices from computers to medical devices to cell phones. For example, if someone is wearing a pacemaker and has a heart attack, his or her cell phone could automatically dial 911.

Transmission is governed by sets of technical standards or rules called **protocols**. The protocols take care of how the connection is set up between devices. Protocols also establish security procedures. You do not have to think about these factors because they are embedded in the communications software. For information on standards-setting organizations, visit ConsortiumInfo.org.

■ USES OF TELECOMMUNICATIONS AND NETWORKING

The linking of computers and communications devices via telecommunications lines into networks of all sizes has made many things possible. A complete list is beyond the scope of this text. Networking allows such things as the electronic linking of health departments in a National Health Information Network for Public Health Officials. This linking permits the sharing of information, which can be important in containing potential epidemics. The successful sharing of information will only take place if the computers are interoperable.

■ THE EXPANSION OF WIRELESS TECHNOLOGY: CELL PHONES, GLOBAL POSITIONING SYSTEMS, WI-FI, AND PERSONAL DIGITAL ASSISTANTS (PDAs)

During the last few years, the use of wireless technologies has expanded. Cell phones, Global Positioning System (GPS) technology, and PDAs with Internet access have become commonplace. In places without electricity and without landlines, wireless networks using cell phones and PDAs are both bringing health information to people and gathering information to track the spread of disease. **Wi-Fi** is a wireless technology that allows you to connect, for example, a PDA (and other devices) to a network (including the Internet) if you are close enough to a Wi-Fi access point. There are currently investigations into the possibility that wireless communication poses a radiation threat.[6]

The most common wireless device is the **cell phone**. The use of GPS technology, which can pinpoint your location to within several feet, is widely available. Radio frequency identification (RFID) tags are becoming more and more common. RFID tags can be incorporated into products; they receive and send a wireless signal. By identifying doorways and other objects, these tags could be used to help people with impaired vision. They can be incorporated into sponges used in surgeries, so that sponges are not left in the patient. They could be incorporated into medication bottles, so that people could more easily locate their medications.[7]

THE INTERNET AND THE WORLD WIDE WEB

The **Internet** (short for *inter*connected *net*work) is a global network of networks, connecting innumerable smaller networks, computers, and users. It is run by a committee of volunteers; no one owns it or controls it. The Internet originated in 1969 as **ARPAnet**, a project of the Advanced Research Projects Agency of the U.S. Department of Defense. The Department of Defense was attempting to create both a national network of scientists and a communications system that could withstand nuclear attack. The network was, therefore, to be decentralized, forming a communications web with no central authority. The protocol that eventually governed ARPAnet and continues to govern the Internet today is public domain software called **transmission-control protocol/Internet protocol (TCP/IP)**. Any computer or network that subscribes to this protocol can join the Internet.

Intranets/Extranets

Private corporate or hospital networks that use the same structure as the Internet and TCP/IP protocols are called **intranets**. Software called a **firewall** is used to protect the intranet from unauthorized users. What the user sees looks like a Web page. Companies can use the intranet to distribute information to employees in an easy, attractive format, for training videos, or to post job openings. If the intranet in one organization is linked to other intranets in other organizations, it becomes an **extranet**.

Internet Services

Once you are connected, what services are available? You can access reliable, peer-reviewed medical information databases, such as MEDLINE using a search engine called **PubMed** (http://www.ncbi.nlm.nih.gov/PubMed/). MedlinePlus is a fairly reliable site for consumers of health care information. However reliable the site, the information should be reasonable and should be checked. For example, the Food and Drug Administration (FDA) can provide a great deal of health information; however, much of its drug approval project budget comes from the drug companies it regulates. Drug companies provide "more than 50 percent of the Center for Drug Evaluation's budget."[8,9] Be very careful of any information you find, whatever the source. Try to check it with another source.

You can find support groups and information on almost any disease, medication, hospital, and treatment. The information, which may or may not be accurate, can be so up to date that your physician may not even be aware of it. Internet support groups may help people cope with illness and isolation.

The **World Wide Web (WWW)** or **Web** is the part of the Internet that is most accessible and easiest to navigate. The Web is made up of information organized as documents (pages). The information on the Web is stored in files called **Web sites**. To browse the Web, you need a connection to the Internet and software called a **Web browser**. Finding what you are looking for on the Web can be challenging. If you know the address **(uniform resource locator [URL])**, you can just type it in. If you, however, are just looking for information on a particular topic, you can use a program called a **search engine**.

The Internet and Web provide an enormous amount of information—some of it reliable, some not. The lack of regulation, the freewheeling quality, is also an attraction but may bring some negative consequences. *Any* information may find its way onto the Internet, and there are no safeguards for accuracy. How do you judge the reliability of medical information on the Net? There are health Web sites that rate services. These rating services, however, are not subject to regulation or quality control either. Recognizing the difficulty of sifting through the health information and advice on the Internet, in 1997, the Federal Department of Health and Human Services created Healthfinder (http://www.healthfinder.gov), a listing of "sites 'hand-picked' . . . by health professionals." Most of the sites it recommends are "government agencies, non-profit and professional organizations, universities, libraries," although it does list a few commercial sites. Along with a listing, **Healthfinder** provides the source of the information and a summary.

The lack of regulation applies not only to speech and information but also to commerce. Web sites promote and sell worthless remedies. These sites play on fear—for example, promoting protection from severe acute respiratory syndrome (SARS), which first appeared in February 2003.

IN THE NEWS

Excerpt from, "Like Having a Secretary in Your PC"

by David Pogue

TESTING, testing, one two three. Is this thing on?

Well, I'll be darned. It's really on and it's really working. I'm wearing a head-set, talking, and my PC is writing down everything I say in Microsoft Word. I'm speaking at full speed, perfectly normally except that I'm pronouncing the punctuation (comma), like this (period).

Let's try something a little tougher. Pyridoxine hydrochloride. Antagonistic Lilliputians. Infinitesimal zithers.

Hm! Not bad.

(continued)

Excerpt from, "Like Having a Secretary in Your PC" *(continued)*

O.K., back again. The software I'm using is Dragon NaturallySpeaking 9.0 (www.nuance.com), the latest version of the best-selling speech-recognition software for Windows. This software, which made its debut Tuesday, is remarkable for two reasons.

Reason 1: You don't have to train this software. That's when you have to read aloud a canned piece of prose that it displays on the screen—a standard ritual that has begun the speech-recognition adventure for thousands of people.

I can remember, in the early days, having to read 45 minutes' worth of these scripts for the software's benefit. But each successive version of Naturally Speaking has required less training time; in Version 8, five minutes was all it took. . . .

I gave it a test. After a fresh installation of the software, I opened a random page in a book and read a 1,000-word passage—without doing any training.

The software got 11 words wrong, which means it got 98.9 percent of the passage correct. Some of those errors were forgivable, like when it heard "typology" instead of "topology." . . .

The best part is that these are the lowest accuracy rates you'll get, because the software gets smarter the more you use it—or, rather, the more you correct its errors.

You do this entirely by voice. You say, "correct 'typology,'" for example; beneath that word on the screen, a numbered menu of alternate transcriptions pops up. You see that alternate 1 is "topology," for example, so you say "choose 1." The software instantly corrects the word, learns from its mistake and deposits your blinking insertion point back at the point where you stopped dictating, ready for more. . . .

For this reason, it doesn't much matter whether or not you skip the initial training; the accuracy of the two approaches will eventually converge toward 100 percent.

NatSpeak 9 is remarkable for a second reason, too: it's a new version containing very little new.

Yes, they've eliminated the training requirement. And yes, the new NatSpeak is 20 percent more accurate than before if you do the initial training. Then again, what's a 20 percent improvement in a program that's already 99.4 percent accurate—99.5? That's maybe one less error every 1,000 words.

(Nuance has done some clever engineering to wring these additional drops of accuracy out of the program. For example, the program has always used context to determine a word's identity, taking into account the two or three words on either side of it to distinguish, say, "bear" from "bare." The company says that Version 9 scans an even greater swath of the surrounding words.). . .

CHAPTER SUMMARY

Chapter 1 introduces the reader to the concepts of IT and computer literacy and their significance. It also deals with computer hardware and software and how they interact to accept data as input, process the data, and produce information as output. This chapter familiarizes you with networking and connectivity, telecommunications, the Internet, and World Wide Web and gives you the basic information you need for appreciating the significance of these developments in medicine.

- IT includes not only computers but also communications networks and computer literacy.
- Computer literacy is knowledge of computers and their functions.
- A computer is an electronic device that can accept data as input, process the data, and produce information as output following step-by-step instructions called a program.
- Inside a digital computer, all data and information are represented by combinations of binary digits (bits).
- Physical components of a computer are called hardware.
- Input devices digitize data, so that the computer can process the data.
  - Input devices include keyboards and direct-entry devices.
  - Direct-entry devices include pointing devices, scanning devices, smart cards, optical cards, sensors, and human-biology input devices.
- The system unit includes the CPU, which is comprised of the arithmetic-logic unit and the control unit, and memory, which temporarily stores the work you are currently doing. The CPU and memory work together following the instructions of a program to process data into information.
- Output devices (printers and monitors) present the processed information to the user.
- Secondary storage devices (drives) and media (diskettes, hard disks, optical disks, Zip disks, magnetic tape, and solid-state memory devices) allow you to store information permanently.
- Software (programs) is comprised of the step-by-step instructions that tell the hardware how to process data.
- Software is classified as system software, which controls the basic operation of the hardware, and application software, which completes tasks for the user.
- When computers are connected in networks, the data that are transmitted travel over a path or medium.
- Data transmission is governed by technical standards or rules called protocols.
- Wireless transmission is becoming more and more common with the widespread use of cell phones and other wireless devices.
- The connection of computers and communications devices into networks makes many things possible, including telemedicine.
- The Internet is a global network of networks, which makes vast amounts of information available.

- The World Wide Web is part of the Internet, organized as documents with links to other documents.
- Speech-recognition software is getting better and better.

KEY TERMS

application software
arithmetic-logic unit
ARPAnet
automatically
    recalculated
binary digits (bits)
biometrics
Bluetooth
booted
cell phone
central processing unit
    (CPU)
communications
    software
compact disks (CDs)
computer
computer literacy
connectivity
control unit
database management
    software
digital video disks
    (DVDs)
digitize
direct-entry devices
electronic spreadsheets
embedded computer
expansion boards
expansion slots
extranet
firewall
firmware
graphical user interface

hard copy
hardware
Healthfinder
information
    technology (IT)
input devices
Internet
intranets
keyboards
local area networks
    (LANs)
magnetic disk
main circuit
    board (or
    motherboard)
memory
monitors
mouse
network
open architecture
operating system
optical disks
output devices
personal digital
    assistants (PDAs)
plotters
ports
printers
processing unit
processor
program
protocols
PubMed

radio frequency identi-
    fication (RFID) tags
random-access memory
    (RAM)
read-only memory
    (ROM)
scanning devices
search engine
secondary storage devices
sensor
soft (digital) copy
software
solid-state memory
    devices
system software
system unit
telecommunications
    networks
transmission-control
    protocol/Internet
    protocol (TCP/IP)
uniform resource
    locator (URL)
user interface
Web browser
Web sites
wide area networks
    (WANs)
Wi-Fi
word processing
    software
World Wide Web
    (WWW) or Web

REVIEW EXERCISES

Multiple Choice

1. A computer literate person _____.
   A. can use a computer to perform tasks in his or her field
   B. is generally familiar with what a computer can do
   C. can program a computer
   D. A and B

2. Binary digits (ones and zeroes) are used to represent _____ inside the computer.
   A. words
   B. music
   C. graphics
   D. All of the above

3. A/An _____ is a computer that can solve complex scientific equations and may be used for worldwide weather forecasting.
   A. supercomputer
   B. mainframe
   C. embedded computer
   D. microcomputer

4. A/An _____ can generate a payroll for a large business. Several hundred users can access terminals at the same time.
   A. supercomputer
   B. mainframe
   C. embedded computer
   D. microcomputer

5. The type of input device that collects data directly from the environment and sends the data to the computer is called a _____. It is used in clinical monitoring devices.
   A. scanner
   B. sensor
   C. mouse
   D. keyboard

6. Pointing devices include the _____.
   A. mouse
   B. trackball
   C. light pen
   D. All of the above

7. An input device that reads printed text aloud is the _____.
   A. keyboard
   B. mouse
   C. digitizing tablet
   D. Kurzweil scanner

8. The actual manipulation of data inside the computer is performed by the _____.
   A. input devices
   B. output devices
   C. processing unit
   D. secondary storage devices

9. Wi-Fi _____.
   A. is a wireless technology
   B. allows you to connect to the Internet
   C. Both A and B
   D. None of the above

10. In areas of the world that lack electricity and landlines, _____ bring health information and help track the spread of disease.
    A. cell phones
    B. desktop computers
    C. PDAs
    D. Only A and C

11. During the past few years, the use of _____ technology (including cell phones and PDAs) has expanded.
    A. wired
    B. wireless
    C. Both A and B
    D. None of the above

12. Standards governing communications are called _____.
    A. standards
    B. protocols
    C. conventions
    D. rules

13. The _____ is a global network that connects many smaller networks.
    A. intranet
    B. extranet
    C. Internet
    D. None of the above

14. The part of the Internet comprised of pages with hyperlinks to other pages is referred to as the _____.
    A. public information utility
    B. bulletin board system
    C. World Wide Web
    D. None of the above

15. The _____ directs the operation of the computer in accordance with the program's instructions.
    A. arithmetic-logic unit
    B. control unit
    C. printer
    D. All of the above

True/False Questions

1. Embedded computers can be embedded in humans as well as appliances. _____
2. IT includes not only computers but also networks and computer literacy. _____
3. Information from reliable sites (such as the FDA) does not need to be checked. _____
4. A computer manipulates data by following the step-by-step instructions of a program. _____
5. Hardware refers to the physical components of the computer. _____
6. Another word for hardware is programs. _____
7. Solid-state memory devices include flash memory cards. _____
8. The main circuit board of a computer is also called the motherboard. _____
9. Application software controls the basic operations of the computer hardware including input and output. _____
10. The operating system must be booted for the computer to work. _____
11. If you are using a computer to create a budget, you would need a word processing program. _____
12. The binary number system uses two digits: 0 and 1. _____
13. RFID tags can be incorporated into products; they send a wireless signal. _____
14. Hospitals may use broadband connections for real-time consultations. _____
15. You are sure to get reliable medical information from the Web. _____

Critical Thinking

1. What input devices do you foresee being used in the health care field? Comment on how such devices as sensors and speech-recognition devices are especially relevant to your discipline.
2. What measures can be taken to help assure the quality of medical information one receives over the World Wide Web?
3. Critically examine the issue of implanting RFIDs into humans.
4. Critically examine the issue of conflict of interest. Discuss the FDA. Does a conflict of interest necessarily corrupt information from the organization?

NOTES

1. Anjana Ahuja, "Doctor, I've Got This Little Lump in My Arm . . . Relax, That Tells Me Everything," timesonline.co.uk, July 24, 2006, http://www.timesonline.co.uk/tol/comment/columnists/anjana_ahuja/article691731.ece (accessed November 12, 2007).
2. Richard Waters, "U.S. Group Implants Electronic Tags in Workers," ft.com, February 12, 2006, http://www.ft.com/cms/s/2/ec414700-9bf4-11da-8baa-0000779e2340.html (accessed November 12, 2007).
3. David Pogue, "Like Having a Secretary in Your PC," nyt.com, July 20, 2006, http://www.nytimes.com/2006/07/20/technology/20pogue.html?partner=rssnyt&emc=rss (accessed November 12, 2007).
4. Jeffrey Winters, "Communicating by Brain Waves," *Psychology Today,* http://psychologytoday.com/articles/PTO-20030724-000002.html (accessed November 12, 2007).

5. Steve Lohr, "Microsoft to Offer Software for Health Care Industry," nyt.com, July 27, 2006, http://www.nytimes.com/2006/07/27/technology/27soft.html?ex=1311652800&en=2e589acf4a87ba92&ei=5090&partner=rssuserland&emc=rss (accessed November 12, 2007).

6. "WiFi could be Health Risk at Schools," PhysOrg.com, http://www.physorg.com/news96519690.html (accessed November 12, 2007).

7. John Peifer, "Mobile Wireless Technologies for Rehabilitation and Independence," *Journal of Rehabilitation Research & Development* 42, no. 2 (March/April 2005): vii–x.

8. Manette Loudon, "The FDA Exposed: An Interview with Dr. David Graham, the Vioxx Whistleblower," Newstarget.com, August 30, 2005, http://www.newstarget.com/011401.html (accessed November 12, 2007).

9. Sidney Wolfe, "How Independent Is the FDA?" *Frontline*, November 13, 2003, http:// www.pbs.org/wgbh/pages/frontline/shows/prescription/hazard/independent.html (accessed November 27, 2007).

ADDITIONAL RESOURCES

Anderson, Sandra. *Computer Literacy for Health Care Professionals.* Albany, NY: Delmar, 1992.

Austen, Ian. "A Scanner Skips the ID Card and Zeroes In on the Eyes." nyt.com, May 15, 2003. http://topics.nytimes.com/2003/05/15/technology/circuits/15howw.html (accessed August 17, 2006).

Baase, Sara. *A Gift of Fire: Social, Legal, and Ethical Issues in Computing.* Upper Saddle River, NJ: Prentice-Hall, 1996.

Beekman, George. *Computer Confluence: Exploring Tomorrow's Technology.* 5th ed. Upper Saddle River, NJ: Prentice Hall, 2002.

Bureau of Labor Statistics. *Occupational Outlook Handbook (OOH), 2006–07 Edition.* http://www. bls.gov/oco/ (accessed November 12, 2007).

Divis, Dee Ann. "Bill would Push Driver's License with Chip." March 17, 2003, *The Washington Times,* May 1, 2002.

Eisenberg, Anne. "When the Athlete's Heart Falters, a Monitor Dials for Help." nyt.com, January 9, 2003. http://query.nytimes.com/gst/fullpage.html?res=9B03E0DE113EF93AA35752C0A9659C8B63 (accessed November 12, 2007).

Evans, Alan, Kendall Martin, and Mary Anne Poatsy. *Technology in Action.* Upper Saddle River, NJ: Prentice Hall, 2006.

Feder, Barnaby. "Face-Recognition Technology Improves." nyt.com, March 14, 2003. http://query.nytimes.com/gst/fullpage.html?res=9805E0D9103EF937A25750C0A9659C8B63 (accessed November 12, 2007).

Fein, Esther B. "For Many Physicians, E-Mail is the High-Tech House Call." *The New York Times,* November 20, 1997, A1, B8.

Harmon, Amy. "U.S., in Shift, Drops Its Effort to Manage Internet Addresses." *The New York Times,* June 6, 1998, A1, D2.

Markoff, John. "High-Speed Wireless Internet Network Is Planned." nyt.com, December 6, 2002. http://query.nytimes.com/gst/fullpage.html?res=9807EEDB133BF935A35751C1A9649C8B63 (accessed November 12, 2007).

Oakman, Robert L. *The Computer Triangle.* 2nd ed. New York: Wiley, 1997.

Petersen, Melody. "A Respiratory Illness: Cashing in; The Internet Is Awash in Ads for Products Promising Cures or Protection." nyt.com, April 14, 2003, http://query.nytimes.com/gst/fullpage.html?res=950DE5DA133BF937A25757C0A9659C8B63 (accessed November 12, 2007).

Race, Tim. "What Do They Mean by Digital, Anyhow?" *The New York Times,* March 19, 1998, G11.

Senn, James A. *Information Technology in Business: Principles, Practices, and Opportunities.* 2nd ed. Upper Saddle River, NJ: Prentice Hall, 1998.

Stewart, Angela. "Health Departments will Link Up to Share Data." *Star-Ledger,* July 18, 1998.
Stewart, Angela. "A Shot-in-the-Arm Microchip could Save Your Life." nj.com, August 7, 2006. http://www.nj.com/news/ledger/jersey/index.ssf?/news/ledger/stories/microchip_0807.html (accessed November 12, 2007).
"What Is Bluetooth?" Palowireless. http://www.palowireless.com/infotooth/whatis.asp (accessed November 12, 2007).

RELATED WEB SITES

The following Web sites provide research information on medical matters. We cannot, however, vouch for the accuracy of the information.

Healthfinder.gov (http://www.healthfinder.gov), for a government listing of nonprofit and government organizations that provide you with health-related information.
HealthTouch Online (http://www.healthtouch.com), for information on medications.
MedicineOnLine (http://www.meds.com), for information on pharmaceutical and medical device companies.
OncoLink (http://www.oncolink.upenn.edu), for information on cancer.
PubMed (http://www.ncbi.nlm.nih.gov/PubMed), for access to reliable medical information databases.
U.S. National Library of Medicine (http://www.nlm.nih.gov/). Services include Health Information, MEDLINE/PubMed, MEDLINEplus, NLM Gateway, Library Services, Catalog, Databases, Historical Materials, MeSH, Publications. Description: The world's largest medical library.

CHAPTER 2

Medical Informatics: The Health Information Technology Decade

CHAPTER OUTLINE

- Learning Objectives
- Medical Informatics
- The Health Information Technology Decade
- The Health Insurance Portability and Accountability Act of 1996: A Brief Introduction
- The Patient Information Form
- The Paper Medical Record
- The Electronic Medical Record
- The Electronic Health Record
- Regional Health Information Organizations
- The Indian Health Service Electronic Health Record
- Computer Information Systems in Health Care
- Does Computerization Improve Patient Outcomes?
- The Introduction of Computer Systems
- In the News
- Chapter Summary
- Key Terms
- Review Exercises
- Notes
- Additional Resources

LEARNING OBJECTIVES

After reading this chapter, the student will be able to

- Define medical informatics.
- Define the decade of health information technology (HIT).
- Define the electronic medical record (EMR) and electronic health record (EHR) and discuss the differences between the two.
- Define interoperability.

- Define regional health information organizations (RHIOs) and discuss their role in interoperability.
- Discuss the EMR developed by the U.S. Indian Health Service.
- Describe computer information systems used in health care settings.
  - Hospital information systems (HIS)
  - Financial information systems (FIS)
  - Clinical information systems (CIS)
  - Pharmacy information systems (PIS)
  - Nursing information systems (NIS)
  - Laboratory information systems (LIS)
  - Radiology information systems (RIS)
  - Picture archiving and communication systems (PACS)
- Discuss the issues raised by several studies of the computerization of health records.
- Discuss the introduction of and resistance to computer systems in health care environments.

MEDICAL INFORMATICS

Medical informatics is a rapidly expanding discipline. It has a thirty-five year history in which it has sought to improve the way medical information is managed and organized. Medical informatics is located at the "intersection of information technology and medicine and health care."[1]

Medical informatics has many definitions. The common emphasis in all definitions is on the use of technology to organize information in health care. That information includes patient records, diagnostics, expert or decision support systems, and therapies. The stress is not on the actual application of computers in health care, but the theoretical basis. **Medical informatics** is an interdisciplinary science "underlying the acquisition, maintenance, retrieval, and application of biomedical knowledge and information to improve patient care, medical information, and health science research." The tool used to perform these tasks is the computer.[2] Medical informatics focuses on improving all aspects of health care. Some of the aspects it focuses on include improving the clarity of diagnostic images, improving image-guided and minimally invasive surgery, developing simulations that allow health care workers to improve treatments without practicing on human subjects, developing low-cost diagnostic tests, treating physical handicaps, providing consumers with information, coordinating international medical reporting, developing and improving information systems used in health care settings, and developing decision-support systems.

There are several subspecialties of medical informatics. A few are bioinformatics that uses computers to solve biological problems; dental informatics that combines computer technology with dentistry to create a basis for research, education, and the solution of real-world problems in dentistry; and nursing informatics that uses computers to support nurses.[3] Public health informatics uses computer technology to support public health practice, research, and learning.[4]

Currently one important focus of medical informatics is the integration of **hospital information systems (HIS)**, so that radiological images, for example, are available in real time in the operating room. Once the system in one institution is integrated, another important focus of medical informatics is creating regional, then national (and even international) **interoperability** (the connection of people and diverse computer systems). The application of computer technology continues to contribute to the achievement of these goals.

This entire book is about medical informatics; in this chapter, we will focus on the health information technology (HIT) decade, electronic medical record (EMR), the electronic health record (EHR), and various **computer information systems** used in hospitals. In the next chapter, we will focus on accounting in a health care environment. In the rest of the book, specific clinical applications will be emphasized. All of these applications are the focus of medical informatics.

THE HEALTH INFORMATION TECHNOLOGY DECADE

The U.S. government is attempting to make the EHR and electronic prescribing (e-prescribing) universal by 2014. It is calling 2004–2014 the Health Information Technology decade. It has established an Office of the National Coordinator of Health Information Technology (ONCHIT) whose mission is to "provide leadership for the development and nationwide implementation of an interoperable health information technology infrastructure to improve the quality and efficiency of health care and the ability of consumers to manage their care and safety."[5,6]

The ONCHIT asserts that "every doctor, outpatient office, hospital and nursing home" needs to computerize. It predicts that HIT will save money, reduce errors, allow the easy tracking of public health data, and protect privacy.[7]

The Bush administration (2001–2009) requested $169 million for HIT for 2007, including $116 million for ONCHIT. The specific tasks proposed for 2007 include the following: promote interoperability; find ways to improve collecting public health surveillance data; find ways for patients to keep their own medical records; "define key elements of basic EHRs"; increase e-prescribing; attempt to solve privacy and security issues.[8] With computerized physician order entry (CPOE), a doctor enters a prescription electronically and it is checked against a hospital database of patients' allergies and drug interactions. Using bar code medication administration, each patient is given a bar code, which is scanned to identify the patient. Each medication is also bar coded. E-prescribing is seen as a way to reduce medication errors. It is discussed in Chapter 8 on pharmacy. A short definition of **e-prescribing** is the use of computers and software to enter prescriptions and send them to pharmacies electronically. At the present time (2006), fewer than 20 percent of doctors make use of e-prescribing.[9,10] Today, information is gathered manually in most health care facilities.

Health records and the privacy of health information have been under the jurisdiction of state governments for many years. However, the federal government was interested in some aspects of health; note such agencies as the Centers for Disease Control (CDC). With health information crossing state lines routinely since the 1990s, HIPAA, which regulates some aspects of health care, was passed by the U.S. Congress.

THE HEALTH INSURANCE PORTABILITY AND ACCOUNTABILITY ACT OF 1996: A BRIEF INTRODUCTION

The Health Insurance Portability and Accountability Act of 1996 (HIPAA) was passed by the U.S. Congress and signed into law in 1996. Its goal was to make health insurance portable from one job to another and to secure the privacy of medical records. Its privacy provisions went into effect gradually in 2003 and the Enforcement rule went into effect in 2006. Its primary purpose is to protect the privacy of individually identifiable health information. Basically, patients must be aware of the privacy policy of the health care provider and be notified when their information is shared (with major exceptions detailed in the Patriot and Homeland Security acts). Patients are guaranteed the right to see and request changes and corrections in their medical records. The information may be used for research, but software exists to remove all personal identifiers. Staff must be trained to respect the privacy of patients; they should not discuss patients in a public area. Measures must be taken to ensure that only authorized people in the office see the record. These measures may include **biometrics** (using body parts to identify the user), **encryption**, and password protection. When data is sent over the Internet it is encrypted using software; that is, it is scrambled; it can only be seen by someone with a decryption key.[11,12] (For a more detailed discussion of HIPAA, see Chapter 12.)

THE PATIENT INFORMATION FORM

At or before a patient's first visit, he or she fills out a patient information or registration form. It includes personal data like name, address, home, cell and work phones, date of birth, Social Security number, and student status. The patient is also asked to fill in information about his or her spouse or partner.

Medical information is required: allergies, medical history, and current medications. The patient is also asked for the reason for the visit, such as accident or illness, and the name of a referring physician.

In addition, the patient is asked to provide insurance information for him or herself and a spouse or partner. This information includes the name of the primary, secondary, and tertiary insurance carriers, name and birth date of the policyholder, the co-payment, and policy and group numbers.

THE PAPER MEDICAL RECORD

The information on the patient information forms will then be entered onto the patient's record. The traditional patient record was on paper, stored in one doctor's office. One of the problems with paper records is that they may be illegible, which can lead to serious errors in diagnosis, treatment, and billing. There is only one copy of a paper record leading to difficulty in sharing patient information and the possibility of misplacing the record. There can be a time delay between the examination and the completion of the doctor's notes on the record. A transcribed record or a record typed using a word processor may include human errors also. A paper record is hard to search for specific information. The use of electronic records may help solve some of these problems.

THE ELECTRONIC MEDICAL RECORD

In a computerized office, the information that was gathered and entered onto a patient information form will then be entered into a computer into EMRs. This will form the patient's medical record. Encouraged by HIPAA and the federal government, the EMR is very gradually replacing the paper record. The federal government has set a goal of 2014 for universal adoption of electronic records and e-prescribing. However, only 14 percent of group practices are currently using e-prescribing. The EMR may be stored in a hospital's private network. But it may be kept on the Internet. Patients may establish their own records through the iHealth Record. The **iHealth Record** is a personal medical record that the patient can create and maintain at no cost. It is available at some doctors' offices.[13]

New software has been developed that makes it possible to store medical information on cell phones. The records include prescribed medications, insurance, and names of doctors among other relevant data. It also contains digital photo identification.[14]

THE ELECTRONIC HEALTH RECORD

The information on a patient's EMR will form the basis of the electronic health record (EHR) (Figure 2.1 ■). Although the terms EMR and EHR are used interchangeably, their meanings are not the same. According to the Healthcare Information Management Systems Society, an organization that promotes the expansion of the use of information technology in health care, "[t]he Electronic Health Record (EHR) is a longitudinal electronic record of patient health information generated by one or more encounters in any care delivery setting. Included in this information are patient demographics, progress notes, problems, medications, vital signs, past medical history, immunizations, laboratory data, and radiology reports. The EHR automates and streamlines the clinician's workflow. The EHR has the ability to generate a complete record of a clinical patient encounter, as well as supporting other care-related activities directly or indirectly . . ."[15]

There are specific differences between the EMR and EHR. The EMR belongs to one health care institution—a doctor's office or hospital; it must be interoperable (be able to communicate and share information with the other computers and information systems) within that institution only. Ideally the EHR is not the property of any one institution or practitioner. Eventually, it must be interoperable nationally and internationally.[16] It is the property of the patient who can access the

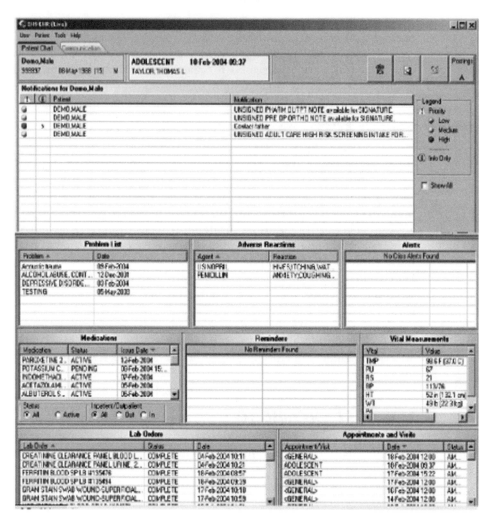

■ **FIGURE 2.1**   Electronic Health Records. The electronic record used by the Indian Health Service includes windows for the Problem, Adverse Reactions, Alerts, Medications, Reminders, Vital Measurements, Lab Orders, and Appointments. Courtesy of the U.S. Department of Health and Human Services.

record and add information. It must include information from all the health care providers and institutions that give care to the patient. It thus eases communication among many practitioners and institutions. It is a source for research in clinical areas, health services, patient outcomes, and public health. It is also an educational source.[17,18] A fully developed EHR automatically sends an alert to a doctor, for example, to warn of any adverse drug interactions. It will also send reminders to a patient who needs a particular test. EHRs also provide decision support in the form of medical references.[19]

There are many benefits predicted from the EHR: As records become interoperable your record will be available anywhere there is a computer on the network; this helps guarantee continuity of care; each of your health care providers will know your full medical history and can therefore provide better care. If you are in an accident in New Jersey, for example, but live in California, your record is a mouse click away. The EHR is legible and complete. Despite its benefits, the EHR raises serious privacy issues. Any network can be broken into, and your medical information can be stolen and misused; a great deal of medical information is private. No one wants their psychiatric diagnosis, HIV status, or children's head lice infestation broadcast to the neighborhood. HIPAA provides the first federal protection for medical records. (See Chapter 12 for a full discussion of HIPAA and the privacy of medical information.)

According to the U.S. Department of Health and Human Services (HHS), the EHR has been shown to improve health care—(although it cites no actual studies to support this assertion)—and should be universally adopted.[20] However, by 2005 fewer than 20 percent of group practices used the EHR.[21] In hospitals, computerization of all aspects of patient care is also progressing slowly.

Some of the obstacles in the way of introducing the EHR are the initial cost, resistance from medical personnel, and the absence of convincing proof that the EHR improves health care (patient outcomes). HHS recommends that personnel be well-trained and convinced of the necessity of introducing the EHR, that the cost of introducing it be shared among health care providers and others, that EHRs be certified to guarantee their quality, and that the use of EHRs in rural areas be increased. HHS emphasizes that eventually EHRs must be completely interoperable (be able to communicate with each other nationally). "Unless EHR systems can communicate, they are simply islands of data where patient information does not flow seamlessly from one clinical setting to the next."[22]

REGIONAL HEALTH INFORMATION ORGANIZATIONS

A first step toward national interoperability would be regional interoperability. Regional cooperation is being fostered through the establishment of **regional health information organizations (RHIOs)** in which data could be shared within a region. The **national health information network (NHIN)** is the infrastructure that would allow communication between RHIOs. Finally a nationally interoperable system would be established, where any patient record would be available anywhere on the national network.

In order to move toward its goal of fully interoperable EHRs, HHS puts out Requests for Proposals (RFPs) that lead to contracts between private, nonprofit groups and HHS. For example, in 2005 three of the contracts that were awarded dealt with some of the problems blocking the adoption of EHRs. Some of the issues these partnerships will address include standardizing health information, evaluating products, and dealing with privacy and security issues.[23]

THE INDIAN HEALTH SERVICE ELECTRONIC HEALTH RECORD

The Indian Health Service of the Department of HHS of the federal government is responsible for health services for Native Americans and Alaskans. It has developed an EHR with a graphical user interface, which interacts with the resource and patient management system (RPMS) database of health care applications. Each patient's record is made up of several screens or pages of information including: a notifications page that displays information for the provider, such as new lab reports; a problem list page, which lists a patient's problems with **International Classification of Disease (ICD) codes**, and is easy to add to, delete from, and modify. The health care provider can use the problem list to generate a purpose of visit (POV), by picking a problem from a variety of POV lists and the patient's problem list. An adverse reactions page lists all the adverse reactions a patient has had to medications. A page of medications interacts with the pharmacy information system. The system also includes a page to list reminders, and a page for crisis alerts. The lab orders page lists all of a patient's lab orders and the status of each order. The lab results page lists lab results and also allows the user to graph results. The appointments and visits page lists all of a patient's appointments and visits to the health care provider. Each patient has a page of vital measurements listing such things as the patient's temperature and blood pressure. The system provides a reports section in which the provider can create any needed report. The notes page allows the provider to both review old notes and create new ones. Medications, lab tests, and images can be ordered from one screen (the enter orders screen). Superbills of any kind can also be generated. This EHR is customizable; it can be set to open to any screen of choice.[24] This EHR shows how if all the information systems in a hospital are interoperable, they are united in the individual's EHR. For those using this system, the Office of Information Technology of New Mexico publishes a clear online manual at http://www.rpms.ihs.gov/TechSupp.asp (Figure 2.1 ■).

COMPUTER INFORMATION SYSTEMS IN HEALTH CARE

Computerized information systems are used in some hospitals and other health care facilities to help manage and organize relevant patient, financial, pharmacy, laboratory, and radiological information. To receive the full benefits of computer technology, each of these separate information systems needs to be linked under the hospital information system (HIS). Very few hospitals have reached this point of computerization. Issues from the high cost of introducing and maintaining computerized systems, to the resistance of staff to systems for which they are not adequately trained, to the imposition of systems designed without worker participation and knowledge of the work process have to be dealt with.[25]

The first information systems introduced into hospitals (in the 1960s) were used for administrative purposes (managing finances and inventory). Today, the HIS attempts to integrate the administrative and clinical functions in a hospital. Ideally, the HIS includes clinical information systems, financial information systems, laboratory information systems, nursing and pharmacy information systems, picture archiving and communication systems, and radiology information systems. Systems may be technically perfect. However, if the people in the hospital do not use them, they are a failure.[26]

A **financial information system (FIS)** is concerned with the financial details of running a hospital. These include payroll, patient accounting (all charges that a person generates as an inpatient or outpatient); accounts payable, accounts receivable, general ledger and asset, claims, and contract management.[27] FIS are among the oldest and most widely used computerized information systems in health care. Although FIS are not the most important use of computers in health care, because they are so widely used Chapter 3 examines accounting systems in detail.

A **clinical information system (CIS)** uses computers to manage clinical information. This information includes medical history, and other relevant information, which helps health care personnel make decisions.

The information in a computerized information system is legible and accessible. The U.S. government states that these systems will lead to improved patient outcomes by improving decision making using computerized decision support systems and reducing adverse drug events by eliminating handwritten prescriptions. Actual studies are divided on these questions. However, these systems are expensive to adopt, raise privacy questions, and may be resisted by doctors who believe that their workload will increase.[28]

Pharmacy information systems (PIS) monitor drug allergies and interactions, and fill and track prescriptions. They also track inventory and create patient drug profiles. Because the PIS receive prescriptions, they need to be able to interact with the CIS. For billing purposes, they needs to be able to interact with the FIS.[29]

Nursing information systems (NIS) are supposed to improve nursing care by using computers to manage charting, staff scheduling, and the integration of clinical information. NIS are not common and may meet with resistance from nurses. The resistance may stem from a lack of adequate training, the imposition of a system by the management, or the perception (which may be accurate) that the new system will add to their workload.[30]

Laboratory information systems (LIS) use computers to manage both lab tests and their results.[31] Ideally, the LIS can interact with the EHR. However, this is often not the case; lab results are usually mailed or faxed to the doctor's office to be entered into the EHR manually. The California HealthCare Foundation EHR-Lab Interoperability and Connectivity (ELINCS) project is attempting to create "a national standard for the delivery of real-time laboratory results from a lab's information system to an electronic health record."[32]

Radiology information systems (RIS) manage patients in the radiology department including scheduling appointments, tracking film, and reporting results. To add images to a patient's electronic record, the RIS must be able to interact with the EMR.[33]

Picture archiving and communication systems (PACS) manage digital images. Digital images are immediately available on the monitor and can be shared over a network. PACS can enhance images and eliminate film.[34] The standard communication protocol of imaging devices is called digital imaging and communications in medicine (DICOM).

Under the resource and patient management system (RPMS) EHR, the U.S. Department of Health and Human Services Indian Health Service is developing and testing the patient information management system (PIMS) to integrate clinical and administrative functions. PIMS incorporates software that can be used in a hospital setting for admissions, discharge, transfer, outpatient appointments, chart requests, and overseeing the use of patient records deemed "sensitive." Although the system continues to change in response to users' comments, it is currently in use in many hospitals.[35,36]

DOES COMPUTERIZATION IMPROVE PATIENT OUTCOMES?

While HHS mandates the EHR and e-prescribing by 2014 and states that this will improve patient care, it does not cite particular studies. Some studies support HHS' position, others question it. A recent study published in *Health Affairs* did find the EHR and e-prescribing improved health care by decreasing errors caused by illegible handwriting and improving preventive medicine by generating reminders.[37] Another study, completed in 2006 found that alerts led to a "22% relative decrease in prescribing of non-preferred medications."[38] However, the authors point to the fact that not enough providers are using the EHR to see the full benefit of computerization, and an editorial in *Health Affairs* asserted that more testing is needed before "embarking on a widespread program."[39]

With all the positive reports on the effects of IT in health care, there are many dissenting voices. In 2005, research published in *JAMA* and reported in the *New York Times* warns of some unintended and negative consequences; although decreasing some medication errors, computerized order entry systems can introduce other kinds of errors. Among the causes cited are "information on patients' medications was scattered in different places in the computer system. To find a single patient's medications, the researchers found, a doctor might have to browse through up to 20 screens of information." Computer crashes can also cause errors. Another study published in *JAMA* examined one hundred decision support systems. It found "most of the glowing assessments of those clinical decision support systems came from technologists who often had a hand in designing the systems."[40]

THE INTRODUCTION OF COMPUTER SYSTEMS

Computer systems may have the potential of improving the management of health care information, but only if they are accepted by the people who need to use them. There is no one comprehensive study of the introduction of computer information systems into health care environments. However, the studies that do exist suggest that the most successful systems are created with the participation of those who will use them. Systems imposed from above are not as readily accepted. Any system that is perceived to add work or change workflow is resisted. One Canadian study of three hospitals (published in *CMAJ*) found that the response to physician resistance to the introduction of computer systems was a crucial variable. If the response addressed the real issues that physicians were concerned with, resistance dropped. However, a lack of response or antagonistic response increased resistance to the point of having to discontinue the use of the new information systems (in two of the three hospitals studied). A commentary on this article points out that in all three cases the introduction of the new computerized system "meant that clinicians would need to take more time to care for a patient during a particular encounter." The commentary further points out that those systems that reduce or are perceived to reduce workload (for example, PACS) are readily accepted.[41–47]

IN THE NEWS

Excerpt from, "Doctors Join to Promote Electronic Record Keeping"

by Milt Freudenheim

He is a self-described techie, but that did not help Dr. Eugene P. Heslin harness the wonders of electronic medical records. The technology seemed too complicated and expensive for a small medical group like his six-doctor family practice in rural upstate New York.

"The large groups can afford the software," said Dr. Heslin . . . "For the onesies and twosies, small groups like ours, there is no profit margin."

Now, though, in a collaboration with 500 like-minded doctors, as well as hospitals, insurers and employers in two Hudson Valley counties, Dr. Heslin and his partners are clearing barriers that have made modern information technology inaccessible to the hundreds of thousands of small doctors' offices around the nation.

The Hudson Valley effort is being watched as a potential model by federal and state government and industry officials, who say that up to 60 percent of

(continued)

Excerpt from, "Doctors Join to Promote Electronic Record Keeping" (continued)

Americans receive their primary care at small-scale physicians' offices. Unless those small medical practices can adopt the most modern and efficient information technology, millions of Americans may never know the benefits of the most advanced and safest care.

Electronic records, particularly ones that can be shared online by different doctors and hospitals, can improve the quality and safety of patient care by reducing errors that kill tens of thousands of patients each year. That is why . . . big organizations like Kaiser Permanente, the Mayo Clinic and many medical centers across the country are spending billions to convert to electronic records.

. . . [I]n the aftermath of Hurricane Katrina, government and private health care officials were rushing to build an electronic database of prescription drug records for hundreds of thousands of people who lost their records in the storm. Health and Human Services Secretary Mike Leavitt said the chaos wreaked by Katrina "powerfully demonstrated the need for electronic health records."

. . . Dr. Heslin and his regional colleagues, who call their cooperative effort the Taconic Health Information Network and Community, are pooling their resources and knowledge.

A Web-based, central database approach means that doctors need little more than a few standard PC's, a high-speed Internet connection.

Dr. David J. Brailer, the Bush administration's health information technology coordinator, said that programs like the Taconic network are obviously out in front of the rest. "My mantra is to ask, How can we make electronic medical records cheaper and more valuable to the doctor?" Dr. Brailer said . . .

Under the Taconic system, which is being introduced in phases, doctors can log onto a secure Web site to get prompt laboratory and X-ray and other imaging results for their patients from four local hospitals and two big lab companies. Later this year, the doctors will be able to send prescriptions electronically to participating local drugstores or online pharmacies. The biggest part of the push is to start next year: the introduction of electronic health records accessible online to the patient's doctor and, with the patient's permission, to any other medical provider on the network.

Mark Foster, a pediatrician, has already seen the benefit of his electronic lab-results link. When a boy came in recently with a painful swollen knee, Dr. Foster suspected Lyme disease, which is endemic in the county.

"We tested him, and the next morning I looked online and called his mother and got him on antibiotics," Dr. Foster said. "Within 48 hours, his fever was gone. He's absolutely normal now."

CHAPTER SUMMARY

- The Bush administration (2001–2009) has declared 2004–2014 the decade of health information technology (HIT) and established an Office of the National Coordinator of Health Information Technology (ONCHIT) to promote the universal use of the EHR, and e-prescribing.
- The EMR is a computerized record of a patient's health information within one health care facility.
- The EHR is a patient's record of all his or her health care and will eventually be interoperable nationally.
- The first step for national interoperability is to enable regional interoperability through the establishment of RHIOs.
- The Indian Health Service of the Department of HHS of the federal government has developed an EHR with a graphical user interface that interacts with the RPMS database of health care applications.
- Computerized information systems (hospital information systems that should include FIS, CIS, PIS, LIS, and RIS) are used in some hospitals and other health care facilities to help manage and organize relevant information.
- There is not yet a consensus based on studies on the effects of computerization on patient outcomes.
- The introduction of computer systems may be resisted by those who are supposed to use them.
- In order to afford the EHR, some small practices are banding together.

KEY TERMS

biometrics
clinical information
   systems (CIS)
computer information
   systems
encryption
e-prescribing
financial information
   systems (FIS)
hospital information
   systems (HIS)
iHealth Record

International Classification of Disease
   (ICD) codes
interoperability
laboratory information
   systems (LIS)
medical informatics
national health
   information
   network (NHIN)
nursing information
   systems (NIS)

picture archiving and
   communication
   systems (PACS)
pharmacy information
   systems (PIS)
radiology information
   systems (RIS)
regional health
   information
   organizations
   (RHIOs)

REVIEW EXERCISES

Multiple Choice

1. _____ Information Systems use computers to manage both lab tests and their results.
   A. Custom
   B. Financial
   C. Laboratory
   D. All of the above

2. _____ informatics focuses on the use of technology to organize information in health care in order to improve health care; it includes the administrative, clinical and special purpose uses of computers
   A. Financial
   B. Chemo-
   C. Medical
   D. None of the Above

3. _____ informatics uses computer technology to support public health practice, research, and learning.
   A. Public health
   B. Research
   C. Pediatric
   D. Laboratory

4. One important focus of medical informatics is the _____ of HIS, so that the results of one system are immediately available to the others. For example, radiological images would be available in real time in the operating room.
   A. separation
   B. integration
   C. All of the above
   D. None of the above

5. 2004–2014 has been named the _____ decade by the federal government.
   A. public health
   B. health information technology
   C. decade of electronic prescribing
   D. decade of the EHR

6. The _____ is a longitudinal electronic record of patient health information generated by one or more encounters in any care delivery setting.
   A. EMR
   B. EHR
   C. EPR
   D. Both A and B

7. The _____ belongs to one health care institution—a doctor's office or hospital.
   A. electronic medical record (EMR)
   B. electronic health record (EHR)
   C. electronic personal record (EPR)
   D. Both A and B

8. According to the U.S. Department of HHS, the EHR _____.
   A. has no effect on health care
   B. improves health care
   C. has a negative effect on health care
   D. None of the above
9. Some of the obstacles in the way of introducing the EHR are _____.
   A. the absence of convincing proof that EHR improves health care
   B. resistance from medical personnel
   C. the initial cost
   D. All of the above
10. Regional cooperation is being fostered through the establishment of _____ in the United States.
    A. National Health Organizations (NHO)
    B. International Health Organizations (IHO)
    C. RHIOs
    D. None of the above
11. A _____ information system is concerned with the financial details of running a hospital.
    A. clinical
    B. radiological
    C. patient
    D. financial
12. _____ information systems are supposed to improve nursing care by using computers to manage charting, staff scheduling, and the integration of clinical information.
    A. Clinical
    B. Radiological
    C. Nursing
    D. Financial
13. _____ information systems use computers to manage both lab tests and their results.
    A. Laboratory
    B. Radiological
    C. Patient
    D. Financial
14. _____ information systems manage patients in the radiology department including scheduling appointments, tracking film, and reporting results.
    A. Clinical
    B. Radiological
    C. Patient
    D. Financial
15. PACS is a system associated with _____ information systems.
    A. Clinical
    B. Radiological
    C. Patient
    D. Financial

True/False Questions

1. The EHR is the property of any one institution or practitioner. _____
2. The EMR belongs to one health care institution—a doctor's office or hospital. _____
3. There are no specific differences between the EMR and EHR. _____
4. Regional cooperation is being fostered through the establishment of RHIOs. _____
5. In order to move toward its goal of fully interoperable EHRs, the HHS puts out RFPs that lead to contracts between private, nonprofit groups and the HHS. _____
6. One of the problems with paper records is that they may be illegible. _____
7. HIPAA's goal was to make health insurance portable from one job to another and to secure the privacy of medical records. _____
8. At the present time a huge majority of doctors make use of e-prescribing. _____
9. The common emphasis in all definitions of medical informatics is on the use of technology to organize information in health care. _____
10. When medical data is sent over the Internet it is encrypted using software; that is, it is scrambled; it can only be viewed by someone with a decryption key. _____

Critical Thinking

1 and 2. Describe the objectives of the HIT decade.
   How would you create reality out of these plans? Where relevant refer to the selected reading. Address some of the following questions:
   a. How would you convince administrators and doctors that EHR and e-prescribing are worth the cost.
   b. You might design a study of a large institution (veterans hospitals) with an electronic system in place.
   c. How would you deal with the negative aspects of introducing EHR and e-prescribing?
   d. How would you deal with the staff who would have to change work patterns to use EHR and e-prescribing.
3. Define the following
   • Hospital information systems (HIS)
   • Laboratory information systems (LIS)
   • National Health Information Network (NHIN)
   • Nursing information systems (NIS)
   • Picture archiving and communication systems (PACS)
   • Pharmacy information systems (PIS)
   • Radiology information systems (RIS)
4. What does interoperability mean? Why is it crucial for the EHR to be nationally interoperable?
5. What are the differences between the EMR and the EHR? How are they interdependent?

NOTES

1. Daniel C. Davis and William G. Chismar, "Tutorial Medical Informatics," http://www.hicss.hawaii.edu/hicss_32/tutdesc.htm (accessed August 18, 2006).

2. John Gennari, "Biomedical Informatics Is the Science Underlying the Acquisition, Maintenance, Retrieval, and Application of Biomedical Knowledge and Information to Improve Patient Care, Medical Education, and Health Sciences Research," July 22, 2002, http://faculty.washington.edu/gennari/MedicalInformaticsDef.html (accessed November 23, 2007).

3. "Nursing Informatics," 2006, http://www.allnursingschools.com/faqs/informatics.php (accessed July 23, 2006).

4. Public Health Informatics, April 22, 2002, http://www.nlm.nih.gov/archive//20061214/pubs/cbm/phi2001.html (accessed December 22, 2007).

5. "Office of the National Coordinator for Health Information Technology (ONC)—Mission," August 19, 2005, http://www.hhs.gov/healthit/mission.html (accessed November 23, 2007).

6. "Health Industry Insights Survey Reveals Consumers Are Unaware of Government's Health Records Initiative," www.crm2day, February 15, 2006, http://www.crm2day.com/news/crm/117351.php (accessed December 22, 2007).

7. U.S. Department of HHS, Office of the National Coordinator for Health Information Technology (ONC), "Value of HIT," HHS.gov, May 23, 2005, http://www.os.dhhs.gov/healthit/valueHIT.html (accessed January 5, 2008).

8. Scott Weier, "Subcommittee Recommends $98M for ONCHIT in 2007," iHealthbeat, June 15, 2006, http://www.ihealthbeat.org/articles/2006/6/15/Subcommittee-Recommends-98M-for-ONCHIT-in-2007.aspx (accessed December 22, 2007).

9. Jane Sarasohn-Kahn and Matthew Holt, "The Prescription Infrastructure: Are We Ready for ePrescribing?" iHealth and Technology, California HealthCare Foundation, chcf.org, January 2006, http://www.chcf.org/documents/ihealth/ThePrescriptionInfrastructureReadyForERx.pdf (accessed December 22, 2007).

10. Toni Hebda, Patricia Czar, and Cynthia Mascara, *Handbook of Informatics for Nurses and Health Care Professionals*, 3rd ed. (Upper Saddle River, NJ: Prentice Hall, 2005).

11. Laurinda Harman, "HIPAA: A Few Years Later," Online Journal of Issues in Nursing, July 21, 2005, http://www.medscape.com/viewarticle/506841 (accessed December 22, 2007).

12. Kevin M. Kramer, "HIPAA 2006: HHS' HIPAA Enforcement Rule Is Now Effective," April 21, 2006, http://www.gibbonslaw.com/news_publications/articles.php?action=display_publication&publication_id=2033 (accessed December 22, 2007).

13. "eHealth Spotlight: Medem Launches iHealth Record," 2005, http://www.msdc.org/newsEvents/newslineMAY2005/newsline_2005_may_IT_medem_launches_ihealth_record.shtml (accessed December 22, 2007).

14. Roy Whittington, "New Electronic Medical Records Device Can Save Lives in an Emergency," April 24, 2007, http://www.prwebdirect.com/releases/2007/4/prweb520655.htm (accessed November 23, 2007).

15. Healthcare Information Management Systems Society (HIMSS), "EHR: Electronic Health Record," http://himss.org/asp/topics_ehr.asp (accessed February 6, 2008).

16. A. Virginia Sharpe, "Perspective: Privacy and Security for Electronic Health Records," medscape.com, December 19, 2005, http://www.medscape.com/viewarticle/517403 (accessed April 19, 2006).

17. Peter C. Waegmann, "Status Report 2002: Electronic Health Records," http://www.medrecinst.com/uploadedFiles/MRILibrary/StatusReport.pdf (accessed May 20, 2006).

18. Dave Garets and Mike Davis, "Electronic Medical Records vs. Electronic Health Records: Yes, There Is a Difference," A HIMSS Analytics White Paper, January 26, 2006, http://www.himssanalytics.org/docs/WP_EMR_EHR.pdf (accessed December 22, 2007).

19. Richard W. Gartee, *Electronic Health Records: Understanding and Using Computerized Medical Records* (Upper Saddle River, NJ: Prentice Hall, 2007), 6–8.

20. Office of the National Coordinator for Health Information Technology, 2005.

21. Kim Krisberg, "Improved Medical Technology Could Affect Health, Lower Cost," *The Nation's Health*, 1 November, 2005, http://www.medscape.com/viewarticle/515529 (accessed April 19, 2006).

22. Health Information Technology, "Goal 2—Interconnecting Clinicians," 2004, http://www.hhs.gov/healthit/framework.html#interconnect (accessed December 1, 2007).

23. "HHS Awards Contracts to Advance Nationwide Interoperable Health Information Technology," October 6, 2005, http://www.hhs.gov/news/2005pres/20051006a.html (accessed June 29, 2006).

24. "HIS-EHR Walk Through," http://www.ihs.gov/CIO/EHR/pdf/ehr-walkthru-1.pdf (accessed November 23, 2007).

25. Garets and Davis, "Electronic Medical Records vs. Electronic Health Records."

26. Hospital Information System, 2006, http://www.biohealthmatics.com (accessed April 21, 2006).

27. Financial Information System, 2006, http://www.biohealthmatics.com (accessed April 21, 2006).

28. Clinical Information System, 2006, http://www.biohealthmatics.com (accessed April 21, 2006).

29. Pharmacy Information System, 2006, http://www.biohealthmatics.com (accessed April 21, 2006).

30. Nursing Information System, 2006, http://www.biohealthmatics.com (accessed April 21, 2006).

31. Laboratory Information System, 2006, http://www.biohealthmatics.com (accessed April 21, 2006).

32. "ELINCS: Developing a National Lab Data Standard for EHRs," February 2006 http://www.chcf.org/topics/chronicdisease/index.cfm?itemID=108868 (accessed December 22, 2007).

33. Radiology Information System, 2006, http://www.biohealthmatics.com (accessed April 21, 2006).

34. PACS (Picture Archiving and Communication System), 2006, http://www. biohealthmatics.com (accessed April 21, 2006).

35. U.S. Department of HHS Indian Health Service, "RPMS EHR Home Page," http://www. ihs.gov/CIO/EHR/index.cfm (accessed December 22, 2007).

36. U.S. Department of HHS Indian Health Service, "EHR Current Status." April 12, 2006, http://www.ihs.gov/CIO/EHR/index.cfm?module=currentstatus (accessed December 22, 2007).

37. Krisberg, "Improved Medical Technology Could Affect Health, Lower Cost."

38. Kate Ackerman, "EHR Alerts Reduce Prescription Oversights," ihealthbeat.org, June 2, 2006, http://www.ihealthbeat.org/articles/2006/6/2/EHR-Alerts-Reduce-Prescription-Oversights.aspx?a=1 (accessed December 22, 2007).

39. Krisberg, "Improved Medical Technology Could Affect Health, Lower Cost."

40. Steve Lohr, "Doctors' Journal Says Computing Is No Panacea," *New York Times*, March 9, 2005.

41. Liette Lapointe and Suzanne Rivard, "Getting Physicians to Accept New Information Technology: Insights from Case Studies," cmaj.com, May 23, 2006, http://www.cmaj.ca/cgi/content/full/174/11/1573 (accessed December 22, 2007).

42. David Zitner, "Physicians Will Happily Adopt Information Technology," cmaj.com, May 23, 2006, http://www.cmaj.ca/cgi/content/full/174/11/1583 (accessed December 22, 2007).

43. Erica Danielson, "A Qualitative Assessment of Changes in Nurses' Workflow in Response to the Implementation of an Electronic Charting Information System," A thesis presented to the Division of Medical Informatics and Outcomes Research and the Oregon Health & Science University School of Medicine in partial fulfillment of the requirements of the degree of Master of Science, June 2002.

44. John F. Hurdle, "Can the Electronic Medical Record Improve Geriatric Care?" *Geriatric Times*, March/April 2004, http://www.cmellc.com/geriatrictimes/g040425.html (accessed December 22, 2007).

45. Seth Schiesel, "In the E.R., Learning to Love the PC," *New York Times*, October 21, 2004.

46. "Latest News in Minimally Invasive Medicine," 2006, http://sirweb.org/news/newsPDF/Media_Alert_Round-up.pdf (accessed December 21, 2007).

47. "MTCC to Host 5000 Interventional Radiologists in Professional Society's International Meeting," 2006, http://www.google.com/search?q=cache:v6FA0L1ZszEJ:www.mtccc.com/admin/contentEngine/dspDocumentDownload.cfm%3FPCVID%3D41885715-1422-0efc-51ff-674cc3e1d3ec+MTCC+to+Host+5000+Interventional+Radiologists&hl=en&ct=clnk&cd=3&gl=us (accessed December 21, 2007).

ADDITIONAL RESOURCES

Resource and Patient Management System. "Nurses Getting Started Guide User Manual Version 1.0." June 2005. http://www.rpms.ihs.gov/TechSupp.asp (accessed December 22, 2007).

CHAPTER 3

An Introduction to the Administrative Applications of Computers: Accounting

CHAPTER OUTLINE

LEARNING OBJECTIVES

Upon completion of this chapter, the reader will be able to

- Define clinical, special-purpose, and administrative applications of computer technology in health care and its delivery.
- Define telemedicine.
- Discuss the computerization of accounting tasks in the medical office.
  - Define bucket billing.
  - Discuss coding systems, insurance, and the various accounting reports used in the medical office.

INTRODUCTION

As you recall, **medical informatics** refers to the use of computers to organize health-related information to improve patient care. It addresses all aspects of health care. The first (and most widely) used application is financial; many health care facilities have computerized accounting functions.

Traditionally, the application of computer technology in health care is divided into three categories. The **clinical** use of computers includes anything that has to do with direct patient care, such as diagnosis, monitoring, and treatment. **Special-purpose applications** include the use of computers in education, research, and some aspects of pharmacy. **Administrative applications** include office management, scheduling, and accounting tasks. Many programs are specifically designed for medical office management. **Telemedicine**—the delivery of health care over telecommunications lines—includes clinical, special-purpose, and administrative applications.

ADMINISTRATIVE APPLICATIONS OF COMPUTER TECHNOLOGY IN THE MEDICAL OFFICE

Beginning with the computerization of hospital administrative tasks in the 1960s, the role of digital technology in medical care and its delivery has expanded at an ever-increasing pace. Today, computers play a part in every aspect of health care.

As you recall, administrative applications include office management tasks, scheduling, and accounting functions. These are tasks that need to be performed in any office. However, some of these activities are slightly different in a health care environment, so programs are needed that take into account the special needs of a medical office.

Many programs are specifically designed to computerize basic administrative functions in a health care environment—the coding systems, insurance information, and payment information. Such programs allow the user to organize information by patient, by case, and by provider. These programs enable the user to schedule patient appointments with a computer; take electronic progress notes; create lists of codes for diagnosis, treatment, and insurance; submit claims to primary, secondary, and tertiary insurers; and receive payment electronically. These programs must allow the bucket (balance) billing that medical offices must use to accommodate two or three insurers, who must be billed in a timely fashion before the patient is billed. Moreover, because these programs establish **relational databases** (organized collections of related data), information input in one part of the program can be linked to information in another part of the program. Billing information and financial status are easily available. Tables can be searched for any information, and this information can be presented in finished form in one of the many report designs provided, including various kinds of billing reports. If no report design meets the user's need, a customized report can easily be designed and generated by the user. Medical accounting software can be used by medical administrators and office workers, doctors and other healthcare workers, and students. It can ease the tasks of administering a practice using a computer. The amount of data and information a modern practice has to collect and organize is overwhelming. These programs allow the user to computerize tasks performed every day in any medical environment. All the disparate tasks and pieces of data and information need to be well organized, accessible, and easily linked. The user may quickly and easily organize, access, and link information from one part of the program to information in any other part of the program.

A **database** is an organized collection of information. **Database management software (DBMS)** allows the user to enter, organize, and store huge amounts of data and information. The information is then linked, updated, sorted, resorted, and retrieved. To use DBMS efficiently, the user should be familiar with certain concepts and definitions. A database **file** holds all related information on an entity, for example, a medical practice. For instance, the "Doctors' Practice of Anywhere" would store all of its data and information in a database file stored on a computer. Within the file, there can be several tables. Each **table** holds related information; for example, one table might hold information on the doctors working for the "Doctors' Practice of Anywhere"; another holds information on its patients; another on its insurance carriers. All the tables are stored in the practice's file. A table is made up of related **records**; each record holds all the information on one item in the table. Each patient has a record in the practice's patient table. All the information on one patient makes up that patient's record. Each record is made up of related **fields**. One field holds one piece of information, such as a patient's last name, or Social Security number (SSN), or chart number. One field—the **key field**—uniquely identifies each record in a table. The information in that field cannot be duplicated. SSN is a common key field because no two people have the same SSN. Chart number uniquely identifies each patient's chart. In a relational database, related tables are linked by sharing a common field. If a practice is completely computerized, a patient's electronic record may contain several pages for personal information, medical history, insurance information, notes, appointments, radiological images, alerts and reminders, and allergies. The structure of a database makes it possible to enter information in one table (say, the appointments table), and that appointment is automatically entered into the patient's electronic record.

MEDICAL OFFICE ADMINISTRATIVE SOFTWARE—AN OVERVIEW

Medical office administration software allows the user to create one database file for each practice. Within each database, information is organized into tables. The tables are linked by sharing a common field.

Coding and Grouping

Each category of information (personal, medical, and insurance) provided by a patient is entered into a form and becomes part of a record in a table in a database.

Some of it is translated into codes before it is entered. Codes provide standardization, which allows the easy sharing of information. Because codes of diagnoses and procedures are precise and universally used, one physician recognizes another's diagnoses and procedures immediately.

Standard coding systems include **DRG (diagnosis-related group)**. Today, hospital reimbursement by private and government insurers is determined by diagnosis. Each patient is given a DRG classification, and a formula based on this classification determines reimbursement. If hospital care and cost exceed the prospective cost determination, the hospital absorbs the financial loss.

Services including tests, laboratory work, exams, and treatments are coded using CPTs (*Current Procedural Terminology*, Fourth Edition). ICD-9-CM (or ICD-10-CM) provides three-, four-, or five-digit codes for more than one thousand diseases. The **ICD** is the *International Classification of Diseases*, Ninth Edition. These coding systems make electronic claim forms easier to file because each condition or disease, each service, procedure, and diagnostic test is identified by a widely agreed-on several digit number. These codes are standardized, but no practice uses all of them. When a new practice is set up, only codes that relate to its specialty are entered in one of the tables of codes; these tables can always be amended. The **CPT** is used on the **superbill** or **encounter form** (list of diagnoses and procedures common to the specialty) to identify all procedures performed by that practice (Figure 3.1 ■). The codes are also used in the **electronic health record** (discussed in Chapter 2) and in data collection on public health issues (see Chapter 5).

Other coding systems have been developed. **MEDCIN** provides 250,000 codes for such things as symptoms, history, physical exams, tests, diagnoses, and treatments. MEDCIN codes can be integrated with other coding systems. **SNOMED** (Systematized Nomenclature of Medicine) "provides a common language that enables a consistent way of capturing, sharing, and aggregating health data." **LOINC** (logical observation identifiers, names, and codes) standardizes laboratory and clinical codes. The national drug codes (NDC), which were developed by the Food and Drug Administration (FDA), identify drugs.[1]

ACCOUNTING

Many of the computerized tasks in a health care environment have to do with accounting. Therefore, several definitions are required. **Charges, payments**, and **adjustments** are called **transactions**. A charge is simply the amount a patient is billed for the provider's service. A payment is made by a patient or an insurance carrier to the practice. An adjustment is a positive or negative change to a patient account. Transactions are organized around cases. A **case** is the condition for which the patient visits the doctor. This information is entered by the medical office staff and stored in the practice's database tables. There can be several visits associated with one case. The case can be closed when the condition is resolved. And there can be several cases (one for each diagnosis) for one patient.

TEXAS CARDIOLOGY   877 555-1212

| Patient Number | Ticket Number | Service Date | Prior Balance |
| Pat |
Patient Name		Gender	Ins
Address		Phone	Other
SSN	Referring Dr.		Total
Primary Insurance Co.	Policy/Group ID		Paymt
Secondary Insurance Co.	Policy/Group ID		Bal Due

Location
- ☐ _____
- ☐ _____
- ☐ _____
- ☐ _____
- ☐ _____
- ☐ _____
- ☐ _____
- ☐ _____
- ☐ _____
- ☐ _____
- ☐ _____

Cardiologist
- ☐ _____
- ☐ _____
- ☐ _____
- ☐ _____
- ☐ _____
- ☐ _____
- ☐ _____
- ☐ Other: _____

X	Code	Service
		New Patient
	99203	Limited/Simple (30m)
	99204	Comprehensive (45m)
	99205	Complex (60m)
		New Patient Consult
		(Need Referring MD)
	99243	Brief (40m)
	99244	Full Consult (60m)
	99245	Very Complex (80m)
		Established Patient
	99211	Nurse Visit
	99212	Very Brief FU (10m)
	99213	Limited/Simple FU (15m)
	99214	Comprehensive FU (25m)
	99215	Complex FU (40m)
		New Cons. 2nd Opin.
	99274	Moderate 2nd Opinion
	99275	Complex 2nd Opinion
		Home Health
	99375	Home Health 30 days
		Drugs:
	J3420	B-12 Injection
	J1940	Lasix
	90724	Flu (Dx V-04.8)
	G0008	MC Flu Admin Fee
		Misc Rx _____
	90782	IM Injections
	90784	IV Injections
	A4615	O2 Cannula

X	Code	Service
		Office Procedures
	93000	EKG w/ Interp
	93015	Stress Tread w/ Interp
	93040	Rhythm strip w/ Interp
	93307	2D Echo Compl.
	93320	Doppler Compl.
	93325	Color Flow Compl.
	93308	2D Echo F/U
	93321	Doppler F/U
	ES	Stress Echo
	BUB	Echo/Bubble/Doppler
		Event Monitor
	93268	Loop- Non MC
	G0005	Loop - Hookup - MC
	G0007	Loop - Interp - MC
	93012	Chest Plate Tech - Non MC
	93014	Chest Pl - Interp Non MC
	G0016	Chest Pl - Interp MC
		Holter Monitor
	93224	Holter w/ Interp Global
		Other
	92960	Cardioversion
	93734	Pacer Eval - Single
	93735	Pacer Eval - Sngl w/ Prg
	93731	Pacer Eval - Dual
	93732	Pacer Eval - Dual w/ Prg
	99499	Review outside records
	99080	Special Reports

X	Code	Service
		Diagnostic w/o Interp
		(Technical only)
	93005	EKG
	93017	Stress Tread
	93225	Holter Hookup
	93226	Holter Scan
	93307-TC	2D Echo
	93320-TC	Doppler Compl.
	93325-TC	Color Flow
	93308-TC	2D Echo F/U
	93321-TC	Doppler F/U
	93880-TC	Carotid Doppler
	Phys	**Interpretation-Supervision,**
		Interpretation & Report Only
	93010	EKG Interp & Reortt only
	TR	Regular Stress Test–S, I & R
	NU	Nuclear Stress Test–S, I & R
	ES-26	Stress Echocardiogram–S, I & R
	307	Echocardiogram 2-D
	320-26	Doppler Echocardiogram
	325-26	Color Flow
	308	Echocardiogram 2-D F/U
	321-26	Doppler F/U
	227	Holter Monitor - I & R only
	71250-26	UltraFast CT
	XXXXX	**LAB ORDERED**
		(see attached sheet)
	36415	VeniPuncture (non MC)
	99000	Specimen Collection (Lab)

Next Appointment:
Return in: _____ (Wks) (Mo) (Yr)

Before next appointment:
- ☐ Ekg
- ☐ TM
- ☐ Echo
- ☐ Stress Echo
- ☐ Doppler
- ☐ CFD
- ☐ CXR
- ☐ Holter
- ☐ Event Monitor
- ☐ Lab

BI: _____

Hospital Admission:
- ☐ Admit Cath
- ☐ Admit to _____ unit at:
- ☐ BAP ☐ WMC ☐ CMC ☐ SHMC
- ☐ Other: _____

Notes:

Cardiac Diagnoses

■ **FIGURE 3.1**   The Superbill or Encounter Form lists procedures and tests common to the practice.

INSURANCE

Today, many people are covered by medical insurance. Those people who are not covered either pay out-of-pocket or seek care in the local emergency room. A **guarantor** is the person responsible for payment; it may be the patient or a third party. There are a variety of options for those with insurance. Some carriers have a **schedule of benefits**— a list of those services that the carrier will cover. This is called an **indemnity plan**. Indemnity plans are becoming less and less common, because they are **fee-for-service plans** and therefore very expensive. The patient is never restricted to a network of providers and needs no referrals for specialists. After fulfilling a **deductible** (a certain amount the patient is required to pay each year before the insurance begins paying,) every visit to a doctor is paid for by the insurance company. The doctor, not the insurance company, determines necessary care and treatment so there is no financial reason for a health care worker to deny necessary care. **Managed care** also has a schedule of benefits for out-of-network providers. Managed care plans and **preferred provider organizations (PPOs)** may require that the provider get **authorization** before a procedure is performed. This is simply permission by the insurance carrier for the provider to perform a medical procedure.

A patient with PPO insurance can seek care within an approved network of health care providers who have agreed with the insurance company to lower their charges and accept **assignment** (the amount the insurance company pays). The patient may pay a **co-payment**, the part of the charge for which the patient is responsible. The patient may choose, however, to go out-of-network and pay the provider's customary charges. The insurance company may then reimburse the patient a small amount.

There are several government insurance plans. They are administered by the federal **Centers for Medicare and Medicaid Services (CMS)**, formerly the **Health Care Financing Administration (HCFA)**. **Worker's compensation** is a government program, which covers job-related illness or injury. Seventy-four million Americans receive their health care through government insurers—some through fee-for-service plans, some through managed care.[2] According to CMS, **Medicaid** is "jointly funded, federal-state health insurance for certain low-income and needy people. It covers approximately 36 million individuals including children, the aged, blind, and/or disabled, and people who are eligible to receive federally assisted income maintenance payments." Medicaid resembles managed care, in that the patient is restricted to a network of providers, must get a pre-authorization for procedures, and needs referrals to any specialist. **Medicare** serves people aged 65 years and over and disabled people with chronic renal disorders. Medicare allows patients to choose their physicians; referrals are not needed. Some Medicare patients choose to belong to **health maintenance organizations (HMOs)**. Many people supplement Medicare with private fee-for-service plans in which they are not restricted to a network of providers; they do not need referrals to specialists. The patient is required to pay a cost-sharing amount and the provider bills the insurance for the remainder. Starting in 2006, people insured by Medicare will have some minimal coverage for medication ("Medicare Prescription Drug Coverage"). **TRICARE** is the health program for U.S. armed service members and their families. **CHAMPUS** covers medical necessities for those eligible: retired military, dependents of active duty, and retired or dead military. Run by the Department of Veterans Affairs, **CHAMPVA** covers the immediate families of veterans who are totally disabled; surviving spouse and children of a veteran who died from a service-connected disability; widow and children of a veteran who was permanently disabled; and the surviving spouse and children of a member of the military who died in the line of duty.[3]

With managed care, it is the insurance carrier that determines what treatment is necessary and pays for it. There are several forms of managed care. In managed care, patients pay a fixed yearly fee, and the insurance company pays the participating provider.

A patient who uses an HMO pays a fixed yearly fee and must choose among an approved network of health care providers and hospitals. The patient needs a referral from his or her primary care provider to see any specialist. If a patient goes out of network without the HMO's approval, the patient must pay out of pocket. However, this may change in light of a Supreme Court decision of April 2, 2003. Under the ruling, states may require HMOs to open their networks, allowing patients more choice.

In a **capitated plan**, a physician is paid a fixed fee (the capitation), and the physician is paid regardless of the amount of treatment he or she provides. Some patients may seek no treatment; some may visit several times.

Claims

To receive payment for services from an uninsured patient, the practice simply bills the patient. To receive payment for services rendered to an insured patient, the practice must submit a claim to the insurance carrier. A **claim** is a request to an insurance company for payment for services. If an insurance carrier requires a treatment plan, the accounting software you use enables you to create one. There are many claim forms, but the most widely accepted form is the **HCFA-1500** and **UB04** for hospital-based claims. (Because of the change in name of HCFA to CMS, the name of the form has been changed to **CMS-1500** (http://www.cms.hhs.gov/forms). It is accepted by government insurers and most private plans (Figure 3.2 ■).

An **EMC (electronic media claim)** is an electronically processed and transmitted claim. To create a claim to submit to an insurance company, the practice needs to gather certain information: the patient's condition, the physician's diagnosis, and the procedures performed in the office or hospital. The patient record can provide them with personal data, medical history, and insurance information. The provider table can supply information about the physician. Claims are submitted on paper or electronically. Practices that submit electronic claims use a **clearinghouse**—a business that collects insurance claims from providers and sends them to the correct insurance carrier. An insurance company can reject the claim or send a check for partial or full payment. The response to a paper claim includes an **explanation of benefits (EOB)** which explains why certain services were covered and others not; an **electronic remittance advice (ERA)** accompanies the response to an EMC.

The practice records the claim and applies it to the charge. It then bills the secondary insurer; the EOB from the first insurer is sent to the secondary insurer with the bill. The secondary insurer responds with a check and EOB or ERA. After the response is received from the secondary insurer, the tertiary insurance company is

PLEASE
DO NOT
STAPLE
IN THIS
AREA

CARRIER →

PICA

HEALTH INSURANCE CLAIM FORM

PICA

1. MEDICARE   MEDICAID   CHAMPUS   CHAMPVA   GROUP HEALTH PLAN (SSN or ID)   FECA BLK LUNG (SSN)   OTHER   1a. INSUREDIS I.D. NUMBER   (FOR PROGRAM IN ITEM 1)
(Medicare #)   (Medicaid #)   (Sponsoris SSN)   (VA File #)   (SSN or ID)   (ID)

2. PATIENTIS NAME (Last Name, First Name, Middle Initial)

3. PATIENTIS BIRTH DATE   MM   DD   YYYY   SEX   M   F

4. INSUREDIS NAME (Last Name, First Name, Middle Initial)

5. PATIENTIS ADDRESS (No., Street)

6. PATIENT RELATIONSHIP TO INSURED   Self   Spouse   Child   Other

7. INSUREDIS ADDRESS (No., Street)

CITY   STATE

8. PATIENT STATUS   Single   Married   Other

Employed   Full-Time Student   Part-Time Student

CITY   STATE

ZIP CODE   TELEPHONE (Include Area Code)   (   )

ZIP CODE   TELEPHONE (INCLUDE AREA CODE)   (   )

9. OTHER INSUREDIS NAME (Last Name, First Name, Middle Initial)

10. IS PATIENTIS CONDITION RELATED TO:

11. INSUREDIS POLICY GROUP OR FECA NUMBER

a. OTHER INSUREDIS POLICY OR GROUP NUMBER

a. EMPLOYMENT? (CURRENT OR PREVIOUS)   YES   NO

a. INSUREDIS DATE OF BIRTH   MM   DD   YYYY   SEX   M   F

b. OTHER INSUREDIS DATE OF BIRTH   MM   DD   YYYY   SEX   M   F

b. AUTO ACCIDENT?   PLACE (State)   YES   NO

b. EMPLOYERIS NAME OR SCHOOL NAME

c. EMPLOYERIS NAME OR SCHOOL NAME

c. OTHER ACCIDENT?   YES   NO

c. INSURANCE PLAN NAME OR PROGRAM NAME

d. INSURANCE PLAN NAME OR PROGRAM NAME

10d. RESERVED FOR LOCAL USE

d. IS THERE ANOTHER HEALTH BENEFIT PLAN?   YES   NO   *If yes*, return to and complete item 9 a-d.

READ BACK OF FORM BEFORE COMPLETING & SIGNING THIS FORM.
12. PATIENTIS OR AUTHORIZED PERSONIS SIGNATURE I authorize the release of any medical or other information necessary to process this claim. I also request payment of government benefits either to myself or to the party who accepts assignment below.

SIGNED _____   DATE _____

13. INSUREDIS OR AUTHORIZED PERSONIS SIGNATURE I authorize payment of medical benefits to the undersigned physician or supplier for services described below.

SIGNED _____

↑ PATIENT AND INSURED INFORMATION

14. DATE OF CURRENT: MM   DD   YYYY   ILLNESS (First symptom) OR INJURY (Accident) OR PREGNANCY(LMP)

15. IF PATIENT HAS HAD SAME OR SIMILAR ILLNESS. GIVE FIRST DATE   MM   DD   YYYY

16. DATES PATIENT UNABLE TO WORK IN CURRENT OCCUPATION   MM   DD   YYYY   FROM   TO   MM   DD   YYYY

17. NAME OF REFERRING PHYSICIAN OR OTHER SOURCE

17a. I.D. NUMBER OF REFERRING PHYSICIAN

18. HOSPITALIZATION DATES RELATED TO CURRENT SERVICES   MM   DD   YYYY   FROM   TO   MM   DD   YYYY

19. RESERVED FOR LOCAL USE

20. OUTSIDE LAB?   YES   NO $ CHARGES

21. DIAGNOSIS OR NATURE OF ILLNESS OR INJURY. (RELATE ITEMS 1,2,3 OR 4 TO ITEM 24E BY LINE)

1. |___.___   3. |___.___

2. |___.___   4. |___.___

22. MEDICAID RESUBMISSION CODE   ORIGINAL REF. NO.

23. PRIOR AUTHORIZATION NUMBER

24. A DATE(S) OF SERVICE From To MM DD YYYY MM DD YYYY	B Place of Service	C Type of Service	D PROCEDURES, SERVICES, OR SUPPLIES (Explain Unusual Circumstances) CPT/HCPCS MODIFIER	E DIAGNOSIS CODE	F $ CHARGES	G DAYS OR UNITS	H EPSDT Family Plan	I EMG	J COB	K RESERVED FOR LOCAL USE
1										
2										
3										
4										
5										
6										

25. FEDERAL TAX I.D. NUMBER   SSN   EIN

26. PATIENTIS ACCOUNT NO.

27. ACCEPT ASSIGNMENT? (For govt. claims, see back)   YES   NO

28. TOTAL CHARGE $

29. AMOUNT PAID $

30. BALANCE DUE $

31. SIGNATURE OF PHYSICIAN OR SUPPLIER INCLUDING DEGREES OR CREDENTIALS (I certify that the statements on the reverse apply to this bill and are made a part thereof.)

SIGNED _____   DATE _____

32. NAME AND ADDRESS OF FACILITY WHERE SERVICES WERE RENDERED (If other than home or office)

33. PHYSICIANIS, SUPPLIERIS BILLING NAME, ADDRESS, ZIP CODE & PHONE #

PIN#   GRP#

↑ PHYSICIAN OR SUPPLIER INFORMATION

(APPROVED BY AMA COUNCIL ON MEDICAL SERVICE 8/88)   *PLEASE PRINT OR TYPE*   APPROVED OMB-0938-0008 FORM CMS-1500 (12/90),   FORM RRB-1500,
APPROVED OMB-1215-0055 FORM OWCP-1500,   APPROVED OMB-0720-0001 (CHAMPUS)

■ **FIGURE 3.2**   The CMS-1500 is the most commonly used claim form.

billed. It is only after the response is received from all of a patient's carriers that the patient is billed. This is called **bucket billing** or **balance billing**.

From the time a patient is charged for a procedure to the time when all payments have been received and credited to the patient's account, there is a sequence of accounting events that occur. **Accounts receivable (A/R)** include any invoice or any payment from the patient or insurance carriers to the medical practice. The diagnoses and procedures relevant to a patient's visit are recorded on a superbill (also called an encounter form). A superbill is a list of diagnoses and procedures common to the practice. Superbills for each patient on a day's schedule are printed that morning or the night before. Information taken from the superbill is utilized in several medical accounting reports.

ACCOUNTING REPORTS

Medical accounting software allows the user to create various kinds of reports that are generated on a daily, monthly, or yearly basis. Daily reports include a patient day sheet, a procedure day sheet, and a payment day sheet. A **patient day sheet** lists the day's patients, chart numbers, and transactions. It is used for daily reconciliation. A **procedure day sheet** is a grouped report organized by procedure. Patients who underwent a particular procedure such as a blood sugar laboratory test are listed under that procedure. This report is used to see what procedures a health care worker is performing. It also can be used to find the most profitable procedures. A **payment day sheet** is a grouped report organized by providers. Each patient is listed under his or her provider. It shows the amounts received from each patient to each provider.

A **practice analysis report** is generated on a monthly basis and is a summary total of all procedures, charges, and transactions. A **patient aging report** is used to show a patient's outstanding payments. Current and past due balances are listed on this report based on the number of days late. For example, an account can be past due 30–60 days, 60–90 days, and over 90 days.

The administrative and accounting tasks of a health care environment can be computerized using medical accounting software. It allows the user to enter all necessary information into tables, link the information, and present it in one of the many reports it provides. Computerizing the accounting transactions allows the office to avoid being buried in paper and keeps all accounts in an accurate, up-to-date, and well-organized structure.

IN THE NEWS

Excerpt from, "Google and Microsoft Look to Change Health Care"

by Steve Lohr

In politics, every serious candidate for the White House has a health care plan. So too in business, where the two leading candidates for Web supremacy, Google and Microsoft, are working up their plans to improve the nation's health care.

By combining better Internet search tools, the vast resources of the Web and online personal health records, both companies are betting they can enable people to make smarter choices about their health habits and medical care. . . .

It is too soon to know whether either Google or Microsoft will make real headway. Health care, experts note, is a field where policy, regulation and entrenched interests tend to slow the pace of change, and technology companies have a history of losing patience. . . .

Google and Microsoft recognize the obstacles, and they concede that changing health care will take time. But the companies see the potential in attracting a large audience for health-related advertising and services.

Microsoft's software animates more than 90 percent of all personal computers, while Google is the default starting point for most health searches. And people are increasingly turning to their computers and the Web for health information and advice.

If the efforts of the two big companies gain momentum over time, that promises to accelerate a shift in power to consumers in health care, just as Internet technology has done in other industries. . . .

The Google and Microsoft initiatives would give more control to individuals, a trend many health experts see as inevitable. . . . The Web is allowing people to take a more activist approach to health. . . . It is now common, Dr. John D. Halamka, a doctor and the chief information officer of the Harvard Medical School, said, for a patient to come in carrying a pile of Web page printouts. "The doctor is becoming a knowledge navigator," he said. In the future, health care will be a much more collaborative process between patients and doctors.

Microsoft and Google are hoping this will lead people to seek more control over their own health records, using tools the companies will provide. . . .

A prototype of Google Health, which the company has shown to health professionals and advisers, makes the consumer focus clear. The welcome page reads, "At Google, we feel patients should be in charge of their health information, and they should be able to grant their health care providers, family members, or whomever they choose, access to this information. Google Health was developed to meet this need."

A presentation of screen images from the prototype . . . has 17 Web pages including a "health profile" for medications, conditions and allergies; a . . . "health guide" for suggested treatments, drug interactions and diet and exercise regimens; pages for receiving reminder messages to get prescription refills or visit a doctor; and directories of nearby doctors. . . .

At Microsoft, the long-term goal is similarly ambitious. . . . Microsoft will not disclose its product plans, but according to people working with the company the consumer effort will include online offerings as well as software to find, retrieve and store personal health information on personal computers, cellphones and other kinds of digital devices—perhaps even a wristwatch with wireless Internet links some day.

Yet personal health records promise to be a thorny challenge for practical and privacy reasons. . . . The process is complicated, and the replies typically come on paper, as photocopies or faxes.

The efficient way would be for that data to be sent over the Internet into a person's digital health record. But that would require partnerships and trust between health care providers and insurers and the digital record-keepers.

Privacy concerns are another big obstacle, as both companies acknowledge. Most likely, they say, trust will build slowly, and the online records will include as much or as little personal information as users are comfortable divulging. . . .

There are plenty of competitors these days in online health records and information from start-ups like Revolution Health, headed by AOL's founder, Stephen M. Case, and thriving profit-makers led by WebMD.

Potential rivals are not underestimating the two technology giants. But the smaller companies have the advantage of being focused entirely on health, and some have been around for years. . . .

Google and Microsoft are great companies, said Wayne T. Gattinella, WebMD's chief executive, but "that doesn't mean they will be expert in a specific area like health."

Still, 58 percent of people seeking health information online begin with a general search engine, according to a recent Jupiter Research report, and Google dominates the field. "Google is the entry point for most health search, and that is a huge advantage," said Monique Levy, a Jupiter analyst. . . .

CHAPTER SUMMARY

- Medical informatics refers to the use of computers in the management and organization of medical information. Its goal is the improvement of patient care, administration, and research through the use of computers.
- The earliest use of computers was the use of administrative applications including the use of computers in the medical office for accounting.

- Medical accounting programs allow the user to computerize medical office management functions.
  - Bucket billing (or balance billing) is specific to health care office environments, where each insurer must be billed and payment received before the patient is billed.
- In today's medical office, coding systems are used to identify conditions, tests, and procedures.
- Various types of insurance need to be understood.
- Different kinds of accounting reports are used in the medical office.
- Accounting programs allow the user to computerize medical office management functions.

KEY TERMS

accounts receivable (A/R)
adjustments
administrative applications
assignment
authorization
balance billing
bucket billing
capitated plan
case
Centers for Medicare and Medicaid Services (CMS)
CHAMPUS
CHAMPVA
charges
claim
clearinghouse
clinical
CMS-1500
co-payment
CPT
database
database management software (DBMS)
deductible

DRG (diagnosis-related group)
electronic health record
electronic remittance advice (ERA)
EMC (electronic media claim)
encounter form
explanation of benefits (EOB)
fee-for-service plans
fields
file
guarantor
HCFA-1500
Health Care Financing Administration (HCFA)
health maintenance organizations (HMOs)
ICD
indemnity plan
key field
LOINC
managed care
MEDCIN

Medicaid
medical informatics
Medicare
patient aging report
patient day sheet
payment day sheet
payments
practice analysis report
preferred provider organizations (PPOs)
procedure day sheet
records
relational databases
schedule of benefits
SNOMED
special-purpose applications
superbill
table
telemedicine
transactions
TRICARE
UB04
worker's compensation

REVIEW EXERCISES

Define the following terms:
administrative applications
bucket billing
Centers for Medicare and Medicaid Services

Multiple Choice

1. The _____ is a code used by private and government insurers to determine insurance reimbursement.
   A. CPT
   B. DRG
   C. ICD
   D. SWP

2. _____ is defined as the use of technology to organize information in health care.
   A. Computer literacy
   B. Information literacy
   C. Medical informatics
   D. Medical computing

3. Centers for Medicare and Medicaid Services (CMS) administers _____.
   A. Medisoft
   B. Medicare
   C. Medicaid
   D. Both B and C

4. _____ provides 250,000 codes for such things as symptoms, history, physical exams, tests, diagnoses, and treatment.
   A. Medline
   B. Medisoft
   C. Medicode
   D. MEDCIN

5. _____ applications include the use of computers in office management, accounting, scheduling, and planning.
   A. Clinical
   B. Administrative
   C. Special-purpose
   D. None of the above

6. Medicare serves _____.
   A. people 65 years and over
   B. people under 65 years with broken legs
   C. people with chronic renal disorders
   D. Both A and C

7. A _____ is used to show a patient's outstanding payments.
    A. patient aging report
    B. practice analysis report
    C. patient day sheet
    D. procedure day sheet

8. A _____ is generated on a monthly basis and is a summary total of all procedures, charges, and transactions.
    A. patient aging report
    B. practice analysis report
    C. patient day sheet
    D. procedure day sheet

9. A _____ lists the day's patients, chart numbers, and transactions. It is used for daily reconciliation.
    A. patient aging report
    B. practice analysis report
    C. patient day sheet
    D. procedure day sheet

10. A _____ is a grouped report organized by procedure.
    A. patient aging report
    B. practice analysis report
    C. payment day sheet
    D. procedure day sheet

11. A _____ is a grouped report organized by providers.
    A. patient aging report
    B. practice analysis report
    C. payment day sheet
    D. procedure day sheet

12. Practices that submit electronic claims use a/an _____, a business that collects insurance claims from providers and sends them to the correct insurance carrier.
    A. insurance collector
    B. collection agency
    C. clearinghouse
    D. None of the above

13. The insurance company's response to a paper claim includes a/an _____ which explains why certain services were covered and others not.
    A. explanation of benefits (EOB)
    B. electronic remittance advice (ERA)
    C. lawyer's letter
    D. All of the above

14. The health care financing administration (HCFA) is now called _____.
    A. Centers for Medicare and Medicaid Services (CMS)
    B. Centers for Medical Services (CMS)
    C. Centers for Minor Surgery (CMS)
    D. None of the above

15. The insurance company's response to an electronic claim includes a/an _____ which explains why certain services were covered and others not.
    A. explanation of benefits (EOB)
    B. electronic remittance advice (ERA)
    C. lawyer's letter
    D. All of the above

True/False Questions

1. A superbill or encounter form is a list of diagnoses and procedures common to the practice. _____
2. A patient is not responsible for the co-payment. _____
3. Charges, payments, and adjustments are called transactions. _____
4. Under fee-for-service insurance plans, the patient is required to pay a deductible before the insurance company will cover medical costs. _____
5. A patient who uses a health maintenance organization (HMO) pays a fixed yearly fee and can choose among any health care provider or hospital. _____
6. ICD-9-CM provides codes for more than one thousand diseases. _____
7. Today, hospital reimbursement by private and government insurers is determined by diagnosis (DRG). _____
8. Bucket billing is used by medical offices to accommodate two or three insurers, who must be billed in a timely fashion before the patient is billed. _____
9. Doctors who accept assignment require payment by the patient, not the insurance company. _____
10. Medicaid finances health care for more than fifty million low-income people, with money provided by the federal government and the states. _____

Critical Thinking

1. The computerization of medical records has advantages and disadvantages. Comment on this statement. Do the advantages outweigh the disadvantages? Support your answer.
2. Under our current health care system, some medical decisions are being made by insurance companies. How would you design a system where health care practitioners and patients determined necessary treatments?
3. Comment on how the computerization of administrative tasks may affect a medical office. Bear in mind both efficiency and the fact that an office can print out reports that show the most profitable procedures and practitioners.

NOTES

1. *MedcomSoft Record 2006 Standards,* 2006, http://www.medcomsoft.com (accessed July 5, 2006).
2. CMS, September 2002, http://cms.hhs.gov/medicaid/default.asp (accessed April 4, 2003).
3. CHAMPVA Overview, March 25, 2003, http://www.military.com/benefits/veterans-health-care/champva-overview (accessed November 19, 2007); Understanding TRICARE, http://www.military.com/benefits/tricare (accessed November 19, 2007).

ADDITIONAL RESOURCES

Anderson, Sandra. *Computer Literacy for Health Care Professionals.* New York: Delmar Publishers Inc., 1992.

Baase, Sara. *A Gift of Fire: Social, Legal, and Ethical Issues in Computing.* Upper Saddle River, NJ: Prentice Hall, 1996.

Ball, Marion J., and Kathryn J. Hannah. *Using Computers in Nursing.* Norwalk, CT: Appelton-Century-Crofts, 1984.

Burke, Lillian, and Barbara Weill. *MediSoft Made Easy: A Step-by-Step Approach.* Upper Saddle River, NJ: Prentice Hall, 2004.

Davis, Daniel C., and William G. Chismar. "Tutorial Medical Informatics." http://www.hicss.hawaii.edu/hicss_32/tutdesc.htm (accessed August 18, 2006).

Felton, Bruce. "Technologies that Enable the Disabled." *New York Times,* September 14, 1997.

Holland, Gina. "Court Backs Regulation of HMOs." *The Star-Ledger,* April 3, 2003, 43.

Ito, Lloyd. "Medical Insurance." August 3, 1999. http://phys-advisor.com/Insure.htm (accessed November 18, 2006).

MediSoft Training Manual. Mesa, AR: NDC Health.

Newby, Cynthia. *Computers in the Medical Office Using Medisoft.* New York: Glencoe, McGraw-Hill, 1995.

Telemedicine

CHAPTER OUTLINE

LEARNING OBJECTIVES

Upon completion of this chapter, the student will be able to

- Define telemedicine.
- Discuss store-and-forward technology and interactive videoconferencing.
- Define the various subspecialties of teleradiology, telepathology, teledermatology, telecardiology, teleneurology, telestroke, telepsychiatry, and telehome care.
- Discuss the use of telemedicine in prisons.
- Discuss the changing role of the telenurse.
- Discuss the legal, licensing, insurance, and privacy issues involved in telemedicine.

OVERVIEW

Telemedicine uses computers and telecommunications equipment to deliver medical care at a distance. It should be noted at the outset, however, that because the telecommunications equipment (hardware and software), the knowledge and training, and financial resources are not evenly distributed within the nation or throughout the world, telemedicine is not universally available. Many doctors do not use computers. Many of the computer systems that are in use are not compatible or interoperable (cannot talk to each other). Where telemedicine is in place, it is used in various medical specialties.

   Several technologies are used in telemedicine: from plain old telephone service to high-speed dedicated lines, to the Internet. The medical information transmitted can be in any form including voice, data, still images, and video. Telemedicine delivers the whole range of medical care from diagnosis to patient monitoring to treatment. It gives patients remote access to experts who in turn have access to patient information. Today, some doctors have stopped using transcriptionists to type their notes; instead, they send their dictation over the Internet. Some dictation is sent overseas. They are returned by e-mail or downloaded from a web site as a word-processed document.[1] The linking of computers and other devices into networks (discussed in Chapter 1) forms the foundation for telemedicine. The field of telemedicine is growing at a rapid rate. In 2002, the executive director of the American Telemedicine Association (ATA) estimated that about one thousand health care facilities were linked via telecommunications lines. He traces part of this growth to the increased coverage provided by government and private insurers.[2] The production of telehome care products grew more quickly in the 1990s than that of any other medical device. There is no comprehensive current study of the extent of telemedicine in the United States. However, a study of its use in California concluded that 37 percent of health clinics and one-third of hospitals were using videoconferencing. By 2006, the U.S. Department of Veterans Affairs (VA) had spent $20 million to install some 15,000 home health monitors; it expects to have 50,000 in place by 2009. The VA has found the systems cut patient care costs by about one-third.[3] Telemedicine encompasses many subspecialties of medicine including radiology, pathology, oncology, ophthalmology, cardiology, neurology (including stroke), dermatology, and psychiatry. It may involve the sending of still images or real-time conferences, the use of remote monitoring devices, and the remote operation of medical equipment such as microscopes. Varieties of telemedicine are now being used to treat everything from psychiatric disorders (telepsychiatry) to skin rashes (teledermatology) to cancer (teleoncology). Remote surgery is in an early phase and will be discussed in Chapter 7. The field of telemedicine is changing and developing very rapidly. As of 2006, one of the reasons that telemedicine continues to expand is the growth of the prison population; telemedicine is increasingly used in prisons. Telemedicine has the potential of making high-quality medical care available to anyone in an urban or rural area regardless of distance from major medical centers, specialists, physicians, and visiting nurses. It can dramatically decrease the time a patient must wait and the miles the patient must travel to consult a specialist. Telemedicine transfers medical expertise instead of medical experts and patients. Many studies have found that patient satisfaction with telemedicine is high.

Medical consultations and exams at a distance have been attempted from the time that people were able to talk to each other from a distance. Early endeavors were made to send heart and lung sounds to experts over the newly invented telephone. But this failed because of poor transmission. Later, doctors tried to transmit electrocardiograms (ECGs) through the telephone. After World War II, pictures could be transmitted. However, it was only with the development of computers and telecommunications networks capable of transmitting high-resolution digital images and accurate sound that telemedicine could become a practical medical reality. The field is expanding so quickly that it is only possible to touch on major uses of telemedicine here. The following survey introduces the student to basic definitions in the field and presents examples of some of the more interesting uses of distance medicine. It also discusses some of the technical, legal, privacy, and insurance issues that need to be addressed in order for telemedicine to fulfill its promise.

STORE-AND-FORWARD TECHNOLOGY AND INTERACTIVE VIDEOCONFERENCING

Telemedicine projects may be based on store-and-forward technology or interactive videoconferencing. Some projects use both. **Store-and-forward technology** involves sharing information in a time- and place-independent way over the Internet. The information is stored, digitized, and then sent. If a medical specialty is image based, store-and-forward technology may be appropriate. The information may include digital images and clinical information. It may be as simple and inexpensive as attaching an image to an e-mail and sending it over telephone lines. Store-and-forward technology does not require the sophisticated telecommunications links required by videoconferencing, so it tends to be cheaper. The earliest use of store-and-forward technology was in teleradiology.

It is appropriate to specialties where diagnosis is based on images, such as dermatology and pathology. Images can be created by digital camera and sent over the Internet. This technique is used, for example, in some teleophthalmology programs, where others use videoconferencing. Because store-and-forward technology is cheaper and does not require sophisticated equipment or broadband lines, it is being used simply to introduce telemedicine at low cost to developing countries in specialties that had traditionally used videoconferencing. For example, a small tele-neurology program using store-and-forward technology was created between the United Kingdom and Bangladesh. The program was used with twelve patients to deliver expert advice; it was found to be effective.

Interactive videoconferencing or **teleconferencing** allows doctors to consult with each other and with patients in real time, at a distance. A patient may be in his or her primary physician's office with a camera and a telecommunications link to a special-ist's office. All can see and hear each other in real time. It might require only a video-phone and a connection to the Internet. However, the most sophisticated systems involve microphones, scanners, cameras, medical instruments, and dedicated tele-phone lines. One form of video teleconferencing is the remote house call, involving only one medical practitioner and a patient in another location.

TELERADIOLOGY

The oldest form of telemedicine using computers and telecommunications equip-ment is teleradiology. Today, **teleradiology** involves the sending of radiological images in digital form over telecommunications lines. Teleradiology uses store-and-forward technology; the data to be sent are digitized, stored, and transmitted over a telecommunications network. If the image is compressed for storage and transmis-sion, and if, as a result, any data are lost, the consultant is responsible for determin-ing whether the image is useful. The images can be sent any distance—from across the street to across the world. Store-and-forward teleradiology can be combined with interactive videoconferencing for immediate consultation when a problem is detected in pregnancy. The specialist sees the patient and ultrasound on a split screen and controls the exam from miles away. Before telemedicine, a patient might have to wait for a consultation with a specialist and travel long distances. Now, the technology can come to the patient.

Today, many radiological images are telecommunicated to India for interpreta-tion, especially at night. The turnaround time can be as little as thirty minutes. How-ever, there are limits because of licensure issues. "Only those doctors who have relocated from [the] U.S. can do offshoring to America." In other words, a doctor has to be licensed in both the United States and India.[4]

TELEPATHOLOGY

Telepathology is the transmission of microscopic images over telecommunications lines. The pathologist sees images on a monitor instead of under a microscope. Telepathology requires a microscope, camera, and monitor, as well as a connection to a telemedicine system. Telepathology can use real-time videoconferencing for consultation during an operation. But in daily practice, store-and-forward technology is common. Pathology is based on the study of images; diagnosis is based on the study of images on slides from a microscope looking for diagnostic features. If a second opinion is needed from a distant expert, telepathology may be used. The images are taken from the slides by camera. Still images usually are at a higher resolution than those sent in real time. The images and other clinical data are used for a complete case description and then sent, in many cases, over the Internet. One of the problems of store-and-forward telepathology is the choice of images sent. They may not show a complete picture, and this may lead to misdiagnosis.

TELEDERMATOLOGY

Teledermatology (the practice of dermatology using telecommunications networks) is also based partly on the study of images. It uses both videoconferencing and store-and-forward technology. Both methods appear effective. The advantage of the videoconferencing is that it closely resembles the traditional visit to the doctor, but is more expensive. Studies have shown that diagnosis made via videoconferencing agree with face-to-face dermatology visits 59 to 88 percent. A small study comparing store-and-forward teledermatology with face-to-face dermatology found 61 to 91 percent agreement. Certain skin conditions were found to be more difficult to diagnose via teledermatology. Diagnostic confidence was lower and the rate of biopsies higher. The advantage of store-and-forward technology is the high quality of the images and the low cost. To date, there have been no definitive outcomes studies. Some small studies have found that although there are limitations with store-and-forward technology (image quality and lack of patient interaction), teledermatology reduced unnecessary visits to dermatologists by more than 50 percent. In 2005, the "consensus on the diagnostic accuracy and clinical effectiveness of Store and Forward teledermatology appears to be growing, [however,] outcome studies are needed to measure cost effectiveness and patient outcomes."[5]

TELECARDIOLOGY

Prior to the 1800s, a doctor would listen to the heart by placing his ear on the patient's chest. Listening to the heart at a distance has a long history. Since the time of Hippocrates, physicians listened directly to patients' chests as they tried to assess cardiac health. The inventor of the stethoscope, Rene Theophile-Hyacinthe Laennec, relied on this method, too.

> One day, [in 1816] when he needed to examine an obese young woman, Laennec hesitated to put his head to her chest. Remembering that you can hear a pin scraping one end of a plank by putting your ear to the other end, he came up with the idea for a stethoscope prototype. He rolled a stack of paper into a cylinder, pressed one end to the patient's chest, and held his ear to the other end.[6]

Since the invention of the telephone, doctors have attempted to send heart and lung sounds over long distances. But the quality of the sound was not good enough. During the 1960s, it became possible to transmit heart sounds more accurately, and faxes could be used to send ECGs. By the 1990s, echocardiograms could be telecommunicated. Second opinions via telecardiology are one of the most common requests in telemedicine. People come into rural emergency rooms (ERs) with chest pains, and many ER doctors want an expert consultation. Telemedicine is becoming more and more widely used in cardiology. One study evaluated five programs in North America: two use store-and-forward technology and three use real-time videoconferencing. The study concluded that both real-time and store-and-forward tele-echocardiography were effective; both transmit diagnostic quality information.

Other telecommunications technology contributes to cardiac care. The Department of Veteran's Affairs will be able to use an Internet-based service that connects patients wearing pacemakers with their doctors. Patients can use a monitoring device to collect information from the pacemaker by holding an antenna over it. The data are sent by telephone to the CareLink Network. Doctors then have access to it. This system will work anywhere in the United States. Another technology that can be used to connect digital devices is **Bluetooth.** Bluetooth technology can link devices such as a pacemaker and a cell phone.

In 2006, in Japan, a group of scientists began using a mobile phone-based heart monitor. "When a heart discomfort is felt, the patient pushes the data transmission switch . . ." The ECG is sent to a server at the hospital which sends it to a doctor. This system can be used to monitor hospitalized patients and patients at home.[7]

TELENEUROLOGY

Neurology was slower to use telemedicine when compared to other specialties. Now, however, e-mail and videoconferencing are replacing the letter and telephone call. One of the first subspecialties to use telemedicine in neurology is stroke diagnosis.[8]

Telestroke

One of the recognized benefits of telemedicine is saving time. This is essential in treating strokes. There are almost three-quarters of a million new strokes per year in the United States. If the stroke is caused by a clot (determined by a computed tomography [CT] scan), the victim may be helped by the administration of a clot-busting drug called tissue plasminogen activator (tPA) if it is given within a few hours. However, if the stroke is caused by excessive bleeding, tPA can kill the patient. Immediate and accurate diagnosis is crucial. However, many small hospitals do not have experts. One study showed that 70 percent of stroke patients did not receive tPA either because they arrived at the hospital too late or because the hospitals could not provide the correct therapy. Massachusetts General Hospital began a **telestroke** program. Many people die of strokes just because they are taken to small hospitals without the capability of evaluating the stroke quickly. The telestroke program connects small local hospitals with Massachusetts General's stroke experts. When a stroke victim appeared at the local hospital in Martha's Vineyard, the doctors would do CT scans and forward them to stroke specialists at Massachusetts General. Both the local doctors and the specialists would evaluate the tests and interview the patient via a teleconferencing system to determine whether tPA was needed. Other hospitals are currently using this technology. By 2005, Massachusetts passed a law requiring "emergency medical technicians to bring patients exhibiting signs of a stroke to a hospital *that has a neurologist on staff 24 hours a day, bypassing nearby hospitals that might not meet the requirement*" (emphasis added). Telemedicine programs that allow neurologists to consult with the patient and doctor at the remote site via dedicated lines may be used to meet this requirement.[9] By 2006, telestroke in Massachusetts had further expanded. Hospitals in New Jersey, California, Georgia, and Utah also have telestroke programs, and Vermont and New Hampshire are considering instituting such programs.[10] In 2007, in Georgia, using Remote Evaluation of Acute Ischemic Stroke or Reach, tPA was used for about 20 percent of stroke cases.[11] The federal Stop Stroke Act, which was introduced in Congress in 2001 and again in 2005, has not yet (2006) become law. It would provide funding to build telestroke systems.

Telemedicine was also found to be effective in a stroke rehabilitation program. It improved both balance and functioning. Using an e-mail triage system for new referrals halved the number of people attending clinics.[12]

Epilepsy

Teleneurology uses e-mail and videoconferencing for real-time meetings. The patient is with a nurse at one location; the neurologist is at a distant location. Using videoconferencing, the neurologist can take a history and direct and see the physical exam of the patient. The neurologist can also diagnose the patient and create a treatment plan.[13]

A recent study found no difference in the frequency of seizures, hospitalizations, or emergency room visits between patients getting traditional face-to-face care and patients visited via video. A comparison of new patients seen via video "had similar investigation and review rates to patients seen face-to-face."[14]

Teleneurology helps to cope with some common problems of people with epilepsy. Many live in areas with no or little access to neurologists. Restrictions on driving for people with epilepsy can limit care. So teleneurology, which brings the care to the patient, is crucial. A study was completed of a system where a distant neurologist managed epileptic patients at a local rural hospital. Each patient was accompanied by a nurse case manager who managed medication, compliance, and reinforced the neurologist's advice. When this group was compared to a traditionally managed group, it was found that "telemedicine provided an acceptable alternative."

E-mail and Digital Cameras in Teleneurology

Low-cost teleneurology programs can make use of e-mail for referral. In one study, two groups were compared, one referred by e-mail and one in the traditional way.

The study concluded that "teleneurology by e-mail is sustainable . . . and . . . that it is safe, effective and efficient."[15]

Digital cameras that can produce high-quality video clips were successfully used to study gait. The video clips were sent to neurologists via e-mail. It was concluded that "Adequate-quality video clips of movement disorders can be produced with low-cost cameras and transmitted by e-mail for teleneurology purposes."[16]

■■■■■ TELEPSYCHIATRY

Telepsychiatry involves the delivery of therapy using teleconferencing. It usually makes use of some sort of hardware that can transmit and receive both voice and picture. However, to cut costs, psychiatrists are trying to find out if a poor image—or no image at all—makes therapy less effective. Experts warn that therapy at a distance is not a substitute for the human contact involved in face-to-face counseling. However, sometimes it is the only choice, for example, in rural areas where there are very few therapists and patients would have to travel long distances to see them.

During the 1960s, the first telepsychiatry sessions were conducted at the Nebraska Psychiatric Institute. Researchers found that the fact that the therapist was not physically present had little effect on group therapy. Studies of psychiatric consults between primary care providers and psychiatrists in New Hampshire came to the same conclusion—that videoconferencing and face-to-face consults were similar. A study of telemedicine for diagnosing patients with obsessive-compulsive disorder found it as successful as face-to-face therapy. A small study compared video-conferencing and face-to-face cognitive behavioral therapy in treating childhood depression and found them equally effective.[17] Some studies have found patients more comfortable talking to a distant psychiatrist. Others found that using a telenurse and a traditional psychiatrist improved depression more than only a psychiatrist, although there was no improvement in the numbers of clients taking their medication properly. Telepsychiatry was also found to be successful in delivering therapy to the family of a girl suffering from anorexia. It contributed to her recovery. The family was satisfied with the teletherapy.[18] In Australia, telepsychiatry is being used to treat panic disorders with cognitive behavioral therapy. So far, the project is "as effective as . . . therapy."[19] However, there are some negative aspects to telepsychiatry: the technology limits the therapist's perception of nonverbal clues and the equipment can be distracting; the therapist has to be sensitive to distortions in eye contact and the fact that a patient can appear to have stopped speaking when in fact he or she has not. That is, eye contact must be maintained with the camera, not the monitor, and the patient's mouth may stop moving before the patient has stopped speaking. One eighteen-month study of telepsychiatry in a prison setting found that patients were comfortable with the technology, but that many of the therapist's recommendations were not followed by prison personnel. This was a unique situation: the psychiatrist did not have some of the clients' medical records and so some recommendations (that a woman in a wheel-chair ride a bike) could not be carried out. Other recommendations were not carried out either because the doctor had little knowledge of prison rules and routines or because the doctor had no relationship with prison personnel. The psychiatrist had never been to the prison, and the medical records (which were paper records) had to stay at the prison. This points out some of the limitations of telepsychiatry—the clues that would be easily available in person are not obvious via telecommunications lines.[20]

Telepsychiatry continues to grow, partly because in eighteen states it is covered by Medicaid, and some states require private insurers to cover it. The problems of poverty, drug abuse, child abuse, and suicide plague rural as well as urban areas. Rural areas still lack psychiatrists; for example, in one U.S. county there is not one psychiatrist for 69,000 people, although its suicide rate is twice the national average. Telepsychiatry is also expanding with the prison population. It is cheap, reimbursed, and safer for the doctors.[21]

There are questions of whether telepsychiatry is appropriate for some forms of serious mental illness. For example, can it make schizophrenia worse by reinforcing the delusion that the television is talking to the patient?

REMOTE MONITORING DEVICES

Remote monitoring devices make it possible for patients to be monitored at home. A **telespirometry** system can be used at home by asthmatic patients; it is designed to transmit over the telephone to a remote location. A portable fetal monitor allows test results to be transmitted to a remote location. A miniature ECG Telemetry system allows wireless remote **arrhythmia monitoring**. Remote monitoring devices are also used in ambulances. The condition of the patient can be directly transmitted to the emergency room so that care can begin immediately on arrival. In September 1998, a "smart stretcher" was introduced. Weighing 135 pounds, but only 5 inches high, the stretcher includes a respirator, heart machine, intravenous drugs, and monitors that transmit all the data they gather immediately to the hospital. Using the smart stretcher means that no time needs to be wasted transporting the patient. Monitoring and treatment can begin immediately. The Defense Advanced Research Projects Agency of the U.S. Defense Department has created a smart t-shirt, which can monitor vital signs at a distance. Distance monitoring of blood glucose levels has improved outcomes in diabetes patients. In 2002, the Food and Drug Administration (FDA) approved an implantable cardiac device that enables a doctor to evaluate a patient over the Internet. Not all distance monitoring is successful, however. Distance monitoring of high-risk pregnancies has been a failure.[22]

Many of the newest, still experimental, monitoring devices use sensors embedded in fabric. The Wearable Health Care System (WEALTHY) has completed several years of research. These wearable systems are comfortable. Sensors, electrodes, and advanced signal processing techniques are embedded in the yarn. One wearable system monitors blood oxygen during sleep. One detects sleep apnea. Another measures ECG. Other wearable systems can measure respiration and temperature.[23–25]

▬▬▬ TELEHOME CARE

Telehome care involves the monitoring of vital signs from a distance via telecommunications equipment and the replacement of home nursing visits with videoconferences. It is usually used to manage chronic conditions such as congestive heart failure and diabetes, but it should be noted that it is beginning to be used for remote monitoring by intensive care unit (ICU) doctors at home. The cost of medical care for chronic conditions represents about 75 percent of medical costs in the United States, and some believe that home monitoring can lower these costs. The number of insurers that cover home monitoring is up from three in 2000 to twenty at the end of 2002. Some large hospitals have received grants from the Centers for Medicare and Medicaid Services (CMS) to expand telehome care. Some of this money will be used for demonstration projects and randomized trials.

The American Telemedicine Association (ATA) conducted a survey that showed "that commercial reimbursement of 'telemed' services other than teleradiology is more widespread than even many industry participants had thought." Many payers cover telemedicine, but payments for e-visits remain in their infancy.

Telehome care involves a link between the patient's home and a hospital or central office that collects the data. Equipment ($2,000–$6,000 per unit) is installed in the patient's home. It links the home or nursing home via telecommunications lines with a central office. The units differ from one another, but generally allow the patient and nurse to see and hear each other and allow the patient to push a button on the monitor, enabling the nurse to hear heart, lung, and bowel sounds; another button allows the nurse to monitor blood pressure. The machines also assess blood–oxygen level and pulse rate. Many units give voice reminders to take medication and ask the patient questions. For example, HANC (home-assisted nursing care) yells more and more loudly until the patient responds. The most sophisticated units show a doctor on the screen to check the patient's vital signs. The patient is able to aim a camera at an injury so that the doctor can advise how to dress and care for it. Some of the programs include extensive education about home management of chronic illness and even provide a telesocial worker for end-of-life planning. The Veterans Administration planned to have 20,000 patients on telehome care in 2007. There have not been any large-scale randomized studies of telehome care. Pilot studies have indicated that telehome care does increase access to health care in rural areas and that it may decrease unnecessary hospital and emergency room visits. It allows a nurse to make many more visits in a day—fifteen to twenty instead of five to six. A small United States-United Kingdom study concluded that 45 percent of U.S. home visits could be remote. Many small studies have found both nurses and patients like the video visits and one study found that telehospice care was quite cost-effective. A study in Italy found home telemonitoring for patients with severe respiratory illness decreased hospital admissions; patients were satisfied. The study concluded that telemonitoring can provide high-quality home care.[26] Another small study found telemedicine effective in reducing hospital admissions for patients with congestive heart failure; patients had their vital signs and general appearance telemonitored, while maintaining regular video contact with health care professionals who offered advice on drug use and diet. In California, a study compared the use of face-to-face therapy with videoconferencing in control and intervention groups. No differences in medication compliance, knowledge of disease, and ability for self-care were found. Patients were satisfied with the videoconferencing. Further, it costs less to treat patients via teleconferencing than face-to-face therapy.[27] A study by Kaiser Permanente found that using telehome care reduced hospital stays by 200 days from 1996 to 1997. One Visiting Nurse Association found a 29 percent reduction in ER visits and a 37 percent reduction in hospitalizations for patients using telehome care.[28] A pilot study of another home monitoring system (E-Care) used to manage patients with chronic illness by keeping track of activity, temperature, pulse, blood pressure, and glucose, using sensors was done in 2003–2004. The system also includes medication reminders and checks current data against the patient's record. "Users praised its practicability, reliability, effectiveness and patient acceptance."[29] Several factors retard the adoption of telehome care, including the attitudes of home health agencies, the initial cost of the equipment, reimbursement rates, and the few studies demonstrating that it is cost-effective.

In 2006, the Visiting Nurse Service of Western New York found that using home monitoring devices reduced rehospitalizations. The national rate of rehospitalization for patients with chronic illnesses is 26 percent; in western New York it dropped by 50 to 13 percent.[30]

In Warren County, New York, small (alarm clock sized) home monitors greet thirty-one patients with "Good morning. It is now time to record your vital signs." The device monitors the patients and transmits its findings via the telephone line. Among these thirty-one patients, hospital visits have dropped by over 70 percent.[31] Other pilot programs found telehome care reduces travel time, improves patient outcomes, and decreases hospitalizations and ER visits. An experimental program is being used to help veterans with spinal cord injuries.[32–34]

TELEMEDICINE IN PRISON

Telemedicine is now widely used in state prisons in Arizona, Iowa, Maryland, Texas, Massachusetts, Virginia, Pennsylvania, and New York, and in the federal prison system. In 2006, South Carolina introduced the use of telepsychiatry.[35] The stated reasons for introducing telemedicine are cost-containment, security, and enhanced medical care for inmates. A recent study of teleophthalmology in prisons found it to be cost-effective and to reduce blindness caused by diabetic retinopathy.[36]

Telemedicine is used to provide specialist care, not primary care, which is delivered onsite. Although no comprehensive study exists, there are some comparisons of traditional to telemedical care in specific areas. The Arizona Department of Corrections did a cost-benefit analysis in FY 2000 and found a $200.89 savings per case, which came to a total savings of $156,694.20. A review of the literature on Texas indicates that both patients and providers are satisfied with the care and that the vast majority of systems experienced reductions in travel and security costs. One preliminary study found that 95 percent of the telemedical consults had saved a trip to a clinic. A teleconsult clinic for human immunodeficiency virus (HIV)-positive inmates was established in Texas in 1999: it was found to cut costs, but has no effect on outcomes. Massachusetts also introduced a telemedicine program for HIV-positive prisoners and found no significant differences in health outcomes. But, HIV patients became increasingly concerned about privacy. Further study of this project is planned. There seems to be a consensus that telemedicine in prisons saves money and increases security by decreasing off-site visits. Survey data also indicate that both prisoners and prison administrators are satisfied with telemedicine. It may be that more prisoners seek treatment because they do not have to travel; in states like Texas, a visit to a clinic can mean four days of travel shackled in a truck. However, there are no comprehensive studies on the effect on the health of prisoners.

OTHER TELEMEDICINE APPLICATIONS

In 1996, the federal government funded nineteen pilot projects in telemedicine. Many are now taken-for-granted aspects of telemedicine: attempts to bring health care to rural areas and attempts to link small hospitals with medical centers for sharing of information. Others sent medication reminders to the elderly. One tested an Adverse Drug Event monitor; these programs are now in common use and will be discussed in Chapter 8. One of the more interesting and highly successful programs is **Baby CareLink**. Baby CareLink was originated in Massachusetts. Its purpose was to compare high-risk, premature infants receiving traditional care with an experimental group, which in addition to traditional care received a telemedicine link to the hospital while the babies were hospitalized and for six months after. The families could see and hear their babies in the nursery, although they were at home. They could log on to a secure Web page with up-to-date information about their babies. Once home, the families had access to the nursery and experts and could ask any question they pleased. The doctor or nurse could see the baby and reassure the parent. One purpose of Baby CareLink was to see whether parents felt more comfortable and knowledgeable about their babies' care, so that the hospital stay would be shorter. The experimental group did have shorter hospital stays. In a later case study of Baby CareLink in Chicago, it was found that the average length of stay for the experimental group was 2.73 days shorter, only 18 percent were readmitted (less than the expected 40 percent), medical staff were happy with the program, and parents were more comfortable with their infants. Baby CareLink is now covered by several state Medicaid programs and at least one private insurer. Baby CareLink is currently established in many hospitals throughout the country.

In 2006, Dr. Darius Moshfeghi began using RetCam™ II Digital Imaging System to diagnose retinopathy of prematurity (ROP), a condition that can leave premature babies blind if not treated early. Almost 20 percent of very premature babies develop signs of ROP; it is one of the leading causes of blindness among babies. Very few doctors can screen for ROP. Using a telemedicine network called SUNDROP (Stanford University Network for Diagnosis of Retinopathy of Prematurity), the doctor can examine his or her patients from afar.[37,38]

In 2006, telemedical devices are being developed to help people with Alzheimer's. Some of the devices include "visual prompts by the telephone that showed . . . the caller's name, picture, relationship, and reminders of their last interaction." Special "Presence" lamps would light up in an adult child's home when the parent sat in her favorite chair. The senior and her family would be able to see a representation of her social network.[39]

In Texas and Kansas, day care centers have brought teledoctors to day care. An onsite nurse uses a video camera and stethoscope and other equipment. A doctor diagnoses the child. In the vast majority of cases, the child is allowed to stay at day care and a prescription is called in. The parent does not have to leave work. In Rochester, New York, a federal grant is helping to set up a telemedicine system serving day care centers. By 2005, the program was considered successful. Studies report that "there has been a 63 percent drop in sickness-related absences at the pilot centers [and] that 92 percent of parents said the program enabled them to go to work when they otherwise would have needed to take their children to a family physician or emergency department."[40]

Telemedicine is currently being utilized in almost every aspect of health care: One of the more interesting new uses of telemedicine is in Vermont in a teletrauma project that links trauma surgeon's homes with hospital emergency departments, providing immediate expert service at any time.[41]

It is especially common for rural areas to lack high-speed communications, although this varies and there is a lack of hard data on the issue. Presently, several rural states including Alaska, Maine, Nebraska, and Tennessee are using telemedicine applications. In Arkansas, "41 percent of patients who use telemedicine services would not have been able to see a doctor because of a doctor shortage and travel costs."[42]

Telemedicine is being used in weight management, pain management, spinal cord injury, and podiatry. **Teleoncology** systems are helping cancer patients avoid lengthy trips to the doctor and feel more secure because they have a 24-hour link to health care. Telemedicine programs are using motion detectors to monitor elderly people in a nursing home; with the motion detectors, "atypical days" when activity was less than normal could be detected.[43]

In hospitals and even operating rooms, health care personnel (including 17 percent of doctors) are making use of personal digital assistants for writing prescriptions, quickly accessing patient information, and finding facts in online databases of medical articles and journals.

Information is crucial in fighting disease—access to the latest journal articles and newest treatment is necessary. However, in developing countries, access to the best information is limited at best. In 1989, **SATELLIFE** was founded. Its purpose was to deliver journals and other information to health care workers in developing areas. It "meets the . . . needs of health workers where the diseases of poverty are decimating entire communities . . ." In 1994, SATELLIFE began using e-mail and discussion groups. Approximately 100,000 health care workers in 159 countries use SATELLIFE each day.[44]

Telenurses and doctors are using the eICU Smart Alerts® to monitor intensive care patients from afar. In an ICU, onsite personnel are busy and can be distracted.

Remote doctors and nurses can act as adjuncts, spotting patients in trouble immediately and sending alerts to the ICU. According to Terry Davis, an operations director of an eICU, "Because the eICU physician and nurse as are always watching trends for the patient, the remote monitoring decreases the number of complications and . . . the length of stay in the ICU."[45]

Veterans of modern wars have been returning home with myriad injuries. This is because of the nature of the weaponry on one hand and the medical care they receive on or near the battlefield on the other. Blast injuries lead to multiple problems or polytruama: visual and hearing impairments, head trauma, amputations, spinal cord injuries, and posttraumatic stress disorder. There are so many forms of rehabilitation these people need, that only telemedicine can keep track of them.[46–47]

In July 2006, the FDA approved a wireless electronic capsule to help diagnose stomach disorders. The capsule that is small enough to be easily swallowed is used to diagnose gastroparesis—a condition that causes the stomach to empty slowly. The capsule transmits to a receiver that the patient wears while it travels through the intestinal tract. "When [it] is passed, the patient brings the cell-phone-sized receiver back to the physician, who downloads the data to a computer."[48]

THE TELENURSE

Telemedicine is changing the role of the nurse. **Telenursing** involves teletriage and the telecommunication of health-related data, the remote house call, and the monitoring of chronic disease. Teletriage starts with a call from a worried patient or parent with a question to the nurse. Software helps the nurse ask a series of questions to aid in diagnosis and make a recommendation to the patient. Telenursing increases access to medical advice by making it available in the home. Nurses may be in more autonomous positions in telemedicine programs. In England, there is a 24-hour telephone line staffed by nurses. The nurses use diagnostic software and are linked to databases, hospitals, primary care providers, and ambulances. The nurses staffing these lines need to know how to use the software and how to get the correct information; the nurse also needs knowledge of local health care services. In the United States, the VA telephone care program is staffed by Registered Nurses (RNs) only. The nurses have access to the patient records and to the primary care provider through e-mail. Patients appreciate the immediate attention from an expert. One study of patients whose doctors allowed secure e-mail found 90 percent of patients who used it rated their doctors as good, very good, or excellent, compared to 80 percent of a group which did not use e-mail. Those using e-mail found it to be convenient and felt free to talk about more personal issues.[49]

In teleconferencing, the nurse takes the patient's vital signs from a distance and assesses the patient via a monitor. Although the televisit is similar to the actual visit, it is not identical. Nurses lead many telemedicine programs. In some programs, nurses perform diagnostic services. Nurses need to be familiar with computerized equipment and comfortable using it. When telemedicine is used in schools, the school nurse becomes responsible for the referral and follows up on home care. Nurses involved in a study of the role of **telehealth** in psychiatry needed knowledge of management of depression, medication, counseling, and the ability to provide emotional support. In a telemedicine project examining diabetes, the nurse case manager performed weekly consultations and the doctor monthly consultations. The nurse would recommend changes in diet and exercise and participate in the doctor's monthly consult.

ISSUES IN TELEMEDICINE

For telemedicine to fulfill its promise, certain technical, legal, insurance, and privacy issues need to be addressed. On the technical side, an appropriate telecommunications infrastructure must be in place. The Telecommunications Act of 1996 proposes that access be increased, but does not specify how. Certain aspects of telemedicine require high-speed, broadband media, because the files transmitted may be so huge (greater than one gigabyte). This applies particularly to the utilization of real-time interactive video teleconferencing, which transmits voice, sound, images, text, and motion video.

In addition, legal issues such as licensing, medical liability, and privacy concerns need to be addressed. Furthermore, there are problems of insurance. Currently, there is some insurance coverage for telemedicine, although this is changing. If the Medicare Remote Monitoring Services Coverage Act becomes law, Medicare would cover the remote house call. Currently, Medicare and most private insurers cover only face-to-face medical care, with exceptions. As of January 1, 1999, the Balanced Budget Act of 1997 required that Medicare pay for telemedical services in medically underserved areas. However, after two years of this expanded reimbursement, Medicare had only reimbursed $20,000 for 301 teleconsultation claims. In an attempt to expand coverage further, the Congress passed the Medicare, Medicaid, and State Children's Health Insurance Program (SCHIP) Benefits Improvement and Protection Act. It went into effect in October of 2001. Twenty state Medicaid programs now cover some telemedicine services, as do some private insurers. In California, Texas, and Louisiana, it is illegal for insurers to discriminate between face-to-face and telemedical services.

One of the most serious legal obstacles to the development of telemedicine is state licensing. Medical personnel are required to be licensed by the state in which they practice. Acquiring a license is a costly and time-consuming process. Practicing without a license is a crime. Licensing laws are different in each state. Some states allow consultations across state lines. However, the American Medical Association supports requiring physicians to be licensed in any state in which they practice telemedicine. Some states have reciprocity agreements with other states. Some states require telemedicine providers to be separately licensed in each jurisdiction. Not all the states have agreements that make it easier for nurses to practice across state lines.

Telemedicine raises many privacy issues; medical information routinely crosses state lines, some of it via e-mail, which is not private. There are typically nonmedical personnel involved including technicians and camera operators. According to the Final Health Insurance Portability and Accountability Act Privacy (HIPAA)

Rules, several privacy issues are relevant: Under HIPAA, "Federal laws preempt state laws that are in conflict with regulatory requirements or those that provide less stringent privacy protections. But those states that have *more* stringent privacy laws would preempt Federal law." This leads to a "patchwork" of different standards. In a telemedical consultation, many people (both medical and nonmedical) may be present—but not apparent to the patient. Telemedicine requires greater concern with patient privacy and more complicated consent from patients.

The laws concerning telemedicine today are ambiguous; legal liability is not clear. It is not even clear what pieces of equipment used in a telemedical consult or exam are considered medical devices and are therefore subject to regulation by the FDA. Some of the legal ramifications are made clear by the following:

- If a doctor in one state sends an X-ray to a specialist in another state and the specialist misreads it, leading to the death of the patient, who is liable?
- If a reporter gains access to a database, finds records of a telepsychiatric consult, and publicizes them, who is liable?

The answers to these questions are not yet clear.

IN THE NEWS

Excerpt from, "TV Screen, Not Couch, Is Required for This Session"

by Kirk Johnson

FLAGSTAFF, Ariz.—Dr. Sara Gibson looked into the television screen and got right down to it.

"What's keeping you alive at this point?" she asked her patient, a middle-aged woman who asked to be identified only as D. D grimaced, looked down, then to the side and finally into Dr. Gibson's face, which filled the screen before her in a tiny clinic three hours east of here in the Arizona desert.

"Nothing," said D, who Dr. Gibson says suffers from bipolar disorder and post-traumatic stress from the sexual abuse she suffered as a child.

It is Wednesday in the hinterlands of rural Arizona, and the psychiatrist is in. Sort of.

Actually, Dr. Gibson was here in Flagstaff in a closet-size office of a nonprofit medical group, with a pale blue sheet behind her as a backdrop and a cup of tea at her side. She is one of a growing number of psychiatrists practicing through the airwaves and wires of telemedicine, as remote doctoring is known.

Psychiatry, especially in rural swaths of the nation that also often have deep social problems like poverty and drug abuse, is emerging as one of the most promising expressions of telemedicine. At least 18 states, up from only a handful a few years ago, now pay for some telemedicine care under their Medicaid programs. . . .

Growing prison populations have a lot to do with the trend. Since reimbursement for prison care is easy and safety issues for doctors are significant, many telemedicine programs, notably an ambitious one in Texas, started there. . . .

Dr. Gibson rides a disembodied circuit through this terrain. On Wednesdays, she sees patients in the tiny community of Springerville near the New Mexico border through a firewalled T1 data line, and on Thursdays in St. Johns. Each side of the exchange has its own television-mounted camera, angled so that doctor and patient can maintain the illusion of looking into each other's eyes in real time.

Dr. Gibson, 44, was a pioneer in the field. She has been seeing patients only this way for 10 years and is still one of a handful of doctors in the country who practice telepsychiatry exclusively. . . .

The American Psychiatric Association says on its Web site that it supports telemedicine, "to the extent that its use is in the best interest of the patient," and practitioners meet the rules about ethics and confidentiality. But in places like Apache County, where the alternative is no treatment at all, most mental health workers say that every new wire and screen is to be deeply cheered.

"Basically, doctors can do, surprisingly, almost everything," said Don McBeath, the director of telemedicine and rural health at the Texas Tech University Health Sciences Center in Lubbock. "The difference is they can't touch you or smell you."

Dr. Gibson said the lack of smelling and touching, at least when it comes to psychiatry, has proved to be a good thing. Being physically in the presence of another human being, she said, can be overwhelming, with an avalanche of sensory data that can distract patient and doctor alike without either being aware of it. . . .

She worries, sometimes, about the children she sees . . . "Do they understand that the TV doesn't always talk to them?" Dr. Gibson said. . . .

Some things did not happen as expected. Dr. Gibson predicted, for example, that at least one patient would incorporate the teleconferencing technology into his or her delusions. . . .

What Dr. Gibson's patients imagine of her life and what she is like when she is not on camera is unknown. . . . She speculated that telemedicine has probably in some ways amplified and enlarged her image in the minds of some patients. . . .

She has been to Apache County once, for a "meet the psychiatrist" event in St. Johns years ago. Many of the patients who showed up remarked, she said, about how much shorter she was than they had expected.

CHAPTER SUMMARY

- Chapter 4 introduces the reader to the field of telemedicine and some of its subspecialties. In addition, its effectiveness and some of the issues that must be addressed for telemedicine to fully develop are discussed.
- Telemedicine uses computers and telecommunications technology to deliver health care including diagnosis, patient monitoring, and treatment at a distance. As such, it has the potential of making high-quality health care available to anyone regardless of distance from major medical centers. It may use store-and-forward technology for transmission of still images or interactive videoconferencing for real-time consultations.
- It encompasses subspecialties such as teleradiology, telepathology, telecardiology, teleneurology, telestroke, telehome care, and telepsychiatry, as well as the use of remote monitoring devices and remote operation of medical equipment.
- Remote monitoring devices allow patients to be monitored at home or in an ambulance; the information is transmitted to a remote location.
- Telemedicine is changing the role of the nurse.
- Telemedicine is currently being evaluated, and the assessments tend to be positive. It is used in prison settings where its efficacy is being judged. Several studies have been completed and more are underway. The federal government has funded several projects to be evaluated.
- For the promise of telemedicine to be fulfilled, certain problems have to be solved. These include the establishment of adequate high-bandwidth communications lines, barriers posed by state licensing, the lack of insurance coverage in many instances, and the insecurity of the electronic medical record. HIPAA addresses some of the privacy problems posed by telemedicine.
- Telepsychiatry is a necessary part of the health care system in sparsely populated areas with few therapists.

KEY TERMS

arrhythmia monitoring
Baby CareLink
Bluetooth
interactive
    videoconferencing
remote monitoring
    devices
SATELLIFE

store-and-forward
    technology
teleconferencing
teledermatology
telehealth
telehome care
telemedicine
teleneurology

telenursing
teleoncology
telepathology
telepsychiatry
teleradiology
telespirometry
telestroke

REVIEW EXERCISES

Multiple Choice

1. Telemedicine involves _____.
   A. the linking of doctors and patients at a distance
   B. the transmission of radiologic images via telecommunications lines
   C. the transmission of patient data in any form
   D. All of the above
2. The technology used in teleradiology is called _____.
   A. send-and-receive
   B. receive-and-send
   C. store-and-forward
   D. None of the above
3. Before telemedicine can deliver high-quality medical services at a distance _____.
   A. a reliable broadband telecommunications network has to be in place
   B. state licensing barriers have to be overcome
   C. every patient needs to own a printer
   D. A and B only
4. The transmission of microscopic images over telecommunications lines is called _____.
   A. teleradiology
   B. telepsychiatry
   C. telepathology
   D. remote monitoring
5. Telemedicine projects in prisons have been found to _____.
   A. improve health care
   B. cut costs
   C. improve security
   D. All of the above
6. _____ allows doctors and patients to consult in real time, at a distance.
   A. Telepathology
   B. Teleradiology
   C. Teleoncology
   D. Interactive videoconferencing
7. In which of the following cases would face-to-face medical care be less expensive than telemedicine? _____
   A. Therapy for depression
   B. Medical care for prisoners
   C. Surgery
   D. Telemedicine is always less expensive
8. Telemedicine is used in some way in the treatment of _____.
   A. psychiatric disorders
   B. cancer
   C. skin rashes
   D. All of the above

9. Remote medical consultations and exams were first tried _____.
   A. after World War II
   B. in 1997
   C. as soon as the telephone was invented
   D. in 1977
10. A remote house call by a visiting nurse is an example of _____.
    A. telepathology
    B. teleradiology
    C. video teleconferencing
    D. None of the above
11. _____ technology is used to link electronic devices (e.g., a pacemaker with a cell phone).
    A. Telephone
    B. Bluetooth
    C. Video teleconferencing
    D. Store-and-forward
12. The _____ program at Massachusetts General diagnoses quickly and can determine if tPA should be used in treatment.
    A. telestroke
    B. telecardiology
    C. telenurse
    D. teledoctor
13. One of the most successful telemedicine programs links hospitalized premature infants with their parents at home. It is called _____.
    A. telebaby
    B. computer parenting
    C. telepreemie
    D. Baby CareLink
14. Many telemedicine programs have been found to be effective. But _____ is not.
    A. distance monitoring of problem pregnancies
    B. telehome care
    C. telemedicine in prisons
    D. teletriage programs run by telenurses
15. In Vermont, a _____ project links trauma surgeon's homes with hospital emergency departments.
    A. telestroke
    B. teletrauma
    C. telecardiology
    D. teleoncology

True/False Questions

1. Medical insurance is beginning to cover telemedicine. _____
2. The broadband links are in place to deliver telemedicine all over the world. _____

3. State licensing of doctors is an obstacle to the development of telemedicine. _____
4. The electronic patient record is absolutely secure. _____
5. The oldest form of telemedicine is teleradiology. _____
6. Telemedicine has the potential of giving immediate access to specialists regardless of distance. _____
7. Establishing a telemedicine site is so inexpensive that any clinic can afford it. _____
8. Telepsychiatry is the recommended therapy for anyone regardless of mental disorder. _____
9. In 2006, in Japan, a group of scientists began using a mobile phone-based heart monitor. _____
10. Remote monitoring devices make it possible for patients to be monitored at home. _____

Critical Thinking

1. Cite some examples of the current usage of aspects of telemedicine technologies in the diagnosis and treatment of patients. Can you suggest future uses of telemedicine that would improve health care?
2. How can patient confidentiality be safeguarded, given the establishment of a vast national database of medical records?
3. Discuss who should be held accountable for mistakes in diagnosis and treatment when there are several parties involved including (but not limited to) the onsite physician, remote specialist and other medical personnel, and telecommunications equipment manufacturer.
4. Should medical personnel involved in telemedicine be licensed in every state or licensed nationally? Discuss the advantages and disadvantages of each.
5. Today, medical personnel need to be retrained in certain telemedicine technology areas. How would you convince them to retrain?

NOTES

1. "Computers in Medicine Online," January 4, 2006, http://www.brickellresearch.com/news.shtml (accessed January 28, 2006).
2. Julie Jette, "A Life-Saving Link: Stroke Patients Can Connect with Mass General," May 16, 2002, http://www.massgeneral.org/stopstroke/newsStory051602.aspx/ (accessed November 28, 2007).
3. Josie Henderson and Will Engle (eds), "Telemedicine and Telehealth News," August 2, 2006, http://telemed.org/news/#item1380 (accessed August 22, 2006).
4. "Indian Docs Read CT Scans from U.S.," March 28, 2006, http://sify.com/finance/fullstory.php?id=141171542 (accessed March 30, 2006).
5. Gunter Burg, "Store-and-Forward Teledermatology," August 25, 2005, http://www.emedicine.com/derm/topic560.htm (accessed August 22, 2006).
6. "History of Stethoscopes and Sphygmomanometers," October 7, 2003, http://www.hhmi.org/biointeractive/museum/exhibit98/content/b6_17info.html (accessed August 19, 2006).

7. J. Iwamoto, Y. Yonezawa, H. Maki, H. Ogawa, I. Ninomiya, K. Sada, S. Hamada, A. W. Hahn, and W. M. Caldwell, "A Mobile Phone-Based ECG Monitoring System," Abstract, 2006, http://www.ncbi.nlm.nih.gov/pubmed/16817611?ordinalpos=2&itool= EntrezSystem2.PEntrez.Pubmed.Pubmed_ResultsPanel.Pubmed_RVDocSum (accessed December 28, 2007).

8. Victor Patterson and Richard Wooten, "How Can Teleneurology Improve Patient Care?" medscape.com, July 17, 2006, http://www.medscape.com/viewarticle/540191 (accessed August 4, 2006).

9. "Telemedicine Helps Victims of Stroke," August 9, 2005, http://www.networkworld.com/news/2005/052305-stroke.html (accessed December 28, 2007).

10. Liz Kowalczyk, "Going the Distance in Stroke Treatment," *Boston Globe*, April 3, 2006, http://www.boston.com/yourlife/health/diseases/articles/2006/04/03/going_the_distance_in_stroke_treatment/ (accessed December 28, 2007).

11. Susan Jeffrey, "Telemedicine System May Increase tPA Use in Stroke," July 17, 2007, http://www.medscape.com/viewarticle/559914 (accessed December 28, 2007).

12. Patterson and Wooten, "How Can Teleneurology Improve Patient Care?"

13. Victor Patterson and Ena Bingham, "Telemedicine for Epilepsy: A Useful Combination," *Epilepsia* 44, no. 5 (2005): 614–15.

14. Patterson and Wooten, "How Can Teleneurology Improve Patient Care?"

15. V. Patterson, J. Humphreys, and R. Chua, "Teleneurology by Email," *Journal of Telemedicine and Telecare* 9, no. 2 (2003): S42–3, http://www.ncbi.nlm.nih.gov/sites/entrez?cmd=Retrieve&db=PubMed&list_uids=14728758&dopt=AbstractPlus (accessed December 28, 2007).

16. Kerrie L. Schoffer, Victor Patterson, Stephen J. Read, et al., "Guidelines for filming digital camera video clips for the assessment of gait and movement disorders by teleneurology," *Journal of Telemedicine and Telecare* 11, no. 7, October 2005: 368–71(4), http://www.ingentaconnect.com/content/rsm/jtt/2005/00000011/00000007/art00008 (accessed February 7, 2008).

17. E. L. Nelson, M. Barnard, and S. Cain, "Treating Childhood Depression over Videoconferencing," *Telemedicine Journal and e-Health Spring* 9, no. 1 (2003): 49–55, http://www.ncbi.nlm.nih.gov/sites/entrez?db=pubmed&uid=12699607&cmd=show detailview (accessed December 28, 2007).

18. G. S. Goldfield and A. Boachie, "Delivery of Family Therapy in the Treatment of Anorexia Nervosa Using Telehealth: A Case Report," Abstract, 2003, http://www.ncbi.nlm.nih.gov/sites/entrez?db=pubmed&uid=12699614&cmd=show detailview (accessed December 28, 2007).

19. Kenneth Lane, "Telemedicine News," *Telemedicine and e-Health* 12, no. 2 (2006): 81–84.

20. Jeanine Turner, "Telepsychiatry as a Case Study of Presence: Do You Know What You Are Missing?" *JCMC* 6, no. 4 (2001), http://jcmc.indiana.edu/vol6/issue4/turner.html (accessed December 24, 2007).

21. Kirk Johnson, "TV Screen, Not Couch, Is Required for This Session," nyt.com, June 8, 2006 (accessed December 28, 2007).

22. Carol Lewis, "Emerging Trends in Medical Device Technology: Home Is Where the Heart Monitor Is," FDA Consumer, May–June 2001, http://www.fda.gov/Fdac/features/2001/301_home.html (accessed December 28, 2007).

23. "'Smart' Fabrics to Keep Patients Healthy." March 16, 2005, http://www.medicalnewstoday.com/articles/21338.php (accessed December 28, 2007).

24. Sarah Wright, "Media Lab Hosts Workshop on Body Sensors," mit.edu, April 12, 2006, http://web.mit.edu/newsoffice/2006/media-sensors.html (accessed December 24, 2007).

25. S. Milior, "A Wearable Health Care System Based on Knitted Sensors," Abstract, September 2005, http://www.ncbi.nlm.nih.gov/sites/entrez?orig_db=PubMed&db= PubMed&cmd=Search&TransSchema=title&term=A%20Wearable%20Health%20Care %20System%20Based%20on%20Knitted%20Sensors (accessed December 28, 2007).

26. C. Maiolo, E. I. Mohamed, C. M. Fiorani, and A. De Lorenzo, "Home Telemonitoring for Patients with Severe Respiratory Illness: the Italian Experience," *Journal of Telemedicine and Telecare* 9, no. 2 (2003): 67–71, http://www.ncbi.nlm.nih.gov/sites/entrez?db=pubmed&uid=12699574&cmd=showdetailview (accessed December 28, 2007).

27. B. Johnson, L. Wheeler, J. Deuser, and K. H. Sousa, "Outcomes of the Kaiser Permanente Tele-Home Health Research Project," Abstract, January 2000, http://tie.telemed.org (accessed August 22, 2006).

28. Candace Choi, "Screen Presents a Picture of Health," *Star Ledger,* March 15, 2006, 25.

29. "Remote Healthcare Monitoring Not So Distant," March 21, 2005, http://www.medicalnewstoday.com/articles/21599.php (accessed December 28, 2007).

30. "Monitoring Devices Help Reduce Rehospitalizations," ihealthbeat.org, June 26, 2006, http://www.ihealthbeat.org/articles/2006/6/26/Monitoring-Devices-Help-Reduce-Rehospitalizations.aspx?topicID=53 (accessed December 28, 2007).

31. Lane, "Telemedicine News."

32. Marinella Galea, Janine Tumminia, and Lisa Garback, "Telerehabilitation in Spinal Cord Injury Persons: A Novel Approach," *Telemedicine and e-Health* 12, no. 2 (2006): 160–2.

33. Stanley M. Finkelstein, Stuart M. Speedie, and Sandra Potthof, "Home Telehealth Improves Clinical Outcomes at Lower Cost for Home Healthcare," *Telemedicine and e-Health* 12, no. 2 (2006): 128–36.

34. Thomas S. Nesbitt, Stacy L. Cole, Lorraine Pellegrin, and Patricia Keast, "Rural Outreach in Home Telehealth: Assessing Challenges and Reviewing Successes," *Telemedicine and e-Health* 12, no. 2 (2006): 107–13.

35. "Upstate Prison to Use Telemedicine for Mentally Ill Inmates," August 8, 2006, http://www.wistv.com/Global/story.asp?S=5256538 (accessed November 28, 2007).

36. Noriaki Aoki, Kim Dunn, Tsuguya Fukui, J. Robert Beck, William J. Schull, and Helen K. Li, "Cost-Effectiveness Analysis of Telemedicine to Evaluate Diabetic Retinopathy in a Prison Population," *Diabetes Care* 27 (2004), 1095–101, http://care.diabetesjournals.org/cgi/content/abstract/27/5/1095/ (accessed December 10, 2007).

37. "Using Telemedicine to Save Babies' Vision," businesswire.com, April 11, 2006, http://www.genengnews.com/news/bnitem.aspx?name=356247 (accessed December 24, 2007).

38. "Clarity Medical Systems Announces Major Move into Adult Eye Care Market: Company to Introduce New Technology Aimed at Revamping How Eye Exams Are Performed," June 23, 2006, http://www.claritymsi.com/news/060623.html (accessed December 24, 2007).

39. Henderson and Engle, "Telemedicine and Telehealth News."

40. "Rochester Expands Use of Telemedicine in Day Care Centers," May 5, 2005, http://www.ihealthbeat.org/index.cfm?Action=dspItem&itemID=110905 (accessed August 22, 2006).

41. M. A. Ricci, "The Vermont Tele-Trauma Project: Initial Results," Abstract, April 2003, www.liebertonline.com (accessed August 22, 2006).

42. Nancy Ferris, "The Missing Last Mile," April 17, 2006, http://www.govhealthit.com/print/3_7/news/94029-1.html (accessed December 28, 2007).

43. Ryoji Suzuki, Sakuto Otake, Takeshi Izutsu, Masaki Yoshida, and Tsutomu Iwaya, "Monitoring Daily Living Activities of Elderly People in a Nursing Home Using an Infrared Motion-Detection System," *Telemedicine and e-Health,* 12, no. 2 (2006), http://www.liebertonline.com/doi/abs/10.1089/tmj.2006.12.146 (accessed November 20, 2007).

44. "Harnessing the Power of ICT for health," May 2005, http://www.i4donline.net/may05/healthNet.pdf (accessed December 28, 2007).

45. Mark Cantrell, "Nurses Keep Watch for Miles Away of at the Bedside," January 10, 2005, *Nursing Spectrum,* http://community.nursingspectrum.com/MagazineArticles/article.cfm?AID=13378/ (accessed December 1, 2007).

46. Stephen Spotswood, "Blast Injury Programs at VA Targets Source," usmedicine.com, January 2006, http://usmedicine.com/article.cfm?articleID=1238&issueID=83 (accessed December 28, 2007).

47. Erik Eckholm, "The New Kind of Care in a New Era of Casualties," nyt.com, January 31, 2006, http://www.nytimes.com/2006/01/31/national/31wounded.html (accessed December 28, 2007).

48. "E-Messaging Enhances Patient Satisfaction, Research Shows," August 15, 2005, http://www.health-itworld.com/newsletters/index_08172005.html (accessed January 18, 2008).

49. "FDA Approves Electronic Capsule for Stomach Disorder," iHealthBeat.org, July 21, 2006, http://www.ihealthbeat.org/articles/2006/7/21/FDA-Approves-Electronic-Capsule-for-Stomach-Disorder.aspx?topicID=53 (accessed November 28, 2007).

ADDITIONAL RESOURCES

American Heart Association. "Stroke Treatment and Ongoing Prevention Act: Fact Sheet." Americanheart.org, after December 2003 (accessed August 19, 2006).

"American Indian Diabetic Teleophthalmology Grant Program." http://tie.telemed.org/funding/default.asp?return=record&type=program&genus=State&id=22 (accessed August 22, 2006).

Austen, Ian. "For the Doctor's Touch, Help in the Hand." nyt.com, August 22, 2002. http://query.nytimes.com/gst/fullpage.html?res=9A0CE2DD163CF931A1575BC0A9649C8B63 (accessed December 28, 2007).

Baby CareLink in the News. "Clinician Support Technology Announces Major Enhancements in 2003 Release of Baby CareLink." April 1, 2003. http://www.babycarelink.com/news (accessed August 22, 2006).

Baby CareLink In the News. "Clinician Support Technology Helps Colorado Develop New Infant Care Program for Hospitals." 2002. http://www.babycarelink.com/news (accessed August 22, 2006).

Baby CareLink In the News. "Iowa Hospitals to Use CST's Baby CareLink to Improve Care of Premature Infants." December 3, 2002. http://www.babycarelink.com/news (accessed August 22, 2006).

Baby CareLink In the News. "Medicaid Case Study: Mount Sinai Hospital in Chicago." 2002. http://www.babycarelink.com/news (accessed August 22, 2006).

Baby CareLink In the News. "More than a Baby Monitor." CBS News, 2002. http://www.babycarelink.com/news (accessed August 22, 2006).

Barbara, Rohland M., Shadi S. Saleh, James E. Rohrer, and Paul A. Romitti, "Acceptability of Telepsychiatry to a Rural Population," May 2000, http://psychservices.psychiatryonline.org/cgi/content/full/51/5/672 (accessed November 20, 2007).

Bates, James, Barbara R. Demuth, Christine M. Trimbath, et al. "Telemedicine Versus Traditional Therapy in the Management of Diabetes." PPT presentation, April 2003. http://www.americantelemed.org/news/selected2003.htm#diabetes (accessed December 24, 2007).

Brown, Nancy, and Robert Roberts. "Telemedicine Information Exchange News." March 13, 2003. http://tie.telemed.org/news/partnerships.asp (accessed December 28, 2007).

Chin, Tyler. "Remote Control: The Growth of Home Monitoring." amednews.com, November 18, 2002. http://www.ama-assn.org/amednews/2002/11/18/bisa1118.htm (accessed December 24, 2007).

"The Comprehensive Telehealth Act of 1997." Arent Fox, 1997, 1–2. http://www.thecre.com/fedlaw/legal17/105.htm (accessed December 28, 2007).

"Computers Broaden Capabilities in Medicine." *Doctor's Guide Medical and Other News,* June 18, 1997, 1. http://www.pslgroup.com/dg/2CB4A.htm (accessed August 22, 2006).

"Department of Corrections Brief History." http://www.vadoc.state.va.us/about/history.shtm (accessed December 24, 2007).

Doolittle, G. C., A. Allen, C. Wittman, E. Carlson, and P. Whitten. "Oncology Care for Rural Kansans via Telemedicine: The Establishment of a Teleoncology Practice (Meeting Abstract)." asco.org, 1996. http://www.asco.org/portal/site/ASCO/template.ERROR/; jsessionid=H1NrHhql9VtMhGpGZZF7qCs2GZP7rT2VfZyfhQY7QWz9Bc0xTpyq!-1886814676 (accessed January 18, 2008).

Doolittle, G. C., A. R. Williams, and D. J. Cook. "An Estimation of Costs of a Pediatric Telemedicine Practice in Public Schools." *Medical Care* 41, no. 1 (2003): 100–9. http://www.ncbi.nlm.nih.gov/sites/entrez?db=pubmed&uid=12544547&cmd=showdetailview (accessed December 24, 2007).

"Federal Legislative Issues Update—July 2005." The Stop Stroke Act, July 27, 2005. http://www.arota.org/pdfs/July2005legupdate.pdf (accessed August 19, 2006).

"Federal Telemedicine Legislation 105th Congress." Arent Fox. http://www.thecre.com/fedlaw/legal17/105.htm (accessed December 28, 2007).

Fischman, Josh. "Bringing Doctors to Day Care." May 27, 2002. http://www.usnews.com/usnews/newsletters/healthsmart/hs020522.htm (accessed December 28, 2007).

Garshnek, V., et al., "The Telemedicine Frontier: Going the Extra Mile." http://www.quasar.org/21698/knowledge/telemedicine_frontier.html (accessed August 22, 2006).

Gray, James E., Charles Safra, Roger B. Davis et al. "Baby CareLink: Using the Internet and Telemedicine to Improve Care for High-Risk Infants." *Pediatrics* 106, no. 6 (2000): 1318–24 (accessed December 28, 2007).

"Great-West Insurer First Commercial User of CST's Baby CareLink Neonatal Care Programme." *Virtual Medical Worlds Monthly,* October 21, 2002. http://www.hoise.com/vmw/02/articles/vmw/LV-VM-11-02-21.html (accessed December 28, 2007).

Hafner, Katie. "'Dear Doctor' Meets 'Return to Sender.'" nyt.com, June 6, 2002. http://query.nytimes.com/gst/fullpage.html?res=9C0CE1DC1F3AF935A35755C0A9649C8B63 (accessed December 28, 2007).

Hoffmann, Allan. "Is There a Doctor in the Net." *Star-Ledger,* April 6, 1998, 21, 25.

Joseph, Amelia M. "Care Coordination and Telehealth Technology in Promoting Self-Management Among Chronically Ill Patients." *Telemedicine and e-Health* 12, no. 2 (2006): 156–9.

Kim, Hyungjin, Julie C. Lowery, Jennifer B. Hamill, and Edwin G. Wilkins. "Patient Attitudes Toward a Web-Based System for Monitoring Wounds." *Telemedicine Journal and e-Health* 10, no. 2 (2004): S-26–S-34. http://www.liebertonline.com/doi/abs/10.1089/tmj.2004.10.S-26 (accessed December 28, 2007).

"Latest News in Minimally Invasive Medicine." Society of Interventional Radiology, March 23, 2006. http://www.newswise.com/articles/view/518995/ (accessed December 28, 2007).

Lesher, Jack L., Jr., L. S. Davis, F. W. Gourdin, D. English, and W. O. Thompson. "Telemedicine Evaluation of Cutaneous Diseases: A Blinded Comparative Study." *The Journal of the American Academy of Dermatology* 38, no. 1 (1998). http://www.ncbi.nlm.nih.gov/sites/entrez?db=pubmed&uid=9448201&cmd=showdetailview (accessed December 28, 2007).

"Literature Review on Aspects of Nursing Education: The Types of Skills and Knowledge Required to Meet the Changing Needs of the Labour Force Involved in Nursing." December 14, 2001. http://www.dest.gov.au/archive/highered/nursing/pubs/aspects_nursing/1.htm (accessed August 22, 2006).

Maddox, Peggy Jo. "Ethics and the Brave New World of E-Health." November 21, 2002. http://www.nursingworld.org/MainMenuCategories/ANAMarketplace/ANAPeriodicals/OJIN/Columns/Ethics/Ethicsandehealth.aspx (accessed December 28, 2007).

Montana Office of Rural Health. "Rural Community-Based Home Health Care and Support Services—a White Paper." Abstract, August 2001. http://ruralwomenshealth.psu.edu/resources.html (accessed January 18, 2008).

Murphy, Kate. "Telemedicine Getting a Test in Efforts to Cut Costs of Treating Prisoners." *New York Times,* June 8, 1998, D5.

Nacci, Peter, US Department of Justice Office of Justice Programs, National Institute of Justice. "Telemedicine." March 1999. http://www.ncjrs.gov/telemedicine/toc.html (accessed August 22, 2006).

Ng, C. H., and J. F. Yeo. "The Role of Internet and Personal Digital Assistant in Oral and Maxillofacial Pathology." July 2004. http://annals.edu.sg/pdf200409/V33N4p50S.pdf (accessed December 28, 2007).

"NLM National Telemedicine Initiative Summaries of Awards Announced October 1996." October 1996. http://www.nlm.nih.gov/research/initprojsum.html (accessed December 28, 2007).

Office of Health and the Information Highway, Health Canada, "How Canadian eHealth Initiatives Are Changing the Face of Healthcare: Success Stories," August 2002, http://www.hc-sc.gc.ca/hcs-sss/pubs/ehealth-esante/2002-succes/index_e.html (accessed November 28, 2007).

Office of Telemedicine, Department of Corrections, Virginia. Virginia.edu (accessed May 17, 2003).

Ohio Department of Rehabilitation and Correction Technology, Telemedicine. January 8, 2001. drc.state.oh.us (accessed August 22, 2006).

Paar, David. "Telemedicine in Practice: Texas Department of Criminal Justice," UTMB Correctional Managed Care, May 2000. http://www.aegis.com/pubs/hepp/2000/HEPP2000-0501.html (accessed December 28, 2007).

Pyke, Bob. "Research, Training, & Practical Applications: A Look at Developing Programs at the University of Texas Medical Branch at Galveston." Interview with Vincent E. Friedewald, 2003. http://www.telehealth.net/interviews/friedewald.html (accessed August 22, 2006).

Raimer, Ben G., Patti Patterson, and Oscar Boultinghouse. "Correctional Health Care in the Texas Department of Criminal Justice." August 16, 2006. http://www.utmb.edu/cmc/Publications/articles_press/CorrectionalHealthCare.asp (accessed August 22, 2006).

Ramo, Joshua Cooper. "Doc in a Box." *Time,* Fall 1996, 55–57.

"Secretary Shalala Announces National Telemedicine Initiative." 1996. http://www.nih.gov/news/pr/oct96/nlm-08.htm (accessed August 22, 2006).

Shepard, Scott. "Telemedicine Brings Memphis Healing to Third-World Patients." January 17, 2003. http://memphis.bizjournals.com/memphis/stories/2003/01/20/story4.html (accessed December 28, 2007).

Struber, Janet C. "An Introduction to Telemedicine and Email Consultations." July 2004. http://ijahsp.nova.edu/articles/Vol2number3/telemedicine_Struber.htm (accessed August 22, 2006).

Telecardiology. *Telemedicine Today.* 2002. www2.telemedtoday.com (accessed August 22, 2006).

"Telehealth Update: Final HIPAA Privacy Rules." February 20, 2001. http://www.hrsa.gov/telehealth/pubs/hippa.htm (accessed December 28, 2007).

"Telemedicine for Psychiatry." medgadget.com, June 9, 2006. http://medgadget.com/archives/2006/06/telemedicine_fo_1.html (accessed December 28, 2007).

"Telemedicine Programs Database." 2003. http://telemed.org/programs/ (accessed August 22, 2006).

"Telemedicine Report to Congress." January 31, 1997. http://www.ntia.doc.gov/reports/telemed/intro.htm (accessed October 9, 2003).

"Telepathology Page." http://www.hoslink.com/telepathology.htm (accessed August 22, 2006).

Tufts University Department of Medicine. "Massachusetts Telehealth Access Program." 2001. http://www.ntia.doc.gov/otiahome/top/research/exemplary/tufts.htm (accessed August 22, 2006).

Turisco, Fran, Tania Shahid, and Lauri Paoli. "Technology Use in Rural Health Care: California Survey Results." chcf.org, April 2003. http://www.chcf.org/documents/hospitals/RuralHealthCareSurvey.pdf (accessed December 24, 2007).

Tye, Larry. "A High-Tech Link to Boston Aids Vineyard Stroke Victims." July 10, 2001. http://www.massgeneral.org/stopstroke/newsStory071001.aspx (accessed December 24, 2007).

VA Technology Assessment Program Short Report. "Physiologic Telemonitoring in CHF." January 2001. http://www.va.gov/vatap/telemonitorchf.pdf (accessed December 24, 2007).

Wachter, Glenn W. "HIPAA's Privacy Rule Summarized: What Does It Mean For Telemedicine?" February 23, 2001. http://tie.telemed.org/articles/article.asp?path=legal&article=hipaaSummary_gw_tie01.xml (accessed August 22, 2006).

Wachter, Glenn W. "Telemedicine Legislative Issue Summary: Interstate Licensure for Telenursing." tie.telemed.org, May 2002. http://tie.telemed.org/articles/article.asp?path=legal&article=telenursingLicensure_gw_tie02.xml (accessed December 24, 2007).

RELATED WEB SITES

The American Telemedicine Association (http://www.atmeda.org) is a non-profit association "promoting greater access to medical care via telecommunications technology." It provides almost unlimited information on the latest developments in telemedicine.

Arent Fox (http://www.arentfox.com) is an excellent source of information on legislative matters relating to telemedicine.

The Center for Telemedicine Law (http://www.ctl.org), a non-profit organization, "distributes information and serves as a resource on legal issues related to telemedicine."

The National Library of Medicine (http://www.nlm.nih.gov) can provide you with access to a great deal of information including bibliographies.

Telemedicine and Telehealth Networks: the Newsmagazine of Distance Healthcare (http://www.telemedmag.com) is a journal covering the field. Online access to past issues is free.

The University of Iowa's Telemedicine Resource Center coordinates the National Laboratory for the Study of Rural Telemedicine.

CHAPTER 5

Information Technology in Public Health

CHAPTER OUTLINE

LEARNING OBJECTIVES

After reading this chapter, you will be able to

- Define the field of public health and public health informatics.
- Discuss the impact of inequality on health.
- Discuss the use of computers in the study of disease.
- Define epidemics and pandemics, and the role of computers and statistics in their study.
- Define computer modeling of disease.
- Define global warming and its effects.
- Discuss Hurricane Katrina (2005) as a public health issue.

INTRODUCTION

Definition

Public health has many definitions. John M. Barry, writing on the flu pandemic of 1918–1919, states that public health "is where the largest numbers of lives are saved, usually by understanding the epidemiology of a disease—its patterns, where and how it emerges and spreads—and attacking it at its weak points. This can lead to prevention by means of public health measures like better sanitation, or providing cleaner water. It can also lead to the development and widespread distribution of vaccinations."[1] **Epidemiology** refers to "the study of diseases in populations by collecting and analyzing statistical data."[2] The collection of data on infectious diseases and their spatial and temporal patterns is crucial to public health. National Institutes of Health researchers attempted to do this with pocket PCs and Global Positioning Systems (GPS). The data (geographical location, symptoms, digital images, and class status) are automatically sent to a database.[3]

Even simple measures like advising people to wash their hands, to not share eating utensils and dishes, and to cover their mouths when they cough can have an effect on the spread of some diseases. Public measures like decent sanitation can also affect the spread of disease. The effects of quarantine have been questionable in some instances, and effective in others.[4]

The field of public health is very broad. It includes the care of the environment (water, earth, and air). **Public health informatics** supports public health practice and research with information technology. The *New York Times* reported in 2006 "10 Million people [were] at risk from pollution." Those living in the ten most polluted cities in the world are at risk from "poisoning . . . cancers, lung infections, mental retardation." In the Russian city of Dzherzhinsk that was a center of chemical weapons manufacture, the population (300,000) has a life expectancy of forty-two years for men and forty-seven years for women.[5]

Public health includes the health issue of tobacco use, planning for natural disaster, protecting food supply, and the identification and prevention or containment of epidemics. We have chosen to focus on just a few of these areas: using computers to study disease and to model disease, global warming, new diseases that challenge public health systems, and the public health response to hurricane Katrina (2005). It should also be noted that 100,000 Americans per year are killed by infections they have acquired during hospital stays because of hospital errors—a huge public health concern.[6]

Social Inequality, Poverty, and Health

Some definitions of public health stress that public health involves the health of the whole community, even the whole world; not only the medical treatment of individuals. Because social inequality as well as absolute poverty is one important determinant of health, the field of public health goes far beyond the scope of this text. That is, a poor country with a more equal distribution of wealth and income may have a healthier population than a rich country with an unequal distribution of wealth. For example, the United States, which is ranked first in health spending, has a health system that is ranked 37th in the world by the **World Health Organization (WHO)**, which is the directing and coordinating authority for health within the United Nations system (2000).[7] In terms of longevity and infant mortality, statistics show that the United States is not among the top twenty nations in the world.[8] Therefore, to effectively address questions on the health of a local community, a nation, or the international community, one has to minimize or at least decrease social inequality, for example, provide universal health care, day care, subsidies to bring people above the poverty line, and use the tax system to reduce inequality (rather than redistributing income to the top as we have been doing). In the United States, economic and social inequalities have been increasing since 1967. This means that the distribution of income and wealth has been increasingly unequal and the opportunity for social mobility has decreased.[9]

The fact that health depends more on social class and relative inequality than on the availability of medical treatment was recognized in 1975 by Theodore Cooper, then U.S. Assistant Secretary for Health, "It is one of the great and sobering truths of our profession that modern health care probably has less impact on the population than economic status, education, housing, nutrition and sanitation. Yet we have fostered the idea that abundant, readily available high quality health care would be some kind of panacea for the ills of society and the individual. This is a fiction, a hoax".[10] It has been hypothesized that the constant stress on poor people in a highly stratified society may account for higher rates of illness and death. These questions are beyond the scope of this text, but need to be mentioned in any honest discussion of public health. (See discussion of hurricane Katrina later in this chapter.)

▋▋▋ USING COMPUTERS TO STUDY DISEASE

Information technology (IT) can play a significant role in helping infection control practitioners (ICPs) in their "never-ending whirlwind of surveillance tasks, outbreak monitoring . . . and reporting." According to Dr. Gary A. Noskin (Northwestern University Feinberg School of Medicine), IT "can allow for real-time surveillance. . . . If you have targeted organisms, you might not know if there is a patient . . . [with] that organism . . ." but with computerization, the lab can identify and alert you. IT can also identify trends.[11]

Preventing and controlling epidemics is based on accurate statistics. To answer the question "Is there an epidemic?" statisticians need to define the normal distribution of a disease, and the extra, unexpected cases. Models of a disease and how it is transmitted need to be created. Computers are perfect for these tasks.

Computers can create **what-if scenarios** or **simulations** of what would happen to an infectious disease if something else happened (e.g., if air travel increased or decreased, if the temperature rose or fell, if there was an adequate supply of antiviral drugs, or if a vaccine existed or didn't exist). Computers can also do a what-if simulation to predict the growth of tobacco use as a public health issue. According to the cancer atlas, if tobacco use continues to grow as it is growing now, "tobacco will kill a billion people this century, ten times the toll it took in the twentieth century, public health officials said. [It] accounts for one in five cancer deaths, or 1.4 million deaths worldwide each year, according to two new reference guides that chart global tobacco use and cancer." According to the Massachusetts Department of Health, between 2000 and 2006, the level of nicotine in many brands of cigarettes rose by 10 percent. This means it is easier to become addicted and more difficult to stop smoking.[12] The World Health Organization (WHO) predicts that five hundred million people will die from diseases related to tobacco use.[13]

Computational models are the programs that create the simulations. All of these what-ifs are plugged into a model. Models can be built to answer all sorts of different questions about epidemics. "The experiments consist of computer simulations—representations of actual communities based on demographic and transportation information. . . . [T]he researchers can introduce an infectious agent . . . and watch it spread. . . . [T]he scientists start with assumptions about how people interact and how infectious agents spread." Anyone in the community can contract or transmit the disease through contact with other people. Scientists are using a model to see how a person gets infected and then how he or she spreads the disease. They can change variables to yield different results and answer different questions. Two of these variables are the size of the community and the virulence of the infection. Using very powerful computers the models may produce millions of possible outcomes, none of which may develop. Computer simulations or models may help public health officials prepare for outbreaks in states, in nations, and globally. Currently, MIDAS is modeling the flu and asking whether we can contain it at the source. Using model public health officials test such measures as vaccination, the distribution of antiviral medications, the closing of schools, and the quarantining of neighborhoods or infected people. They also study what could happen if the flu spreads, for example in the Unites States, given the amount that people travel.[14]

STATISTICS AND EPIDEMICS: A HISTORICAL OVERVIEW

An **epidemic** is "an excess in the number of cases of a given health problem. . . . To determine what constitutes an excess implies knowing what is normal or to be expected." Thus the very definition of epidemic is based on statistics. The study of epidemics is one of the important areas of the field of public health. Simple spreadsheet software (such as Microsoft Office Excel) can be used to calculate expected rates for past and present epidemics.[15]

The field of public health has been successful in controlling and containing many diseases. "Science had first contained smallpox, then cholera, then plague, then yellow fever, all through large scale public health measures, everything from filtering water to testing and killing rats, to vaccination."[16]

Before modern science, before any understanding of disease and its causes, there were at least two instances of conferring immunity to smallpox. In China, in the tenth century "physicians . . . induced immunity by having patients inhale the dust from a pulverized scab taken from a smallpox lesion." In Constantinople, in the 1500s, peasant women were inserting needles that had been infected with smallpox into veins to prevent smallpox.[17]

The use of vaccinations to confer immunity works on the following principle: Antibodies which help white cells destroy disease are produced naturally by a healthy immune system about two weeks after the start of the infection. The next time that those bacteria attack, the antibodies immediately destroy them. Vaccines can also confer immunity. "A vaccine is a weakened, killed, or incomplete form of a microorganism that cannot cause disease, but will result in the production of antibodies when it is injected into the body."[18] Vaccinations are not effective against all bacteria or viruses. Although Edward Jenner is referred to as the "father of smallpox vaccination," there were several earlier successful attempts by others to confer immunity. As you recall, a smallpox vaccine to immunize people was used in 1774 in England (pre-dating Jenner by more than twenty years). It was developed by Benjamin Jesty and was based on folk wisdom and observation; he had no knowledge of bacteria, or understanding of disease and immunity. It was common folk wisdom in rural areas that people who developed cowpox (a relatively mild disease) did not contract smallpox. Jesty "reasoned that if dairymaids who caught cowpox accidentally were immune to smallpox, then someone who caught cowpox deliberately should be equally immune. He . . . infect[ed] his family. . . . He took infected pus from the udder of a cow. . . . He scratched his wife's arm." He also vaccinated his two sons. They all caught cowpox and recovered. His neighbors expected the whole family to turn into cows. They of course did not and there is evidence that Jesty went on to vaccinate other people.[19] Jenner's vaccine was first given in 1796. Today vaccines are used against such diseases as tetanus, measles, polio, diphtheria, mumps, rubella, and hepatitis. However, the rising cost and number of vaccines has led to a situation in which insurers may refuse to reimburse doctors. This could possibly mean that childhood diseases long held in check, would recur.[20]

Statistics and mapping of a disease progression were used to contain an epidemic for the first time in the nineteenth century. An early example of public health in action involves the London cholera epidemic of 1854. Dr. John Snow (one of the few scientists who hypothesized that cholera was spread through contaminated water) noticed a large cluster (five hundred deaths in ten days) of cholera in one neighborhood. He plotted the cases on a map. The neighborhood got its water from one pump. Snow reasoned that this was the source of the outbreak. The pump handle was removed and the epidemic contained.[21]

By the beginning of the twentieth century, public health measures had successfully contained some epidemic diseases. Vaccination could prevent small pox. The eradication of mosquitoes could stop yellow fever. Clean water could stop cholera. Then in the early twentieth century epidemic polio struck in New York for the first time. It defied explanation: Although, "[f]ilth, poverty, and overcrowding had successfully predicted other infectious infant disease," polio appeared more frequently in suburban and rural areas than in urban slums. This might suggest a relationship between cleanliness and polio; but epidemiologists did not see this.[22] It took the next fifty years to develop a thorough understanding of the virus that causes polio, to see how it was transmitted, and to develop a vaccine. In early 2000, polio cases began to reappear in "21 previously polio-free countries."[23] **Polio** has now reappeared in 26 countries, the latest Kenya.[24] In response to the reappearance of polio, the WHO recommends that countries prepare to launch massive house-to-house polio vaccination campaigns in response to any outbreak.

When diseases are airborne and when people from many neighborhoods, states, and nations, with different immunities are brought together in close contact, diseases spread quickly. The flu pandemic of 1918–1919 killed anywhere from twenty million to one hundred million people worldwide. A **pandemic** is a global disease outbreak to which everyone is susceptible. The flu pandemic killed strong young people fast and spread throughout the world. How did this happen? War brings people of all areas into close contact with each other. World War I was no exception. The new flu virus apparently was first seen in Kansas in 1918. It spread to a Kansas army base, which housed 56,000 soldiers from across the United States; then with the soldiers it spread to Europe, later returning to North America, from where it spread to Europe, Asia, Africa, and the Pacific islands. At the time that the flu first appeared, it was not seen as a public health concern.[25] It was not the killer it would become in the second wave of the disease. During the War, the U.S. government controlled the dissemination of information.[26] The government's focus was on winning the war, not spreading information about the flu. Doctors and nurses worked for the army. Civilian populations lacked medical care.[27]

In Europe and the United States, public health measures were taken to combat spread of the flu. In the United States, the measures varied from state to state, and city to city. Most of the measures grew out of then-current scientific understanding of disease and how it spread. Most of these measures were ineffective. The attempt was to put in place measures that would "prevent those infected from sharing the same air as the uninfected." Patients in hospitals were separated by sheets and slept head to foot. The authorities attempted to limit public meetings, and recommended good ventilation. Some schools were closed, as were movie theatres, bars, and dance halls. Churches were open, but public funerals banned. In New York and Illinois, those with the flu were isolated and quarantined. Of course troop trains and ships were still effectively spreading the disease. The American Public Health Association (APHA) believed that contamination of the hands by sputum, and the sharing of dishes and utensils spread the disease. They attempted to teach the public to be careful when coughing or sneezing and to wash their hands often. They recommended frequent disinfection in hospitals, and that hospital personnel not wear work clothes outside the hospital. In hospitals and among the general public masks were worn that were believed to prevent the spread of the disease. In San Diego, they observed "a rapid decline" in new cases. However, in the Great Lakes, a study of hospital personnel found that "8 percent who used the mask developed the infection 7.75 percent of non-mask wearers did." Gargling with antiseptics was believed to prevent the disease; the APHA thought that because this attacked the mucus barrier to infection, it was of no value.[28] The epidemic ran its course.

THE EMERGENCE OF NEW INFECTIOUS DISEASES AND VECTOR-BORNE DISEASES: AIDS, SARS, BIRD FLU, WEST NILE VIRUS, MAD COW, AND EBOLA HEMORRHAGIC VIRUS

AIDS

By the last quarter of the twentieth century, humanity had apparently conquered infectious disease, by medical and public health measures, at least in the developed countries. However, since 1973 "30 new pathogens, including Ebola and HIV, have appeared."[29] Today infectious diseases are an international public health concern. For the latest information on epidemic and pandemic alert and response (EPR) the WHO maintains a Web page at http://www.who.int/csr/don/en/. WHO now requires the reporting of any disease that could cross an international border.

No one was thinking "about new plagues in the 1970s because it was widely assumed that vaccination, sanitation and antibiotics were making infections obsolete. The retroviruses . . . were . . . of academic interest only."[30] Then the first cases of a new syndrome started appearing in New York City, Los Angeles, and San Francisco in June of 1981.[31] It was named **acquired immune deficiency syndrome (AIDS)** at a meeting of the U.S. Centers for Disease Control (CDC) in 1982.[32–34] AIDS attacked the immune system leading to susceptibility to opportunistic infection and eventually to death. After years of study, it was found that people were infected through body fluids, not casual contact. **Human immunodeficiency virus (HIV)**, the virus that causes AIDS was identified in 1984. However, more than thirty years after the first cases were identified, although there are effective treatments to lengthen life, there is no cure for or vaccination against AIDS. And the treatments are too expensive for most AIDS sufferers. By 2005, over forty million were living with AIDS; the AIDS pandemic had left 13-million children orphans. In 2004, five million new cases of HIV occurred and more than three million died. In the United States alone, the CDC estimated that between 1981 and 2003 1.6 million people were infected with HIV, of which more than 500,000 died. The rates of new infection in the United States and death due to AIDS have declined since the 1980s, and the AIDS surveillance system is one of the best in the country. However AIDS continues to spread in epidemic fashion in much of the rest of the world.[35]

Currently IT allows researchers to look at "all the genes and proteins in the virus and the human genome, as well as . . . every . . . piece of DNA." (See Chapter 8 on IT in pharmacy.) Supercomputers can investigate vaccine-development, and analyze health and population statistics. Several nations are using supercomputers and bioinformatics to help in developing an effective vaccine. Biomedical informatics integrates "health-related data on all levels, such as molecule, cell, tissue, organ, people, and the entire population." Modeling and simulations by supercomputers can contribute to knowledge on prevention and help in designing effective medications.[36]

AIDS in 2006 is not as simple as it was twenty-five years ago when it was untreatable. Some who are infected with HIV do not get sick. Some get sick and die quickly. Although there are effective treatments for many, some patients do not respond and many cannot afford them. There are patients who cannot tolerate the drugs' effects. For others the drugs simply stop working after a time. However, as the death rate due to AIDS (in the United States at least) declines, the number of people living with AIDS increases.[37]

AIDS has not only left millions dead and dying, but has made some important contributions to society and medicine. AIDS is a factor in the push for living wills and health care proxies, for do-not-resuscitate orders and hospice care. AIDS helped create a social movement that not only changed the drug approval process, but also introduced patients who sometimes had as much information as scientists and doctors into scientific meetings.[38]

SARS

Severe acute respiratory syndrome (SARS) first appeared in 2002 in China. The epidemic, caused by a corona virus, appeared at a time in human history when easy international travel could spread disease as well as information about the disease. SARS demonstrated that epidemics need to be fought within the nation as well as internationally. The epidemic was contained through public health (not medical) measures including identifying patients and people with whom they had contact, quarantine, canceling any large public gathering, issuing travel advisories, and checking travelers at borders using thermal scanners to detect fevers. People were advised to wash their hands, and maintain good personal hygiene. Expedient reporting resulted in the isolation of patients more quickly. They were advised to wear masks in areas where SARS was present; however, it is not known whether this helped to contain the disease.[39,40]

Bird Flu

The first human cases of avian flu were confirmed in 1997. The virus called H5N1 or A(H5N1) that causes the disease currently presents itself in the animal population. The virus would have to mutate to spread to humans. The known cases came from birds; human-to-human transmission of this disease is rare or nonexistent (as yet). As of 2006, 191 people had contracted the virus and of those 108 died.[41] If the disease did start to spread from human to human, a pandemic would be inevitable. The CDC is working with the WHO on surveillance of the disease and its spread.

Some countries lack the resources to adequately track the disease. At least one U.S. pharmaceutical company is developing a vaccine. A recent breakthrough is the creation of a smaller dose vaccine that would enable the vaccination of more people.[42–44] In 2007, in Egypt, the WHO found a drug resistant strain of avian flu, one that could possibly mutate and cause a pandemic.[45]

West Nile Virus

West Nile virus first appeared in the 1930s. It is a form of encephalitis or brain inflammation. It cycles between mosquitoes and birds. Infected birds will infect mosquitoes. Mosquitoes can spread the disease to humans. It can be diagnosed by MRIs. There is no treatment or vaccine.[46]

Mad Cow Disease

Mad Cow disease or "bovine spongiform encephalopathy (BSE) is a progressive neurological disorder of cattle that results from infection." Cows contract this by eating infected food. The transmission agent is called a prion. There have been 167 confirmed human cases caused by the consumption of infected meat. All of the cases were fatal. The human form of mad cow disease is called Creutzfeldt-Jakob disease (CJD). It is a fatal progressive neurodegenerative disorder.[47] In 2003, computers were being used to track diseased animals. Radio frequency identification (RFID) tags on cattle can contain all necessary information including the cows' medical history; the tags can be automatically read. These devices can track the animals from birth. Because of the low incidence of mad cow disease in U.S. cattle, the Agriculture Department is drastically cutting back testing. However, in 2007, it announced it has genetically modified cattle to resist mad cow disease.[48–51]

Ebola Hemorrhagic Virus

The **Ebola virus** was first identified in Zaire in 1976. The same disease appeared in Sudan. It has been seen in the United States in monkeys, but no human cases are known to have occurred here. Very little is known about the disease. It appears only sporadically. And it is contracted by direct contact with body fluids, skin, or mucus. It can also be spread through contaminated needles in hospitals. It spreads easily among people in close contact, such as family members and health care workers. Among human beings the mortality rate is 50 to 90 percent. In 1979, the disease appeared again in Sudan at the same site as the previous outbreak. During the second outbreak in Sudan, public health workers were able to track the spread of the disease and prevent panic among the people. It is very difficult to diagnose Ebola early. Usually the symptoms include "fever, headache, joint and muscle aches, sore throat, and weakness, followed by diarrhea, vomiting and stomach pain." Other symptoms—"rash, red eyes, hiccups and internal and external bleeding" may also occur. According to the CDC, scientists need to develop additional diagnostic tools because a person with Ebola has to be isolated immediately; they also need to "conduct ecological investigations of Ebola . . . and monitor suspected areas."[52]

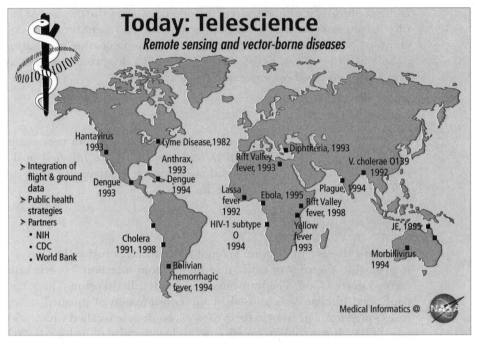

■ FIGURE 5.1   Remote sensing and vector-borne diseases. Courtesy of NASA.

Vector-borne Diseases

A **vector-borne disease** is a disease transmitted to a human or animal host by a tic, mosquito, or other anthropod that carries the bacteria or virus. According to the CDC, vector-borne diseases are emerging and re-emerging. Vector-borne diseases are affected by climate. Some examples of vector-borne diseases are West Nile, malaria, and in the nineteenth century yellow fever (Figure 5.1■).

INFORMATION TECHNOLOGY—COLLECTION MODELING AND SURVEILLANCE OF DISEASE AGENTS

The United States recognizes the importance of public health. The fourth goal of the Office of the National Coordinator for Health Information Technology (ONCHIT) is the improvement of the "health of the entire nation." It proposes the following: "unifying public health surveillance systems" to safeguard against epidemics and unsafe foods. To achieve this it proposes a national interoperable network of health care institutions and public health agencies to gather and disseminate information in a timely manner. A fully interoperable system would connect telehealth activities and the electronic health record.[53] ONCHIT also recommends "standards for quality of care." Research information needs to be disseminated quickly. IT can speed up Food and Drug Administration (FDA) review of clinical trials.[54]

There are registries, which are organized "system[s] for the collection, storage, retrieval, analysis, and dissemination of information" on people with a disease, a predisposition toward a disease, and exposure to anything thought to cause ill health. The information in registries can help define a problem and its size and examine trends over time. A registry may focus on one disease, a group of diseases, or exposure to toxins. Data on individuals can come from doctors and hospital reports, pathology reports, vital statistics, and hospital discharge records. Registries are operated by the federal and state governments, universities, hospitals, nonprofit organizations, or private groups.[55]

Public health also includes the modeling of disease agents—best done by computers. One approach to containing infectious disease that is being explored is called **syndromic surveillance**, which uses "health-related data that precede diagnosis and signal a sufficient probability of a case or an outbreak."[56] Syndromic surveillance can be used, for example, in shelters where there are no medical personnel; people can look out for signs and symptoms (for instance diarrhea) and report them. Public health encompasses the distribution of information, the protection of clean air and water, of the earth, a healthy food supply, and the creation of vaccines for prevention of and medication for treatment of disease. Computers are involved in all of these tasks.

Today with "neighborhoods" worldwide, with easy air travel, and hence the easy spread of infectious disease, one person cannot possibly gather all the statistics on a disease. Computers—from supercomputers to hand-held personal digital assistants (PDAs)—are used for this purpose. In the developing countries of Asia and Africa, **SATELLIFE** PDAs are used for the collection and dissemination of information, warnings, education, etc.[57] Great Britain has established twelve cancer registries that will use new computer systems to generate and collect data.[58] Some U.S. counties are attempting to institute disease-tracking systems.[59] But we are far from having an effective national registry for disease.

The **national electronic disease surveillance system (NEDSS)** (a part of the public health information network) will promote "integrated surveillance systems that can transfer . . . public health, laboratory and clinical data . . . over the Internet." This will be a national electronic surveillance system that will allow epidemics to be identified quickly. Eventually it will automatically collect data in real time.[60–62]

In 2003, the WHO graphed new SARS cases by date and geographic area.[63] There are several epidemiological software tools used to map and predict the spread of diseases. The Joint United Nations Programme on HIV/AIDS (UNAIDS) describes several such tools. The estimation and projection package (EPP) is used "to estimate and project adult HIV prevalence from surveillance data." The data can be used by SPECTRUM, which calculates the numbers infected and deaths from AIDS. The modes of transmission (MoT) spreadsheets predict the number of new infections based on the current infection data and risk patterns. SPECTRUM combines several models.

On May 23, 2005, the WHO approved new rules to control the global spread of disease. The rules went into effect in 2007. They "require member countries to . . . develop . . . capabilities to identify and respond to public health emergencies of international concern and to take routine preventive measures at ports, airports, and border stations." It provides a list of reportable diseases including smallpox, SARS, and polio. Its objectives are to establish global disease surveillance systems and to overcome technical, political, resource, and legal obstacles.[64,65]

The obstacles confronting an effective global response to a new pandemic are daunting. By definition, a pandemic is a *global* outbreak of disease to which every individual in the world is susceptible. Much of the world's population will need medical care, which most nations including our own cannot provide. We are lacking in staff, medication (antiviral drugs), and hospital beds. Our health care system lacks surge capacity (the ability to expand rapidly beyond normal services). There may or may not be a vaccine, at least in the beginning of the pandemic. Economic and social disruption is likely to result from business and school closings, travel bans, and fear of contagion.

With the recognition of the possibility of a new flu pandemic, the department of Health and Human Services is trying to establish stockpiles of flu vaccine by awarding contracts to expand facilities to private drug manufacturers. As of June 2007, two contracts had been awarded.[66] Yet the recommendations that we as citizens read are low-tech. The Department of Health and Human Services recommends that people store food so that they can stay home for a long period, wash their hands correctly, "use safe cough and sneeze techniques," and stay home if they are sick.[67] In July 2007, in a *New York Times* article, Gardiner Harris points out our current lack of preparedness for pandemic flu: "the federal government still has limited capacity to detect a disease outbreak and track its progress."[68]

New York City "unveil[ed] a plan to identify, and contain, a flu outbreak." In the city's worst-case scenario, a flu pandemic would kill fifty-six thousand people, medications would be scarce, and vaccinations nonexistent. The city's health commissioner and mayor advise that "our first line of defense" is "covering your mouth when you cough or sneeze; not going out if you have fever and cough."[69] The Robert Wood Johnson Foundation recommends that everybody prepare a kit containing soap, tissues, paper towels, aspirin, bleach, sports drinks, and a thermometer.

That fighting infectious disease is an international task was recognized at the Group of Eight (G8) summit, which focused on public health in July 2006. They called for increased international cooperation on surveillance and pledged to support programs that fight HIV/AIDS, tuberculosis, malaria, and polio.[70]

COMPUTER MODELING OF DISEASE: HEALTH STATISTICS AND INFECTIOUS DISEASE

Models of Infectious Disease Agent Study

In 2004, the United States funded a plan for researchers to use computers to model diseases called **models of infectious disease agent study (MIDAS)**. The goal of the project is to develop statistical tools to identify and monitor infectious disease. It will (if successful) use electronic health information. According to one of the principal investigators, the grant "will allow us to learn how best to use and combine a variety of electronic health data to detect and monitor infectious disease outbreaks such as pandemic influenza." The researchers are supposed to "devise models of communities of varying size, then simulate the effects of different outbreaks and the potential for success of response options." They will also evaluate the effectiveness of preventive measures, such as vaccination, and containment strategies, such as quarantine. The effect of social networks on the spread of disease will be examined as will outbreaks of disease in "U.S. towns and cities with populations ranging from 2,000 to 48,000. . . . [They] plan to examine the effectiveness of various control methods on smallpox, SARS, pandemic influenza and other . . . biological agents." Eventually these models will help guide policy.[71,72] The models will focus on how many people normally use health care facilities and services, and on detection models that notify the public of potential outbreaks. Models will be evaluated using historical information on real outbreaks and "simulated data based on infectious disease models."

Once the models are created, they will enable public health officials to make more meaningful use of health statistics. Newly gathered statistics will simply be entered into the model. **WHONET** is a microbiology information system developed at Brigham and Women's Hospital in Massachusetts. It is used to monitor antibacterial resistance. MIDAS will take its microbiology data from WHONET (an information system developed to support the WHO's goal of global surveillance of bacterial resistance to antimicrobial agents).[73]

Currently, there is an international attempt to model what would happen if the bird flu began to pass easily between people (not just from birds and animals to people).[74] In the United States, computer experts who use MIDAS and scientists in the flu branch of the CDC are working together to develop simulations that should help to control outbreaks if certain conditions are met including early identification, sufficient supplies of antiviral drugs and the means to get them to those who need them, the ability to enforce quarantine, international cooperation including restricting travel, and sharing antiviral drugs.[75–77] According to Dr. David Heymann, director general of the WHO "The trick with bird flu is to put the funding into areas of work that will strengthen disease detection." This is currently happening.[78]

■ CLIMATE CHANGE: GLOBAL WARMING

According to the Union of Concerned Scientists: *The scientific consensus is in.* Our planet is warming, and we are helping to make it happen by adding more heat-trapping gases, primarily carbon dioxide (CO_2), to the atmosphere. The burning of fossil fuel (oil, coal, and natural gas) alone accounts for about 75 percent of annual CO_2 emissions from human activities. Deforestation, the cutting and burning of forests that trap and store carbon, accounts for about another 20 percent (emphasis added).[79]

A study by the University of New Hampshire has shown that "the northeastern United States has warmed over the past hundred years, and that the rate of this warming is increasing over the past thirty years."[80] According to the American Geophysical Union, which represents 41,000 scientists "Human activities are increasingly altering the Earth's climate . . . add[ing] to natural influences."[81]

Global warming is already having a devastating effect on the earth and on human health: more intense heat waves lead to more heat-related deaths. Asthma and eczema in children have been linked to global warming.[82] More intense storms (witness hurricane Katrina in 2005 in New Orleans) and flooding of major rivers are increasing. A study by the National Academy of Science in 2004 predicted a doubling of heat waves.[83] More intense storms also cause increasing run-off that may pollute water supplies.[84] California depends on the Sierra Nevada snow pack for water. Global warming could cut the snow pack by 29 percent in the next one hundred years.[85] Droughts may increase. When sea levels rise, coastal areas may disappear. Global warming has also contributed to forest fires in California.[86]

In the developing world, global warming is having a devastating effect. Drought has destroyed crops. Rising sea levels could threaten seventy million with floods by 2080. "More than a quarter of the habitats for African wildlife risked destruction."[87]

One of the concrete steps that could be taken to slow global warming is cutting CO_2 emissions. The United States under President Bush opposes this. However, an agreement in California would control CO_2 emissions. It would reduce CO_2 emissions 25 percent by 2020. It would also regulate utilities, oil refineries, cement plants, and automobiles. The controls on cars are under a court challenge.[88]

THE PUBLIC HEALTH RESPONSE TO HURRICANE KATRINA

Hurricane Katrina "slammed into the Gulf Coast on 29 August [2005] . . . [S]everal levees protecting New Orleans failed the following day, and the city, about 80% of which is below sea level, filled with water."[89]

The storm damage can be classified as both a natural disaster (a category five hurricane: winds above 175 miles per hour) and a human-made disaster. (In the words of a scientist who studied hurricanes, "We've had plenty of knowledge to know this was a disaster waiting to happen.") Katrina flooded New Orleans both because it was a "monster hurricane" and because the levees failed; this should not have been surprising. Computers are used to model various hurricanes and their paths and effects. In 2004, "in an exercise simulating a direct hit by a slow-moving category three hurricane [using two different models], both models showed that the levees would not prevent flooding in New Orleans." A report published in May 2006 found that "the levees in New Orleans failed . . . not because the storm was so big, but because of problems in the way they were designed, built, and maintained."[90]

With this knowledge in hand, an adequate public health plan could have been in place before the storm: evacuation plans; the designation of shelters provided with adequate food, clean water, medications, and vaccinations; plans to get all the people to those shelters; and plans to clean up and rebuild the city. Apparently adequate plans were not in place.

Katrina caused the most "massive displacement of a U.S. population" in our history, most of whom were poor, sick, and/or old. A statement on poverty, health, and Katrina that the National Association of County and City Health Officials issued on September 23, 2005 reports, "in New Orleans, areas with significant flooding had lower incomes, higher poverty rates and less education. The overall poverty rate for New Orleans is 28 percent." Their health was significantly worse before the hurricane because "American disease and death rates are not arbitrary."[91] After the hurricane many were "stranded without basic human necessities and exposed to human waste, toxins, and physical violence." Many shelters lacked electricity and air-conditioning.[92] The aftermath of Katrina brought on the possibility of a host of public health problems including sanitation, hygiene, unsafe water, infectious disease, surveillance of health problems, the need for immunization, and lack of access to health care. Shelters lacked basic needs: water, food, and space. This was a perfect situation for the spread of infectious disease. The standing water brought with it the possibility of vector-borne disease, especially viral encephalitis. Systematic syndromic surveillance is needed to identify possible disease. Because shelters do not include health professionals, simple questionnaires should be available to report symptoms; the efforts of the agencies that collect this information (Red Cross, local government, state health departments, or the federal CDC) need to be coordinated. It is necessary to immunize people who have not been vaccinated against preventable disease. Information on immunization could be gathered when people register for a shelter. People with chronic diseases or whose health depends on continual medical care (dialysis, medications for heart disease, HIV, or tuberculosis) are particularly vulnerable. The hurricane disproportionately affected "the economically disadvantaged . . . largely black population of New Orleans whose access to health care was limited before Katrina. . . . In the long run, the destruction of the public health and medical care infrastructure . . . [can be] . . . more devastating to the health of the population than the event itself."[93]

Months after the hurricane, according to a federal mental health agency, such conditions as depression had increased. The agency and Federal Emergency Management Agency (FEMA) have funded counseling centers and a hotline.[94] The number of attempted suicides rose after Katrina.[95] Because people were forced to use gasoline-powered generators, the number of carbon monoxide poisonings rose.[96]

Eleven months after the hurricane, most New Orleans residents were still living with mold and debris. Almost every empty piece of land, including parks and medians, had been turned into trailer parks (with FEMA providing the trailers). The rebuilding of some of the 125,000 structures damaged or destroyed has only now (July 2006) been federally funded.[97] Only three of its eleven hospitals are now open. Many residents get their mail by visiting the post office every ten days. In many neighborhoods there are no dry cleaners, supermarkets, banks, or churches. Garbage that has been attracting rats is now being cleared. Government agencies have removed 17.6 million pounds of garbage. In some neighborhoods, "Electricity is erratic or nonexistent. . . . Water is not safe." Bodies are still turning up. Unemployment insurance benefits are running out, ensuring greater poverty. Neighborhoods are gone, families split up around the country. Most public housing is still closed, and many units are going to be demolished under a federal plan. The population is down from a pre-Katrina 450,000 to 225,000. Revitalization has begun, but it does not begin to address the needs of the poor residents. Thanksgiving 2006 saw three times as many Katrina victims in FEMA trailers (99,000) than Thanksgiving 2005.[98] This was a result of the lack of public health preparedness and planning.

DISCUSSION

Public health involves the protection of the health of whole populations. As the world becomes "smaller" owing to globalization and frequent air travel, public health becomes an international concern. It is clear that global warming requires a global response. Containment of possible epidemics (which can be transmitted across the globe) also requires cooperation between nations with timely reporting of symptoms and diseases. Whether the report is via a PDA from Africa or a phone call from a small-town U.S. physician, every case needs to be counted and mapped. Computers can model disease (MIDAS), prevention, and containment strategies.

Computers can also be used to model natural disasters. If the model points to strategies to minimize damage, perhaps it should be used by policymakers in a timely fashion. Adequate public health plans can be put into place to deal with the aftermath of a predicted disaster. Some "natural disasters" are not merely a product of nature, but also a product of human activity or the lack of it.

IN THE NEWS

Excerpt from, "Hurricane and Floods Overwhelmed Hospitals"
by Sewell Chan and Gardiner Harris

BATON ROUGE, La., Sept. 13—Confusion and desperation permeated the New Orleans hospital system as floodwaters rose, emergency generators failed and dozens of patients died in the three chaotic days after the levees broke, doctors and other witnesses said on Tuesday.

While all of the city's major hospitals had detailed evacuation and emergency plans, officials said, none were prepared for a catastrophic flood. And each responded differently when disaster struck.

At Memorial Medical Center, where 45 bodies were discovered this week, staff members said they could do little more than try to comfort dying patients.

At Memorial, a private 317-bed hospital opened in 1926, "there were patients who were lying on the floor," said Dr. John J. Walsh Jr., a surgeon. Dr. Walsh compared the scene to the railyard hospital for wounded soldiers in "Gone With the Wind," saying: "The nurses were basically standing, and giving them food or water. There were some medications we could give, but nothing like modern medicine. We were back to the 1800s."

A Tenet spokesman, Harry Anderson, acknowledged that the failure of ventilators, dialysis machines and heart-rate monitors contributed to the deaths of patients. The hospital's generators shut down "as part of a general failure of the entire electrical system," not because of low fuel, he said. Of the 45 bodies, 8 to 11 had died before the storm.

The suffering at the hospital played out over four anguished days, as city officials ordered an evacuation of the city, hundreds of residents began streaming into Memorial, in the city's Uptown section, the main power lines to the hospital were disrupted and the backup generators kicked on. By dusk on Monday, most of the people who had taken refuge in the hospital had left. But hundreds of people stayed behind.

On Tuesday morning, the hospital's chief executive, L. René Goux, called an emergency meeting. The administrators decided to evacuate the hospital and not to admit more evacuees from the neighborhood. The telephones had died, and Mr. Goux began sending frantic e-mail messages to Tenet's headquarters in Dallas, requesting assistance.

Meanwhile, workers at Memorial managed to clear up an abandoned landing pad, on top of the Magnolia Street parking garage, for use as a heliport. They strung together extension cords from the generator to the landing pad and shined lights to guide the pilots. . . . At least two helicopters tried to land on the helipad and deliver evacuees to the hospital, which was trying to clear everyone out. Some pilots only wanted to take pregnant women, or babies. Meanwhile, private boats started ferrying away the 1,800 residents who had taken shelter at Memorial.

Around 1:30 a.m. on Wednesday, the generators started to fail. Lights flickered and died.

Dr. Timothy Allen, an anesthesiologist, was astonished. "We were told and we believed that our generators would last six days, and of course they died after two and one-half days, whether because they shorted out or were flooded," he said.

By Thursday morning, doctors were in crisis mode. "We said we had to find a way to get these people out faster," Dr. Allen said. "We could just sense what was coming. It was so hot. We were down to one meal a day. There was no running water or sewage."

"As people died, they were wrapped into blankets," said Dr. Glenn A. Casey, the chief anesthesiologist and one of three doctors who left on the final flight. "We didn't have body bags to put them in."

John J. Finn, president of the Metropolitan Hospital Council of New Orleans, said the chiefs of the city's 20 hospitals had realized late last year in a planning exercise that they should come up with a plan to cope with a devastating hurricane. "We were going to fix those things in our planning," he said. "We just ran out of time."

CHAPTER SUMMARY

This chapter introduced the reader to the field of public health.

- Public health focuses on the health of the whole community: epidemics, pandemics, natural disaster, human-made disaster, environmental health, and any other issue that affects the health of the community.
- Public health measures include education, prevention, vaccination, and any other necessary community health measure.
- Social inequality as well as absolute poverty is one important determinant of health.
- Because statistics are needed to even define an epidemic, computers are vital to the study of public health.
- Computers are also needed to create models of a disease and the path it will take to spread.
- Computers can model global warming, which is already affecting us, and make predictions about future climate change.
- Public health officials still have to deal with unexpected disease outbreaks.
- Hurricane Katrina illustrates how a combination of factors (human-made and natural) can overwhelm a public health system, leading to major disasters.

KEY TERMS

acquired immune
   deficiency syndrome
   (AIDS)
bird flu
Ebola virus
epidemic
epidemiology
global warming
human
   immunodeficiency
   virus (HIV)
mad cow disease

Models of Infectious
   Disease Agent Study
   (MIDAS)
National Electronic
   Disease Surveillance
   System (NEDSS)
pandemic
polio
public health
public health informatics
severe acute respiratory
   syndrome (SARS)

SATTELIFE
simulations
syndromic surveillance
vector-borne diseases
West Nile virus
what-if scenarios
World Health
   Organization
   (WHO)
WHONET

REVIEW EXERCISES

Multiple Choice

1. _____is where the largest numbers of lives are saved, usually by understanding the epidemiology of a disease—its patterns, where and how it emerges and spreads—and attacking it at its weak points.

    A. Surgery

    B. Pharmacy

    C. Public Health

    D. None of the above

2. One major focus of public health is the study of

    A. epidemics

    B. radiological images

    C. All of the above

    D. None of the above

3. A/An _____is a *global* outbreak of disease to which every individual in the world is susceptible.

    A. epidemic

    B. infectious disease

    C. pandemic

    D. None of the above

4. A/An _____ is "an excess in the number of cases of a given health problem."

    A. epidemic

    B. infectious disease

    C. natural disaster

    D. None of the above

5. In 2004, the United States funded a plan for researchers to use computers to model diseases, which was called _____.

    A MIDAS

    B. model informatics

    C. computational informatics

    D. None of the above

6. _____ is a microbiology information system developed at Brigham and Women's Hospital in Massachusetts. It is used to monitor antibacterial resistance.

    A. WHERENET

    B. WHYNET

    C. HOWNET

    D. WHONET

7. _____ are the programs that create the simulations.

    A. Computational models

    B. Syndromics

    C. Pandemic modems

    D. None of the above

8. _____ refers to "the study of diseases in populations by collecting and analyzing statistical data."

    A. Pandemiology

    B. Epidemiology

    C. A and B

    D. None of the above

9. Computers can create what-if scenarios or _____.
   A. pictures
   B. graphics
   C. simulations
   D. None of the above

10. In developing countries in Asia and Africa, _____ PDAs are used for the collection and dissemination of information, warnings, education.
   A. collection
   B. reporting
   C. epidemic control
   D. SATTELIFE

11. Today, some reportable diseases include_____.
   A. smallpox
   B. polio
   C. SARS
   D. All of the above

12. Data can be used by SPECTRUM which calculates the numbers infected with and deaths from _____.
   A. smallpox
   B. polio
   C. AIDS
   D. All of the above

13. In developing countries in Asia and Africa, SATTELIFE PDAs are used for _____
   A. the collection of information, warnings, education . . .
   B. the dissemination of information
   C. health-related education
   D. All of the above

14. Global warming is already having a devastating effect on the earth and on human health; its effects include the following:
   A. more intense heat waves
   B. more intense storms
   C. flooding of major rivers
   D. All of the above

15. The EPP is used to predict_____ from surveillance data.
   A. pandemic flu
   B. SARS
   C. HIV-AIDS
   D. None of the above

True/False Questions

1. The northeastern United States has warmed over the past hundred years; the rate of this warming has been increasing over the past thirty years. _____

2. WHONET is a microbiology information system, used to monitor antibacterial resistance. _____

3. An epidemic is a *global* outbreak of disease to which every individual in the world is susceptible. _____
4. On May 23, 2005, WHO approved new rules to control the global spread of disease. _____
5. Currently there are national standards for the collection of health statistics. _____
6. One goal of the ONCHIT is the improvement of the "health of the entire nation." _____
7. The definition of epidemic is based on statistics. _____
8. An epidemic is "an excess in the number of cases of a given health problem." _____
9. Social inequality as well as absolute poverty are important determinants of health. _____
10. Currently MIDAS is modeling polio. _____

Critical Thinking

1. What goals and procedures would you have in place in the event of a catastrophe such as a terrorist attack, a chemical accident, a pandemic, or an epidemic?
2. How would you make sure that first responders are able to communicate with each other and a command center?
3. In the event of a pandemic or epidemic, how would you ensure that sufficient supplies of vaccinations and antiviral drugs are produced and distributed to the general public? Discuss the following in your answer: funding, what institutions would be involved (e.g., existing pharmaceutical companies, government, or would you set up new institutions).
4. List several effects of global warming.
5. How can we prevent another Katrina-like catastrophe? Deal with the aftermath (death, relocation, destruction, and the failure to rebuild infrastructure), as well as the pre-Katrina crumbling infrastructure (levees).

NOTES

1. John M. Barry, *The Great Influenza* (New York: Penguin, 2005).
2. "Glossary of Mesothelioma Related Terminology," MesotheliomaOnline.com, 2005, http://www.mesotheliomaonline.com/resources/glossary.php (accessed July 24, 2006).
3. Brad Lobitz, "NIH Researchers Track Disease with Pocket PCs," pocketpcmag.com, July 2004, http://www.pocketpcmag.com/_archives/Jul04/NIHResearch.aspx (accessed December 26, 2007).
4. Howard Markel, *When Germs Travel* (New York: Vintage, 2005).
5. "10 Million People at Risk from Pollution," http://nyt.com/, October 18, 2006 (accessed October 18, 2006).
6. Carl Ann Campbell, "Medicare Ends Coverage of Hospital Errors," *The Sunday Star-Ledger*, August 12, 2007, 1, 11.
7. James Lardner and David A. Smith, eds. *Inequality Matters* (New York: The New Press, 2005).
8. Ibid.
9. Ibid.
10. Anita Pereira, "Healthcare Is a Fundamental Human Right," 2004, http://64.233.169.104/search?q=cache:qTHm2FCittMJ:www.law.uconn.edu/journals/

cpilj/contents/archives/vol3/pereira.pdf+health+care+probably+has+less+impact+on+the+population+than+economic+status,+education,+housing,+nutrition+and+sanitation.&hl=en&ct=clnk&cd=1&gl=us (accessed November 28, 2007).

11. Jennifer Schraag, "How Informatics Helps the ICP," infectioncontroltoday.com, January 1, 2006, http://www.infectioncontroltoday.com/articles/611feat4.html (accessed December 26, 2007).

12. "Nicotine Levels Rose 10 Percent in Last Six Years, Report Says," http://nyt.com/, August 31, 2006 (accessed August 31, 2006).

13. Jon Gertner, "Incendiary Device," *New York Times,* June 12, 2005.

14. "MIDAS Fact Sheet," 2007, http://www.nigms.nih.gov/Initiatives/MIDAS/Background/Factsheet.htm (accessed November 28, 2007).

15. Marcelo Bortman, "Establishing endemic levels or ranges with computer spreadsheets," *Pan American Journal of Public Health* 5, no. 1 (January 1999): 1–8(8), Pan American Health Organization (PAHO), http://www.ingentaconnect.com/content/paho/pajph/1999/00000005/00000001/art00001 (accessed January 26, 2008).

16. Barry, *The Great Influenza.*

17. Michael T. Kennedy, *A Brief History of Disease, Science & Medicine* (Portland, OR: Asklepiad Press, 2004).

18. "How We Fight Bacteria: Vaccination (Immunization)," March 2006, http://www.bacteriamuseum.org/niches/hwfbacteria/vaccination.shtml (accessed November 28, 2007).

19. "The First Recorded Smallpox Vaccination," 2000, http://www.thedorsetpage.com/history/smallpox/smallpox.htm (accessed November 28, 2007).

20. Andrew Pollack, "Pediatricians Voice Anger Over Costs of Vaccines," nyt.com, March 23, 2007, http://www.nytimes.com/2007/03/24/business/24vaccine.html?_r=1&oref=slogin (accessed December 1, 2007).

21. Steven Johnson, *The Ghost Map* (New York: Riverhead Books, 2006).

22. Rogers, Naomi, *Dirt and Disease* (New Brunswick, NJ: Rutgers University Press, 1996).

23. Yael Waknine, "Highlights from MMWR: Minimizing Polio Spread in Polio-Free Countries and More," medscape.com, February 17, 2006, http://www.medscape.com/viewarticle/523891 (accessed December 26, 2007).

24. "Kenya: First Case of Polio in Decades." nyt.com, October 18, 2006. http://query.nytimes.com/gst/fullpage.html?res=9B03E0DE1F30F93BA25753C1A9609C8B63&fta=y (accessed December 26, 2007).

25. Barry, *The Great Influenza.*

26. Ibid.

27. Ibid.

28. "The Public Health Response," http://virus.stanford.edu/uda/fluresponse.html (accessed December 11, 2007).

29. Andy Ho, "Why Epidemics Still Surprise Us," nyt.com, April 1, 2003, http://query.nytimes.com/gst/fullpage.html?res=9A03E0D91339F932A35757C0A9659C8B63 (accessed December 26, 2007).

30. Abigail Zuger, "What Did We Learn From AIDS?" nyt.com, November 11, 2003, http://query.nytimes.com/gst/fullpage.html?res=9800E1D71139F932A25752C1A9659C8B63 (accessed December 26, 2007).

31. Sarah Abrams, "The Gathering Storm," July 25, 2006, Harvard.edu/review, 1997, http://www.hsph.harvard.edu/review/the_gathering.shtml (accessed November 2007).

32. Elizabeth Fee and Daniel M. Fox, eds., *AIDS: The Making of a Chronic Disease* (Berkeley: University of California Press, 1991).

33. Jennifer Kates, "HIV Testing in the United States," Kaiser Family Foundation, September 2006, http://www.kff.org/hivaids/upload/6094-05.pdf (accessed December 26, 2007).

34. Jennifer Kates, "The HIV/AIDS Epidemic in the United States," Kaiser Family Foundation, July 2007, http://www.kff.org/hivaids/upload/3029-071.pdf (accessed December 26, 2007).

35. Lawrence K. Altman, "Report Shows AIDS Epidemic Slowdown in 2005," nyt.com, May 31, 2006, http://www.nytimes.com/2006/05/31/world/31aids.html (accessed December 26, 2007).

36. Nicola Mawson, "Supercomputers Accelerate the Search for HIV/AIDS Cure," meraka.org.za, January 23, 2006, http://www.meraka.org.za/news/ Supercomputers_hiv_cure.htm (accessed December 26, 2007).

37. Abigail Zuger, "AIDS, at 25, Offers No Easy Answers," nyt.com, June 6, 2006, http://www. nytimes.com/2006/06/06/health/06aids.html (accessed December 26, 2007).

38. Zuger, "What Did We Learn From AIDS?"

39. David Bell, "Public Health Interventions and SARS Spread, 2003," medscape.com, November, 2004, http://www.medscape.com/viewarticle/490561 (accessed December 26, 2007).

40. D. L. Heymann, "SARS and Emerging Infectious Diseases: A Challenge to Place Global Solidarity Above National Sovereignty," medscape.com, 2006 (accessed July 31, 2006).

41. Patricia Reaney, "Bird Flu Measures Benefit Public Health: WHO," lomasin.com, 2006, http://www.lomasin.com/20060403/Bird-Flu-Measures-Benefit-Public-Health-WHO, 9155/ (accessed December 26, 2007).

42. Denise Grady, "Maker Calls New Bird Flu Vaccine More Effective," nyt.com, July 27, 2006, http://www.nytimes.com/2006/07/27/health/27vaccine.html?_r=1&ref= health&oref=slogin (accessed December 26, 2007).

43. Elisabeth Rosenthal, "Some Countries Lack Resources to Fully Track Bird Flu Cases," nyt.com, June 1, 2006 (accessed July 27, 2006).

44. CDC, "Key Facts About Avian Influenza (Bird Flu) and Avian Influenza A (H5N1) Virus," cdc.gov, June 30, 2006, http://www.cdc.gov/flu/avian/gen-info/facts.htm (accessed December 26, 2007).

45. Donald G. McNeil, Jr., "New Strain of Bird Flu Found in Egypt Is Resistant to Antiviral Drug," nyt.com, January 18, 2007, http://www.nytimes.com/2007/01/18/world/africa/ 18flu.html (accessed November 24, 2007).

46. CDC, "West Nile Virus," cdc.gov, October 6, 2005, http://www.cdc.gov/ncidod/dvbid/ westnile/index.htm (accessed July 31, 2006).

47. CDC, "Prion Diseases," cdc.gov, January 26, 2006, http://0-www.cdc.gov.pugwash.lib. warwick.ac.uk/ncidod/dvrd/prions/ (accessed December 26, 2007).

48. Donald G. McNeil, Jr., "U.S. Reduces Testing for Mad Cow Disease, Citing Few Infections," nyt.com, July 21, 2006, http://query.nytimes.com/gst/fullpage.html?res= 9C0DE6D8173FF932A15754C0A9609C8B63&sec=health&spon= (accessed December 26, 2007).

49. Anthony Faiola, "Japan Says Man Died of Mad Cow Disease," washingtonpost.com, February 5, 2005, http://www.washingtonpost.com/wp-dyn/articles/A64818-2005Feb4. html (accessed December 26, 2007).

50. CBS News, "Better Tracking in Mad Cow Wake?" cbsnews.com, December 31, 2003, http://www.cbsnews.com/stories/2003/12/31/tech/main590915.shtml (accessed December 26, 2007).

51. "Mad Cow Breakthrough? Genetically Modified Cattle Are Prion Free," sciencedaily.com, January 1, 2007, http://www.sciencedaily.com/releases/2007/01/ 070101103354.htm (accessed November 24, 2007).

52. CDC, "Ebola Hemorrhagic Fever Case Count and Fact Sheet," http://www.cdc.gov, October 8, 2002 (accessed November 24, 2007).

53. "Integration of Telehealth Activities and Electronic Patient Records Systems Imperative for Telemedicine Market Growth," biohealthmatics.com, July 6, 2005, http://news. biohealthmatics.com/PressReleases/2005/07/06/000000002350.aspx (accessed December 26, 2007).

54. Office of the National Coordinator for Health Information Technology (ONC), "Goals of Strategic Framework," hhs.gov, December 10, 2004, http://www.hhs.gov/healthit/ goals.html (accessed December 26, 2007).

55. "FAQ on Public Health Registries," May 23, 2007, http://ncvhs.hhs.gov/ (accessed November 25, 2007).
56. "Syndromic Surveillance: An Applied Approach to Outbreak Detection," cdc.gov, January 13, 2006, http://www.cdc.gov/EPO/dphsi/syndromic.htm (accessed December 26, 2007).
57. Andrew Sideman, "Handheld Computers Used to Address Critical Health Needs in Rural Africa and Asia," medicalnewstoday.com, August 21, 2005, http://www.medicalnewstoday.com/articles/29443.php (accessed December 26, 2007).
58. Phil Elliott, newsvote.bbc.co.uk, July 4, 2005 (accessed March 17, 2006).
59. Tony Saavedra, "County System Would Track Disease," www.ocregister.com, December 20, 2005, http://www.ocregister.com/ocregister/news/local/article_904817.php (accessed December 26, 2007).
60. "The Surveillance and Monitoring Component of the Public Health Information Network," CDC.gov (accessed April 21, 2006).
61. "Background on Public Health Surveillance," http://www.cdc.gov/nedss/About/purpose.htm (accessed April 21, 2006).
62. "An Overview of the NEDSS Initiative," http://www.cdc.gov/nedss/About/overview.html (accessed December 26, 2007).
63. "Graphs and Models of SARS Epidemic," sarswatch.org, 2003 (accessed March 29, 2006).
64. "WHO Updates Rules to Prevent the Spread of Disease," May 24, 2005, http://www.cidrap.umn.edu/cidrap/content/bt/bioprep/news/may2405regs.html (accessed December 26, 2007).
65. Michael G. Baker and David P. Fidler, "Global Public Health Surveillance Under New International Health Regulations," cdc.gov, July 10, 2006, http://cdc.gov/ncidod/eid/vol12no07/05-1497.htm (accessed December 26, 2007).
66. "HHS Awards Two Contracts to Expand Domestic Vaccine Manufacturing Capacity for a Potential Influenza Pandemic," June 14, 2007, http://www.hhs.gov/news/press/2007pres/06/pr20070614a.html (accessed November 25, 2007).
67. "HHS Pandemic Leadership Forum Mobilizes Employer, Faith-Based, Health Care and Civic Leaders," June 13, 2007, http://www.hhs.gov/news/press/2007pres/06/pr20070613a.html (accessed November 25, 2007).
68. Gardiner Harris, "Limited Capacity Is Seen in Flu Defenses," July 18, 2007, http://nyt.com/ (accessed July 18, 2007).
69. Diane Caldwell, "City Unveils a Plan to Identify, and Contain, a Flu Outbreak," nyt.com, July 11, 2006, http://www.nytimes.com/2006/07/11/nyregion/11flu.html?fta=y (accessed December 26, 2007).
70. "G8 Commitments to Infectious Disease Can Improve Global Health Security," medicalnewstoday.com, July 18, 2006, http://www.medicalnewstoday.com/articles/47491.php (accessed December 26, 2007).
71. Chris Schneidmiller, "U.S. Funds Computer Modeling of Disease Outbreaks," May 5, 2004, http://www.nti.org/d_newswire/issues/print.asp?story_id=66AA4925-C02D-4439-9AFE-9FDC258F5DD5/ (accessed November 25, 2007).
72. "Computers Combat Disease: New Modeling Grants Target Epidemics, Bioterror," NIH.gov, May 4, 2004, http://www.nih.gov/news/pr/may2004/nigms-04.htm (accessed December 26, 2007).
73. "Mathematics and Statistics Combat Epidemics and Bioterror," terradaily.com, February 2, 2006, http://www.terradaily.com/reports/Mathematics_And_Statistics_Combat_Epidemics_And_Bioterror.html (accessed December 26, 2007).
74. Bell, "Public Health Interventions and SARS Spread."
75. Mayo Clinic, "Threat of Avian Influenza Pandemic Grows, but People Can Take Precautions," sciencedaily.com, December 6, 2005, http://www.sciencedaily.com/releases/2005/12/051206084029.htm (accessed December 26, 2007).
76. "UCI Joins International Effort to Model Influenza Outbreaks," uci.edu, February 1, 2006, http://today.uci.edu/news/release_detail.asp?key=1427 (accessed March 27, 2006).

77. "Researchers Model Avian Flu Outbreak, Impact of Interventions," sciencedaily.com, August 3, 2005, http://www.sciencedaily.com/releases/2005/08/050803172829.htm (accessed December 26, 2007).

78. Reaney, "Bird Flu Measures Benefit Public Health."

79. Union of Concerned Scientists, "Common Sense on Climate Change: Practical Solutions to Global Warming," May 2006, http://ucsusa.org/ (accessed November 25, 2007).

80. Cameron Wake, "Indicators of Climate Change in the Northeast over the Past 100 Years," July 17, 2006, http://www.climateandfarming.org/pdfs/FactSheets/I.2Indicators.pdf (accessed November 25, 2007).

81. "Climate Change," 2006, http://worldwildlife.org/climate/ (accessed December 26, 2007).

82. "Experts Link Asthma to Global Warming," healthandenergy.com, June 22, 2004, http://healthandenergy.com/asthma_&_global_warming.htm (accessed December 26, 2007).

83. Felicity Barringer, "Officials Reach California Deal to Cut Emissions," nyt.com, August 31, 2006, http://www.nytimes.com/2006/08/31/washington/31warming.html (accessed December 26, 2007).

84. Anthony DePalma, "New York's Water Supply May Need Filtering," nyt.com, July 20, 2006, http://www.nytimes.com/2006/07/20/nyregion/20water.html (accessed December 26, 2007).

85. Barringer, "Officials Reach California Deal to Cut Emissions."

86. "Global Warming Linked to Increase in Western U.S. Wildfires," ens-newswire.com, July 12, 2006, http://www.ens-newswire.com/ens/jul2006/2006-07-12-04.asp (accessed December 26, 2007).

87. Gerard Wynn, "Global Warming Major Threat to Humanity: Kenya," abcnews.go.com, 2006 (accessed November 14, 2006).

88. Barringer, "Officials Reach California Deal to Cut Emissions."

89. John Travis, "Hurricane Katrina: Scientists' Fears Come True as Hurricane Floods New Orleans," *Science* 309, no. 5741 (2005): 1656–9, http://www.sciencemag.org/cgi/content/full/309/5741/1656 (accessed December 26, 2007).

90. National Public Radio, "New Orleans: Are the Levees Ready?" npr.org, May 26, 2006, http://www.npr.org/templates/story/story.php?storyId=5434630 (accessed December 26, 2007).

91. Statement of the National Association of County & City Health Officials, "Health Disparities in the Gulf Coast Before and After Katrina: The Public Health Response," September 23, 2005, http://www.umaryland.edu/healthsecurity/mtf_conference/Documents/Additional%20Reading/Session%203/Health%20Disparities%20in%20the%20Gulf%20Coast%20Before%20and%20After%20Katrina.pdf (accessed December 26, 2007).

92. P. Gregg Greenough and Thomas D. Kirsch, "Public Health Response—Assessing Needs," *The New England Journal of Medicine* 353, no. 15 (2005): 1544–6, http://content.nejm.org/cgi/content/full/353/15/1544 (accessed December 26, 2007).

93. Ibid.

94. Cheryl Corley, "Emotional Scars Still Haunt Katrina Survivors," npr.org, June 14, 2006, http://www.npr.org/templates/story/story.php?storyId=5485268 (accessed December 26, 2007).

95. Alix Spiegel, "Suicide Attempts Increase in Katrina's Aftermath," npr.org, November 16, 2005, http://www.npr.org/templates/story/story.php?storyId=5014682 (accessed December 26, 2007).

96. "Carbon Monoxide Poisoning After Hurricane Katrina—Alabama, Louisiana, and Mississippi, August—September 2005," *MMWR Weekly*, October 7, 2005, http://www.cdc.gov/mmwR/preview/mmwrhtml/mm5439a7.htm (accessed December 26, 2007).

97. Ann M. Simmons, "New Orleans Endures the 'New Normal,'" calendarlive.com, July 15, 2006, http://pqasb.pqarchiver.com/latimes/access/1077350371.html?dids=1077350371:1077350371&FMT=ABS (accessed December 26, 2007).

98. "The Morning Edition," National Public Radio, November 23, 2006.

ADDITIONAL RESOURCES

Pérez-Peña, Richard "City Tackles Meningitis in Brooklyn," June 29, 2006, http://nyt.com (accessed August 10, 2006).

RELATED WEB SITES

http://www.cleanair-coolplanet.org/information/pdf/indicators.pdf
http://environment.newscientist.com/channel/earth/climate-change/
www.PandemicFlu.gov
www.AvianFlu.gov

CHAPTER 6

Information Technology in Radiology

CHAPTER OUTLINE

LEARNING OBJECTIVES

After reading this chapter, you will be able to

- Describe the contributions of digital technology to imaging techniques.
- List the uses of traditional X-rays and the advantages of digital X-rays.
- Define the uses of ultrasound.
- Discuss the newer digital imaging techniques of computerized tomography (CT) scans, magnetic resonance imaging (MRIs), functional MRIs, and positron

emission tomography (PET) scans, and single-photon emission computed tomography (SPECT) scans, their uses, advantages, and disadvantages.
- Define picture archiving and communications systems (PACS).
- Describe interventional radiology techniques of bloodless surgery.

INTRODUCTION

The purpose of this chapter is to give students in the health care fields an idea of the extent and impact of information technology in the field of radiology—the branch of medicine that uses imaging techniques to diagnose and radio waves to treat disease. This chapter focuses on digital imaging techniques.

The new imaging techniques use computers to generate pictures of internal organs of the body. A digital image is an image in a form computers can process and store, that is, in binary digits. Computers can make pictures out of mathematical information. The technical methods used by computers to generate the mathematical information are very complex and beyond the scope of this text. The beginning of this chapter presents a short survey of the older imaging techniques like **X-ray** and **ultrasound** and the newer technologies that use computer technology including **computerized tomography (CT)** scan, **magnetic resonance imaging (MRI)**, **single-photon emission computed tomography (SPECT)** scan, and **positron emission tomography (PET)** scan.

Although the focus of the chapter is on digital imaging techniques, radiology is also increasingly concerned with treatment. Interventional radiologists treat disease without surgery; they are now able to open blocked blood vessels and do other procedures. The line between radiology and surgery is changing as bloodless surgery and gamma knife surgery (which does not involve cutting) become more and more widely used. As images become more and more accurate and complete, as they have during the past twenty years, the field of radiology has become increasingly involved with treatment as well as diagnosis. Interventional radiologists currently treat aneurysms and arthrosclerosis and perform bloodless surgeries on tumors. These issues will be touched on briefly below.

Precise, detailed images and image-guided therapies are slowly replacing invasive procedures such as cystoscopies and in the near future colonoscopies. Radiological screening for diseases has decreased the need for exploratory surgeries, leading to more timely diagnosis and treatment. Research continues into more and more sophisticated imaging techniques, which promise to change some aspects of clinical medicine.[1]

X-RAYS

Digital technology is radically transforming the field of radiology. Not only are new imaging techniques (CT scans, MRIs, and PET scans) available, but also older procedures like X-rays and ultrasound are making use of the new technology. A traditional X-ray uses high-energy electromagnetic waves to produce a two-dimensional picture on film. If the X-ray encounters bone, which it cannot penetrate, this appears white on the film. Whatever organ the X-ray passes through appears black on the film. Some soft tissue appears gray. Contrast agents can improve the clarity of the images, but X-rays do not produce good images of all organs and cannot see behind bones at all (Figure 6.1 ■).

Digital images have several advantages over images on film. Digital X-rays do not have to be developed but are immediately available and can be viewed directly on a computer screen, making them accessible to more than one person at a time, that is, to anyone on a computer network. They are more flexible: areas can be enhanced, emphasized and highlighted, and made larger or smaller. The quality of a copy of a digital X-ray is as good as the quality of the original. They can be immediately transmitted over telephone lines for a second opinion. In the future, it is hoped that by taking more than one picture, the X-ray image can be three-dimensional.

X-rays still dominate in several areas. If a broken bone is suspected, an X-ray is likely. Most dentists still depend on traditional X-rays, although digital imaging is becoming more widely used. Digital X-rays use less radiation than conventional X-rays. For a digital X-ray, a highly sensitive sensor containing a microchip is put into the patient's mouth. Because it is so sensitive, less radiation can be used. The data are sent to the computer, which displays an image on the monitor within a few seconds. The image can be manipulated, highlighted, enlarged, and shared on a network. The quality of the image is no better than a traditional X-ray, but it does

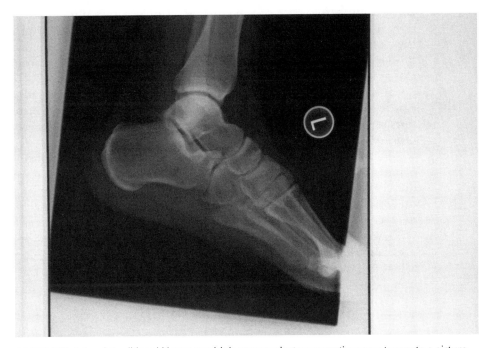

■ **FIGURE 6.1**   A traditional X-ray uses high-energy electromagnetic waves to create a picture on film. Courtesy of Brand X Pictures/Jupiter Images.

expose patients to less radiation. However, the equipment that is required is still quite expensive.

At the present time, a major imaging area dominated by traditional X-rays is mammography, although this may be changing. In 2000, the Food and Drug Administration (FDA) approved the first digital mammography system. Ultrasound, which can distinguish between harmless cysts and tumors, may be used with a mammogram. Other digital imaging techniques may also be used if an abnormality is spotted by a mammogram. But even with the traditional X-ray, computers can play a part: computer software has been developed that can be used to re-examine mammogram films, perhaps decreasing the percentage of women whose mammograms are read by radiologists as cancer free, but who do in fact have malignant tumors. An FDA-approved scanner can further evaluate breast abnormalities found by a mammogram. It is connected to a computer, which displays an image of the breast based on differences in the flow of electricity in normal versus malignant tissue. Today (2007), although digital mammography is not done as a matter of course, it can pinpoint tumors; radiation doses can be adjusted by tracking the tumor.

ULTRASOUND

Ultrasound technology pre-dates computers by many years. However, it now makes use of computers to create dynamic images. Unlike X-rays, ultrasound uses no radiation. It uses very high-frequency sound waves and the echoes they produce when they hit an object. This information is used by a computer to generate an image, producing a two-dimensional moving picture on a screen. Ultrasound is most closely identified with examining a moving fetus (Figure 6.2 ■).

It is also used to study blood flow and to diagnose gallstones and prostate disease. Ultrasound, like other imaging techniques, is being used to decrease the need for surgical biopsies. Ultrasound has been approved for the treatment of prostate disease.

In 2002, an eleven by six and one-half inch, three-pound handheld ultrasound scanner was developed. The traditional ultrasound is two hundred to three hundred pounds. The handheld scanner has a small liquid crystal display. It is easy to use in a doctor's office or emergency room and can be taken to battlefields and accident scenes.[2]

Recently (March 2006), ultrasound was found useful in diagnosing cancer in pregnant women. A study of twenty-three pregnant women with breast cancer found that mammograms detected the cancer in 90 percent of the cases and ultrasound in 100 percent of the cases.[3]

A three-dimensional ultrasonic endoscope is currently being developed for use in minimally invasive surgery. It has not yet reached the point of testing in human beings. If it is successful, it would give surgeons doing endoscopic surgery (see Chapter 7) a three- instead of a two-dimensional view of the inside of the body and might lead to more precise surgeries.[4]

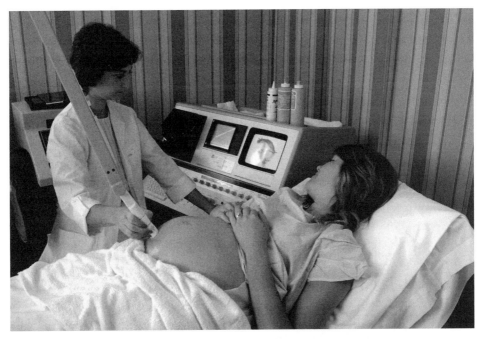

■ **FIGURE 6.2**   One use of ultrasound is to capture an image of a moving fetus. Courtesy of Corbis RF.

A tiny ultrasound device was cleared by the FDA in March 2006. The device is about the size of a silver dollar. It is being used to monitor fetal heart rate.[5,6]

DIGITAL IMAGING TECHNIQUES

Sophisticated imaging machinery uses computers to reduce massive amounts of mathematical data, generated in various ways, to pictures. The pictures that the computer constructs are clearer than traditional X-rays. In addition, the increased use of digital technology has produced kinds of images that were not possible with traditional X-rays, including three-dimensional representations, pictures that clearly distinguish soft tissue within the body, images of function, change, and movement, and of the electrical and chemical processes in the brain.

The machinery needed to produce CT scans, MRIs, and PET scans is very expensive compared to those needed for X-rays and ultrasound. However, by providing a clearer, more detailed, and accurate picture of the inside of the body, sophisticated diagnostic imaging is reducing the need for exploratory surgery, reducing cost and hospital stays, along with pain. When surgery is necessary, it may be less traumatic, because it is guided by precise, accurate images. By allowing a view of the activity in the brain, digital imaging techniques are also improving the understanding of the chemical and physical bases of mental illness and aiding in the development of effective medications. Another form of digital imaging is the

SPECT scan. It, like the PET scan, shows movement. However, SPECT scans are less precise. It is sometimes used because it is less expensive than PET. Both SPECT and PET scans are classified under nuclear medicine.

Computerized Tomography

CT scans use X-rays and digital technology to produce a cross-sectional image of the body. CT scans use radiation passing a series of X-rays through the patient's body at different angles. It is now possible for CT exams to contain thousands of images.[7] The computer then creates cross-sectional images from these X-rays. Soft tissue can be distinguished because it absorbs the X-ray differently. A CT scan produces a more useful image than a traditional X-ray. In addition, CT scans can be used to locate nerve centers, thus helping in the reduction of pain. In enhanced CT scans, a dye is used. Enhanced CT scans are used to show brain tumors: compounds cannot cross normal blood vessels in the brain; abnormal vessels let substances through—including the dye. This can be seen on a CT scan. CT scans help diagnose other conditions, including severe acute respiratory syndrome (SARS). In 2003, a virtual cystoscopy using CT scans was developed to screen for bladder tumors. A traditional cystoscopy is invasive and involves inserting a probe into the bladder; but this does not allow a complete examination. In a virtual cystoscopy, a CT scan of the bladder, an expert uses an image-processing algorithm for help in locating tumors.[8] CT scans are also being used to perform virtual colonoscopies; however, the results still need to be compared to the results of real colonoscopies.

A variation of the traditional CT scan, called the **Ultrafast CT** scan, may be used in place of coronary angiograms to examine coronary artery blockages. Compared to a coronary angiogram, the Ultrafast CT is painless, less dangerous, noninvasive, and less expensive.

Magnetic Resonance Imaging

Magnetic resonance imaging (MRI) machines use computer technology to produce images of soft tissue within the body that cannot be pictured by traditional X-rays (Figure 6.3 ■). Unlike CT scans, MRIs can produce images of the insides of bones. Using a technique called **scientific visualization**, MRI machines use computers and a very strong magnetic field and radio waves to produce pictures. The images are constructed from mathematical data generated by the interaction of radio waves and the protons inside the nuclei of hydrogen atoms in the water and fatty tissue in the human body. The MRI machine creates a magnetic field many times stronger than the earth's; it then generates radio waves. The response of the body's cells is measured by a computer, which uses this data to create an image. MRI can produce accurate and detailed pictures of the structures of the body and the brain and can distinguish between normal and abnormal tissue. MRI is more accurate than other imaging methods for detecting cancer that has spread to the bone, although PET/CT scans find cancer of the lungs more accurately. MRIs may be used for diagnosis and for the treatment of certain conditions that used to require

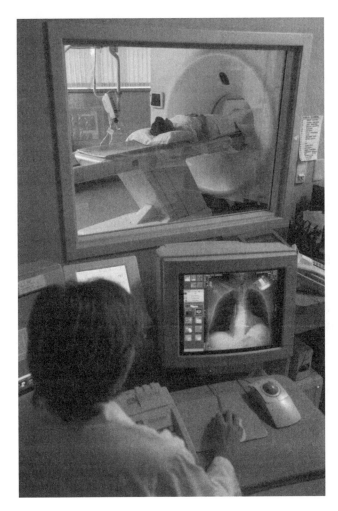

■ **FIGURE 6.3**   MRI machines use computer technology to produce an image of soft tissue within a body. Courtesy of Brand X Pictures/Jupiter Images.

surgery. For example, using MRI, radiologists can now clean or close off arteries without surgery.[9]

MRIs do not use radiation and are noninvasive. MRIs are used to image brain tumors and in helping to diagnose disorders of the nervous system such as multiple sclerosis (MS). MRIs also detect stroke at an earlier stage than other tests. MRIs can help find brain abnormalities in patients suffering from dementia.[10] It is particularly useful with brain disorders because it can distinguish among different types of nerve tissue. In 2003, MRIs were used to study comatose patients and were able to detect normal brain activity.[11] A new technique will attempt to use MRIs in combination with lasers for instant bloodless high-resolution biopsies. High-powered, pulsed lasers are focused on cells. This gives the cells the ability to glow. Computer software is then used to create a picture of the location of the beam and fluorescence of the cells. Any change in the cell is seen. Because this technique cannot see far into the body, MRIs must be used for a complete picture.

Relatively new, **functional MRIs (fMRIs)** measure small metabolic changes in an active part of the brain. fMRI identifies brain activity by changes in blood oxygen. fMRIs can be used to identify brain area by function in the operating room and help the surgeon avoid damaging areas such as those that are associated with speech. Strokes, brain tumors, or injuries can change the areas of the brain where functions such as speech, sensation, and memory occur. fMRIs can help locate these areas and can then be used to help develop treatment plans. They can also help in the treatment of brain tumors and assess the effects of stroke, injury, or other disease on brain function. fMRIs are currently being used to study conditioned response in people—what the brain does when learning to associate a stimulus, such as a bell or an image, with food. They are also being used, along with PET scans, to study schizophrenia.[12]

Another technique modifies the conventional MRI. It is called dynamic contrast-enhanced MRI. This technology is being studied in research institutions. It can take one thousand images of a tumor before a dye is introduced and during and after its introduction. Software analyzes the images. It can reveal new tiny blood vessels and how permeable they are. (Blood vessels that feed tumors are full of holes.) This technique will be able to show the growth of new blood vessels that feed cancerous tumors at an early stage and thus give scientists more information to help develop drugs to inhibit the growth of those blood vessels.[13,14]

A new MRI-related imaging technique is called **diffusion tensor imaging (DTI)**; it can aid in neurosurgery. It shows the white matter of the brain, the connections between parts of the brain, so that these are not damaged during surgery. It has improved brain surgery outcomes, according to the director of neuroradiology at Johns Hopkins in Baltimore.[15] DTI is also used to show brain dysfunction in stroke, MS, dyslexia, and schizophrenia.[16]

Positron Emission Tomography

PET scans use radioisotope technology to create a picture of the body in action. PET scans use computers to construct images from the emission of positive electrons (positrons) by radioactive substances administered to the patient. PET scans—unlike traditional X-rays and CT scans—produce images of how the body works, not just how it looks. PET scans may help detect changes in cell function (disease) before changes in structure can be seen by other imaging techniques.[17,18] PET scans create representations of the functioning of the body and the mind. They are used to study Alzheimer's, Parkinson's, epilepsy, learning disabilities, moral reasoning, bipolar disorder, and cancer. PET scans are also used to diagnose arterial obstructions. They are accurate and can avoid invasive catheterization.[19,20]

In a recent study, PET scans were compared with more common diagnostic tests for breast cancer. The two techniques disagreed in 25 percent of the cases; PET scans provided the correct diagnosis 80 percent of the time as compared with 12 percent using conventional imaging techniques. "PET scans found 6 'true positives' that were not found with conventional imaging tests. As a result those women began more aggressive treatment. Otherwise they would not have received treatment at that particular time."[21] A study published in 2006 concluded that whole-body PET scans could help determine whether breast cancer had spread before surgery.[22]

A recent study has found that PET scans can measure an esophageal cancer patient's response to chemotherapy and radiation therapy before surgery. PET scans can detect metastases that other imaging techniques could not see. They can be used to predict survival rates.[23]

Additionally, PET scans can show the functioning of the brain by measuring cerebral blood flow. PET scans produce a picture of activity, of function. A person is administered a small amount of radioactive glucose. The area of the brain, which is active, uses the glucose more quickly, and this is reflected in the image that the computer constructs. Neuroimaging techniques using PET can present a picture of brain activity associated with cognitive processes like memory and the use of language. PET scans are used to study the chemical and physiological processes that take place in the brain when a person speaks correctly or stutters. PET can show the specific brain activity associated with schizophrenia, manic depression, posttraumatic stress disorder, and obsessive-compulsive disorder. They have shown the precise area of the brain that malfunctions in certain mental illnesses and the effects of both drugs such as Prozac and traditional talking therapy on nerve cells. With PET, a picture of a drug's effect on brain function can be developed. They can now predict which patient will be helped by which medication. Because these pictures are anatomically and physiologically exact, they should help in the development of new psychiatric drugs.

In a study in 2002, Dr. Lewis Baker compared the effects of psychotropic medications and talk therapy on patients with obsessive-compulsive disorder. Using PET scans of the brain, he found that the two very different treatments produce similar effects on brain function.[24]

PET scans have even been used to shed light on an issue that philosophers have been concerned with for centuries: moral reasoning. In 2002, a study surveyed the areas of the brain involved in solving moral dilemmas. When a group of people were asked if they would throw a switch that would kill one person to save five others, most said yes. But when asked if they would personally push one person to his death to save five others, most said no. PET scans showed that depending on how the question was phrased, different areas of the brain were brought into action. The first question was stated impersonally, and the reasoning part of the brain was engaged. The second question was asked personally, and the emotional part of the brain was engaged.[25]

Software packages help researchers study the effects of drugs by combining PET and MRI, allowing them to correlate the functional information from PET scan images of brain activity with the anatomical details acquired by MRIs. Studies of the effects of certain drugs (including alcohol and cocaine) on the brain may make use of the precise image of brain structure that MRI produces and the picture of the functioning of the brain that PET can give us.

Brain imaging techniques, including both PET scans and fMRIs, are aiding in the comprehension of schizophrenia. People with schizophrenia are tormented by auditory hallucinations; their suffering is so great that sometimes it results in suicide. Until now some psychiatrists ignored the voices and the content of the messages. In 2003, scientists began using fMRIs to correlate the hallucinations to the activity of specific areas of the brain. They found increased activity in areas involved in hearing, speech, emotion, and memory. This has led to a discussion of new theories about schizophrenia. One new treatment has been developed. The treatment involves sending low-frequency magnetic pulses to areas of the brain identified by MRIs as active during hallucinations. It gives temporary relief to patients who do not respond to standard medications.[26]

The newly approved Given® Diagnostic Imaging System does not fit into any of our categories. It is a capsule with a video camera, lights, transmitter, and batteries. The patient swallows the capsule, which takes pictures of the small intestine, sending them to a small recorder on the patient's belt. After eight to seventy-two hours, the capsule passes out of the digestive track, and the health care provider analyzes the pictures. This device cannot be used on anyone wearing an implantable medical device like a pacemaker.

SPECT Scans

Like PET scans, SPECT scans are a part of nuclear medicine. However, the machinery needed is much cheaper and available at hospitals that lack the technology for PET scans. Where PET injects the patient with radioactive glucose and measures the response, SPECT depends on gamma radiation. SPECT's image is not as good as PET's. SPECT can be used to study blood flow, stress fractures, infection, and tumors. SPECT is used in a majority of heart imaging and some bone scanning.[27,28] One study found that in patients who went to an emergency room, SPECT scans resulted in a 10 percent reduction in unnecessary admissions.[29]

Currently, CT scans (which show anatomy) are being combined with both PET and SPECT scans, and the result is better diagnostic accuracy. For example, in heart imaging, CT scans show only anatomy. SPECT or PET scans show blood flow and can pinpoint the defective artery.[30]

Bone Density Tests

Osteoporosis is a condition of weak bones. Bones lose mineral content or density. Osteoporosis increases the risk of hip and spine fractures. Some bone loss is a normal accompaniment of aging. Several kinds of tests can be done to diagnose this condition. A bone density scan or **dual X-ray absorptiometry (DEXA) scan** is a special kind of low-radiation X-ray that shows changes in the rays' intensity after passing through bone. Doctors can see small changes in bone density from the amount of change in the X-ray. Quantitative CT creates a three-dimensional image of a skeleton. CT scans are used to measure the amount by which beams of radiation lose power (attenuate) as they pass through matter. This measures the mineral content of bones. Quantitative ultrasound is used but is not as accurate a test.

OTHER IMAGING TECHNOLOGY

Two imaging systems have recently been approved by the FDA. In March 2006, it approved the **LUMA Cervical Imaging System** to help detect cervical cancer. It will be used with colposcopy which magnifies the cervix of women who have had abnormal Pap tests. Colposcopy can detect many precancerous lesions. LUMA shines a light on the cervix and analyzes how it responds. It creates a color-coded map for the doctor. The map may help identify more suspicious areas to biopsy.

In March 2006, the FDA also approved a digital flat panel biplane imaging system (Innova 3131[IQ] and 2121[IQ]). According to General Electric (GE), which makes **Innova**, it is "capable of imaging the finest vessels and cardiovascular anatomy (and producing) three-dimensional images of the vascular system, bone and soft tissue." The system is capable of imaging "the full size of the patients lateral and frontal anatomy simultaneously" and can be used for many interventional, image-guided procedures.[31]

SoftScanR which "has the potential to improve diagnosis and effective treatment of breast cancer" is now used in clinical trials. It is meant to be a diagnostic tool which will complement mammography. It may be able to diagnose tumors as benign or malignant.[32]

PICTURE ARCHIVING AND COMMUNICATIONS SYSTEMS

The transformation of radiology from a discipline working with chemicals and film to one working with computers and monitors has also made images available almost instantaneously. **Picture archiving and communications system (PACS)**, "a picture archiving and communication system (PACS) is an electronic and ideally filmless information system for acquiring, sorting, transporting, storing, and electronically displaying medical images." PACS is a server. The standard communication protocols of imaging devices are called **DICOM** (digital imaging and communications in medicine).[33] The use of PACS to transmit and store digital images offers new speed in the transmission of digital images. The "copy" is available as soon as the original. There is no need to move patients to a facility that has the better imaging equipment. PACS moves the images and makes the images available to any authorized physician. It also reduces hospital stays, by speeding up diagnosis.[34,35]

PACS, however, is not yet integrated into surgery. Computer-assisted surgery is largely image directed. Ideally the development of a surgery PACS (S-PACS) "would focus on intraoperative imaging, with real-time and multidimensional visualization."[36]

INTERVENTIONAL RADIOLOGY: BLOODLESS SURGERY

The effects of digital technology on the practice of medicine cannot be overestimated. As images become more precise, they can guide surgeons better, and thus operations are less invasive. In addition, conditions that once required surgery may be amenable to treatment by interventional radiology. Some biopsies can now be done with a needle instead of surgically. Stereotactic breast biopsies make use of digital X-rays to locate the abnormality and use a needle to extract tissue. They are less invasive than surgical biopsies, but not as accurate and cannot be used with all patients.

Among the developments in radiology is radiosurgery. On the borderline between radiology and surgery, **stereotactic radiosurgery (gamma knife surgery)** is a noninvasive technique that is currently used to treat brain tumors in a one-day session. The use of the gamma knife for brain surgery has grown exponentially over the last few years. It is appropriate for brain tumors because the head can be immobilized. It may be used to treat other parts of the body in a different form called fractionated stereotactic radiosurgery; this is delivered over weeks of treatment.[37] Radiosurgery can be performed by a modified linear accelerator, which rotates around the patient's head and delivers blasts of radiation to the tumor or by a gamma knife. Called a painless, bloodless surgical device, the gamma knife works by delivering focused beams of radiation directly at the tumor. This kills the tumor and spares the surrounding tissue. The procedure makes use of three-dimensional imaging that locates the tumor in the body and uses computerized targeting to make sure that the center of the tumor gets the most radiation. One published review of the cases of fifty-five patients found radiosurgery to be quite effective. The newest interventional radiography equipment allows nonsurgical repair of some thoracic abnormalities. The gamma knife is appropriate for some benign brain tumors and all malignant brain tumors. It is also being used to treat neuralgia, intractable pain, Parkinson's, and epilepsy. Some of the advantages of gamma knife surgery involve its relatively low cost, the lack of pain to the patient, the elimination of the risks of hemorrhage and infection, and short hospital stay. Patients are able to resume daily activities immediately. However, as the procedure grows in popularity, some doctors are questioning its safety and efficacy. What will the effects of high doses of radiation be in the long run? Although it is recognized as effective in treating some brain tumors, they question its widespread use.[38] The newer **cyber knife**, because it compensates for patient movement, can be used to treat brain and spinal tumors with radiosurgery.

Research is being done on the effects of ultrasound on malignancies. **Focused ultrasound surgery** does not involve cutting, but the use of sound waves. Studies involve the use of ultrasound to stop massive bleeding and to treat cancer. By focusing a high-powered ultrasonic beam, the temperature of cancerous tissue at the focal point can be raised to nearly boiling. Within seconds, the tissue dies. The main disadvantage is that it cannot be focused through bone.[39]

The uses of **interventional radiology** continue to expand. A procedure called radiofrequency ablation (RFA) can be used on cancerous tumors on the liver or lungs. An ablation needle is inserted into the tumor. An electric current heats the tumor and kills it. In chemoembolization, a catheter is used to deliver drugs into a liver tumor. Stronger chemotherapy can be used with fewer side effects, because there is less circulation of drugs in the blood. According to the Society of Interventional Radiology, a three-year study "may challenge surgery" as treatment for early-stage small tumors.[40,41]

At the thirty-first annual meeting of the Society of Interventional Radiology in March and April, 2006, research into many new uses of interventional radiology was presented, including the use of treating blocked carotid arteries in patients who do not exhibit stroke symptoms and the use of an improved embolization procedure to treat and reverse male infertility. Lasers are being used to treat children with painful vascular malformations. Interventional radiology is being tested as a treatment for uterine fibroids with a 92 percent success rate. In a study of complications after the surgical versus nonsurgical treatment of uterine fibroids, the interventional radiology group had no major complications; the surgical group had 6.3 percent major complications, including death. Nonsurgical techniques can be used to treat painful cancerous chest tumors, by heating or freezing the cells, killing both the cells and the nerve endings.[42,43]

Some of the most recent findings of interventional radiologists include: (i) stenting of the carotid artery improves memory and thinking ability, (ii) a three-year study indicates that interventional radiology may be as effective as surgery for early liver cancer, and (iii) interventional radiology (embolization) can be successfully used to treat fibroid tumors in 92 percent of postmenopausal women.[44]

IN THE NEWS

Excerpt from, "Treating Troubling Fibroids Without Surgery"

by Lawrence K. Altman

. . . For most women, fibroids, consisting of muscle and fibrous tissue, are no bother. But for millions of others, fibroids can be so large (in some cases, the size of a melon) or so numerous that they cause discomfort, severe bleeding, anemia, urinary frequency and other symptoms. . . .

For decades, major surgery—a hysterectomy to remove the uterus or a myomectomy to remove selected fibroids while leaving the uterus in place—was the main therapy . . . About 30 percent of the 600,000 hysterectomies performed in the United States each year are for fibroids.

(continued)

Excerpt from, "Treating Troubling Fibroids Without Surgery" *(continued)*

With the introduction of technologies like ultrasound, C.T. scans, magnetic resonance imaging and new drugs, however, doctors have in recent years developed a number of alternative therapies.

This year in the United States, about 13,000 women are expected to choose the embolization technique, which is less invasive than surgery. French doctors first reported the embolization procedure in 1995. . . .

Embolization involves injecting pellets the size of grains of sand, made from plastic or gels, into uterine arteries to stop blood flow and shrink the tumors by starvation. The procedure is so named because the pellets are emboli. . . .

In performing the procedure, interventional radiologists insert a thin tube into an artery in the groin and thread it up to the main uterine artery in the pelvis. A dye is injected that outlines the smaller arterial branches on an X-ray, producing a map that guides injection of pellets through the tube into the arteries that nourish the fibroids. . . .

Although the procedure is safe, "there are still significant uncertainties about the procedure, especially in terms of future fertility and long-term outcomes," said Dr. Evan R. Myers, chief of the division of clinical and epidemiologic research in Duke University's department of obstetrics and gynecology.

Judging the safety and effectiveness of embolization compared with to other therapies is hard because randomized controlled studies are lacking and because earlier studies did not report how different symptoms responded to different treatments, Dr. Myers said.

"It is amazing that for a condition as common as fibroids, that has such significant impact on reproductive-age women, there is not a lot of high-quality scientific evidence for many of the things that are done for fibroids," Dr. Myers said. . . .

Dr. Myers directs a registry that the Society of Interventional Radiology has created to monitor the outcome of 3,000 women who have undergone the embolization procedure. He said that the effectiveness and complication rates for embolization seem comparable to surgery. . . .

In very rare cases—less than 1 percent—fibroids are cancerous. The cancers usually develop among postmenopausal women and the embolization procedure is not recommended for that group . . .

"That small risk has to go into the counseling before the embolization procedure," said Dr. Howard T. Sharp. . . .

Dr. Sharp said he believed that there were probably more cases of cancer than the single report in the medical literature, because doctors often "don't report the bad outcomes."

While some researchers are trying to study the embolization procedure further, others, like Dr. Elizabeth Stewart of the Brigham and Women's Hospital in Boston, are testing another fibroid treatment, the ExAblate 2000 System, that won approval from the Food and Drug Administration last month.

The system, made by InSightec Ltd. of Israel, uses ultrasound to destroy the fibroids with heat and M.R.I. to map the uterine anatomy and monitor the degree of fibroid destruction . . .

The patient remains in an M.R.I. machine for about three hours and then can go home. Initial studies found that serious side effects occurred in 2 percent of cases, compared with 13 percent among women who underwent a hysterectomy, Dr. Stewart said.

November 23, 2004. Copyright © 2004 by The New York Times Company. Reprinted by permission.

CHAPTER SUMMARY

- During the past twenty years, imaging techniques have become more precise and accurate because of computer technology. X-rays, which image bones and ultrasound, which shows moving images, have been supplemented by computer-based techniques.
- The CT scan takes many images and combines them in a two- or three-dimensional slice.
- The MRI uses magnetism to image soft tissue. Functional MRIs can see small metabolic changes in the brain and can be used to map brain function.
- The PET scan images function. PET can allow the radiologist to see the difference between normal and cancerous cells and can be used to study brain function in normal and mentally ill patients. PET can watch the brain think and judge.
- The SPECT scan is used for most heart imaging.
- The combination of PET with CT and SPECT with CT scans improves diagnosis.
- The use of these detailed and accurate images has made diagnosis more accurate and made exploratory surgery rare.
- Information technology in the form of the PACS system has made accurate digital images available anywhere.
- Radiology has moved from diagnosis to treatment, using radiosurgery to treat brain tumors and focused ultrasound to treat other kinds of tumors. Interventional radiology is a growing discipline, treating many conditions including cancers, pain, and male infertility.
- The reading of radiological images is beginning to be outsourced.
- Fibroid tumors can now be treated by interventional radiologists using an embolization technique, instead of surgery.

KEY TERMS

computerized tomography (CT)

cyber knife

digital imaging and communications in medicine (DICOM)

diffusion tensor imaging (DTI)

dual X-ray absorptiometry (DEXA) scan

focused ultrasound surgery

functional MRIs (fMRIs)

gamma knife surgery

Innova

interventional radiology

LUMA Cervical Imaging System

magnetic resonance imaging (MRI)

picture archiving and communications system (PACS)

positron emission tomography (PET)

scientific visualization

single-photon emission computed tomography (SPECT)

SoftScanR

stereotactic radiosurgery

ultrafast CT

ultrasound

X-ray

REVIEW EXERCISES

Multiple Choice

1. Which of the following uses sound waves and the echoes they produce when they encounter an object to create an image?
   A. X-rays
   B. Ultrasound
   C. Positron emission tomography
   D. Magnetic resonance imaging

2. _____ study(ies) brain function by sensing small changes in oxygen levels.
   A. X-rays
   B. CT scans
   C. Ultrasound
   D. Functional magnetic resonance imaging

3. _____ uses small amounts of radioactive materials to create a picture of the body in action.
   A. X-ray
   B. Ultrasound
   C. Positron emission tomography
   D. Magnetic resonance imaging

4. _____ take a series of X-rays at different angles. A computer then creates a cross-sectional image.
   A. X-rays
   B. CT scans
   C. PETs
   D. MRIs

5. _____ can be used to show the functioning of the brain.
   A. X-rays
   B. CT scans
   C. Positron emission tomography
   D. All of the above

6. _____ can image soft tissue and the inside of bones.
   A. X-rays
   B. CT scans
   C. Positron emission tomography
   D. Magnetic resonance imaging

7. An advantage of digital X-rays over traditional film X-rays is _____.
   A. a digital X-ray is available immediately
   B. a digital X-ray can be enhanced
   C. digital X-rays use less radiation
   D. All of the above

8. _____ creates images from data generated by the interaction of radio waves and the protons in hydrogen atoms in the water in the human body.
   A. X-ray
   B. CT scan
   C. Positron emission tomography
   D. Magnetic resonance imaging

9. If you wanted to study the effect of Prozac on the brain you would use _____.
   A. X-rays
   B. CT scans
   C. positron emission tomography
   D. None of the above

10. _____ is used to picture a moving fetus.
    A. X-ray
    B. Ultrasound
    C. Positron emission tomography
    D. Magnetic resonance imaging

11. _____ scanning is used to image the heart in a majority of cases.
    A. SPECT
    B. Ultrasound
    C. Positron emission tomography
    D. Magnetic resonance imaging

12. _____ can be used to diagnose breast cancer in pregnant women.
    A. X-rays
    B. Ultrasound
    C. Positron emission tomography
    D. Magnetic resonance imaging

13. _____ transmits, stores, retrieves, and displays digital images and communicates the information over a network.
    A. SPECT
    B. MEDCIN
    C. DICOM
    D. PACS

14. _____ has a lot in common with other industries that are outsourcing jobs. It has high labor costs, it's growing rapidly, and it's portable.
    A. Rehabilitative device
    B. Radiology
    C. A and B
    D. None of the above
15. A three-year study indicates that interventional radiology may be as effective as surgery for _____.
    A. early liver cancer
    B. breast cancer
    C. appendicitis
    D. All of the above

True/False Questions

1. PET scans can show the different activity in the brain when a person speaks correctly versus when he or she stutters. _____
2. Ultrasound uses radiation to create an image. _____
3. Traditional X-rays image behind bones. _____
4. A disadvantage of PET scans is high cost. _____
5. PET scans are usually used for broken bones. _____
6. Interventional radiology is concerned with the treatment of disease. _____
7. Stereotactic radiosurgery involves removing tumors surgically. _____
8. A gamma knife is used to make incisions. _____
9. Dentists still use X-rays, which may be traditional or digital. _____
10. SPECT scans, like PET scans, show the body in motion. _____

Critical Thinking

1. Using MRIs and PET scans, researchers are studying the functioning of the brain. Comment on the possible positive and negative ramifications this could have from developing more effective psychotropic medications to mind control.
2. Advances in radiology are changing the boundary between radiology and surgery so that at times it is difficult to distinguish between the fields. Bloodless surgery (gamma knife surgery) is now used to treat certain brain tumors. What other uses can you imagine?
3. What are the advantages and disadvantages of using digital X-rays in dentistry?
4. When a mammogram is done, it can be read by a technician, checked by special software, and scanned by a computerized scanner. If the image is misread, who is responsible—the technician, the software publisher, and/or the hardware manufacturer?
5. The new digital imaging equipment is becoming more affordable so that more medical institutions can acquire it. Discuss the advantages and disadvantages of each method (CT scans, MRIs, SPECT, and PET scans).

NOTES

1. Clare Tempany and Barbara McNeil, "Advances in Biomedical Imaging," *JAMA* 285 (2001): 562–7.
2. Michel Marriott, "A Palm-Size Ultrasound Scans Safely in a Flash," nyt.com, October 10, 2002, http://query.nytimes.com/gst/fullpage.html?res=9906E1D91F3BF933A25753C 1A9649C8B63 (accessed December 26, 2007).
3. Kenneth F. Trofatter, Jr., "Breast Cancer Diagnosis During Pregnancy," October 8, 2006, http://www.healthline.com/blogs/pregnancy_childbirth/2006/10/breast-cancer-diagnosis-during.html (accessed November 28, 2007).
4. "3D Ultrasound Device Poised To Advance Minimally Invasive Surgery," Science Daily.com, March 30, 2006, http://www.sciencedaily.com/releases/2006/03/060330161609.htm (accessed November 28, 2007).
5. "Analogic OK'd on Fetal Ultrasound Device," upi.com, March 29, 2006, http://www.upi.com/Health_Business/Analysis/2006/03/29/analogic_okd_on_fetal_ultrasound_device/2684/ (accessed December 26, 2007).
6. "Analogic Corporation Receives 510(k) FDA Clearance for Wide-Beam Fetal Ultrasound Transducer," finance.breitbart.com, March 29, 2006 (accessed July 13, 2006).
7. Guido Vaccari and Claudio Saccavini, "Radiology Informatics and Work Flow Redesign," *PsychNology Journal* 4, no. 1 (2006): 87–101, http://www.psychnology.org/File/PNJ4(1)/PSYCHNOLOGY_JOURNAL_4_1_VACCARI.pdf (accessed December 26, 2007).
8. Jaume Sylvain, Matthieu Ferrant, Benoît Macq, et al., "Tumor Detection in the Bladder Wall with a Measurement of Abnormal Thickness in CT Scans," March 2003, http://people.csail.mit.edu/sylvain/jaume-ieee-tbme03.pdf (accessed August 23, 2006).
9. Heather Babiar, "New Cardiac MRI Pinpoints Closed Arteries Without Surgery," June 27, 2006, http://www.eurekalert.org/pub_releases/2006-06/rson-ncm062006.php (accessed November 21, 2007).
10. "MRI of the Head," 2003, http://www.radiologyinfo.org/en/info.cfm?pg=headmr (accessed August 23, 2006).
11. Carl Zimmer, "What if There Is Something Going on in There," nyt.com, September 28, 2003, http://query.nytimes.com/gst/fullpage.html?res=9503E0D71E3AF93BA157 5AC0A9659C8B63 (accessed December 26, 2007).
12. P. J. Johnston, W. Stojanov, H. Devir, and U. Schall, "Functional MRI of Facial Emotion Recognition Deficits in Schizophrenia and Their Electrophysiological Correlates," February 2005, http://www.ncbi.nlm.nih.gov/entrez/query.fcgi?cmd=Retrieve&db=PubMed&list_uids=16176365&dopt=Abstract (accessed August 23, 2006).
13. Anne Eisenberg, "What's Next; a Budding Tumor Unmasked by the Vessels That Feed It," nyt.com, July 24, 2003, http://query.nytimes.com/gst/fullpage.html?res=9E0CE1D 7153FF937A15754C0A9659C8B63 (accessed December 26, 2007).
14. F. L. Giesel, H. Bischoff, H. von Tengg-Kobligk, et al., "Dynamic Contrast-Enhanced MRI of Malignant Pleural Mesothelioma: A Feasibility Study of Noninvasive Assessment, Therapeutic Follow-up, and Possible Predictor of Improved Outcome," June 2006, http://www.mesotheliomamedical.com/modules.php?name=News&file=print&sid=1677 (accessed August 23, 2006).
15. Angela Stewart, "Seeing into the BRAIN," *The Star Ledger,* March 14, 2006, 33.
16. "Diffusion Tensor Imaging," http://www.sci.utah.edu/research/diff-tensor-imaging.html (accessed December 26, 2007).
17. Mount Sinai, "What Is a PET Study of the Heart?" 2003, http://www.mountsinai.org/hospitals/msh/pet/pet_whatis_c.htm (accessed August 23, 2006).
18. "PET Scan," May 2006, http://www.betterhealth.vic.gov.au/BHCV2/bhcarticles.nsf/pages/PET_scan?Open (accessed August 23, 2006).
19. Sinai, "What Is a PET Study of the Heart?"

20. "Nuclear Medicine," 2000, http://www.mountsinai.org/msh/msh_frame.jsp?url=clinical_services/msh_nucmed.htm (accessed August 23, 2006).

21. "Do PET Scans Help Cancer Patients Live Longer?" November 14, 2007, http://www.healthscout.com/news/1/8017501/main.html (accessed November 28, 2007).

22. "Imaging Technique Helps Predict Breast Cancer Spread Before Surgery," August 23, 2006, http://main.pslgroup.com/news/content.nsf/medicalnews/852571020057CCF6852571D3004958BB?OpenDocument&id=&count=10 (accessed August 23, 2006).

23. "PET Scans Promising for Assessing Treatment Response in Esophageal Cancer," 2006, http://patient.cancerconsultants.com/esophageal_cancer_news.aspx?id=34881 (accessed August 23, 2006).

24. Richard A. Friedman, "Like Drugs, Talk Therapy Can Change Brain Chemistry," August 27, 2002, http://www.forensic-psych.com/articles/artNYTTalkTherapy8.27.02.html (accessed December 26, 2007).

25. Sandra Blakeslee, "Watching How the Brain Works as It Weighs a Moral Dilemma," September 25, 2001, https://notes.utk.edu/bio/greenberg.nsf/0/ed7ab7daf43c355b85256ad3004ba9e0?OpenDocument (accessed August 23, 2006).

26. Erica Goode, "Experts See Mind's Voices in New Light," nyt.com, May 6, 2003, http://query.nytimes.com/gst/fullpage.html?res=9C05EEDC103CF935A35756C0A9659C8B63 (accessed December 26, 2007).

27. Mark Dye, "PET and SPECT: Happy Together," June, 2005, http://www.medicalimagingmag.com/issues/articles/2005-06_01.asp (accessed December 26, 2007).

28. Susan Spinasanta, "Nuclear Imaging: PET and SPECT Scans," December 8, 2004, http://www.spineuniverse.com/displayarticle.php/article231.html (accessed December 26, 2007).

29. Urmilla R. Parlikar, "Heart Imaging Procedure Helps Physicians Evaluate Patients Suspected of Having a Heart Attack," http://www.swedish.org/17697.cfm (accessed December 26, 2007).

30. "Going Beyond CT Angiography—SPECT/CT Heart Study Is SNM's Image of the Year," radiologytoday.com, July 3, 2006 (accessed July 7, 2006).

31. "FDA Clears GE Healthcare's New Innova Digital Flat Panel Biplane Imaging System," March 14, 2006, http://home.businesswire.com (accessed March 18, 2006).

32. "ART Initiates Clinical Trials of the SoftScan 'R' System at the University of California-San Diego as Part of Its North American Pivotal Study," cnnmatthews.com, March 29, 2006 (accessed March 30, 2006).

33. S. H. Becker and R. L. Arenson, "Costs and Benefits of Picture Archiving and Communication Systems," *Journal of the American Medical Informatics Association* 1, no. 5 (1994): 361–71, http://www.pubmedcentral.nih.gov/articlerender.fcgi?artid=116218 (accessed November 28, 2007).

34. "Clinical Information Technology for Better Health," 2007, http://www.connectingforhealth.nhs.uk/newsroom/worldview/protti8 (accessed November 28, 2007).

35. "Hospital Implements Latest Advances in Radiology System," March 22, 2006, http://www.newportnewstimes.com (accessed March 30, 2006).

36. Paula Gould and John C. Hayes, "Informatics Integration Drives Intraoperative Planning," CARS/EuroPACS 2005 Conference Reporter, October 5, 2005, http://www.diagnosticimaging.com/pacsweb/features/showArticle.jhtml?articleID=171202282 (accessed December 26, 2007).

37. "Stereotactic Radiosurgery," 2003, http://www.surgeryencyclopedia.com/St-Wr/Stereotactic-Radiosurgery.html (accessed November 28, 2007).

38. Laurie Tarkan, "Brain Surgery, Without Knife or Blood, Gains Favor," nyt.com, April 29, 2003, http://query.nytimes.com/gst/fullpage.html?res=9A01E2D7133DF93AA15757C0A9659C8B63 (accessed December 26, 2007).

39. "Emerging Technologies Meeting," 2002, http://www.insightec.com/36-66-en-r10/MRgFUS-Technology.aspx nd (accessed November 29, 2007).

40. "Latest News in Minimally Invasive Medicine," newswise.com, March 23, 2006, http://www.newswise.com/articles/view/518995/ (accessed December 26, 2007).
41. Michael Murray, "At MGH, the Stakes Don't Get Any Higher," March 29, 2006, http://www.miningjournal.net (accessed November 21, 2007).
42. "Latest News in Minimally Invasive Medicine."
43. "MTCC to Host 5000 Interventional Radiologists in Professional Society's International Meeting," March 30, 2006, http://www.newswire.ca (accessed November 21, 2007).
44. "Latest News in Minimally Invasive Medicine."

ADDITIONAL RESOURCES

Beardsey, Tim. "Putting Alzheimer's to the Tests." *Scientific American,* February 1995, 12–13.

Cluett, Jonathan. "Do I Need a Bone Density Test?" http://orthopedics.about.com/cs/osteoporosis/a/bonedensitytest.htm#b (accessed August 23, 2006).

Cluett, Jonathan. "What Is a Bone Scan?" http://orthopedics.about.com (accessed August 23, 2006).

"Computed Tomography Images Help Radiologists Diagnose SARS." DGNews, May 14, 2003. http://main.pslgroup.com/news/content.nsf/MedicalNews/8525697700573E1885256D26004E0806?OpenDocument&id= (accessed December 26, 2007).

"Computerized Scanner Double-Checks Suspicious Mammograms." August 1999. http://www.patientnews.net/articles/julyaugust/suspiciousmammograms.html (accessed August 23, 2006).

Eisenberg, Anne. "What's Next; Lasers Set Cells Aglow for a Biopsy Without the Knife." nyt.com, June 26, 2003. http://query.nytimes.com/gst/fullpage.html?res=9C05E5DA163AF935A15755C0A9659C8B63 (accessed December 26, 2007).

"Esophageal Cancer." 2006. http://www.cancer.org/downloads/PRO/EsophagealCancer.pdf (accessed December 26, 2007).

FDA Talk Paper. "FDA Approves First Digital Mammography System." January 31, 2000. http://www.fda.gov/bbs/topics/ANSWERS/ANS01000.html (accessed December 26, 2007).

Foreman, Judy. "Brain Scanning and OCD." June 3, 2003. http://www.myhealthsense.com/F030603_Brain.html (accessed December 26, 2007).

Fox, Peter T., Roger J. Ingham, Janis C. Ingham, Traci B. Hirsch, J. Hunter Downs, Charles Martin, Paul Jerabek, Thomas Glass, and Jack L. Lancaster. "A PET Study of the Neural Systems of Stuttering." *Nature* 382, no. 6587 (1996): 158–62.

"Full Body Scan for Breast Cancer." September 7, 2000. http://www.abc.net.au/science/news/stories/s358885.htm (accessed August 23, 2006).

"Functional MR Imaging (fMRI) - Brain." 2006. http://www.radiologyinfo.org/en/info.cfm?pg=fmribrain&bhcp=1 (accessed August 23, 2006).

"Gamma Knife® Surgery." 2006. http://www.irsa.org/gamma_knife.html (accessed August 23, 2006).

Giger, Maryellen, and Charles A. Pelizzari. "Advances in Tumor Imaging." *Scientific American,* September 1996, 110–12.

Goode, Erica. "Studying Modern-Day Pavlov's Dogs, of the Human Variety." August 26, 2003. http://www.hnl.bcm.tmc.edu/articles/Studying%20Modern-Day%20Pavlov's%20Dogs,%20of%20the%20Human%20Variety.htm (accessed August 23, 2006).

Heiken, Jay P., Christine M. Peterson, and Christine O. Menias. "Virtual Colonoscopy for Colorectal Cancer Screening: Current Status." July 9, 2006. http://2006.confex.com/uicc/uicc/techprogram/P10382.HTM (accessed August 23, 2006).

Hooper, Judith. "Targeting the Brain." *Time,* Special Issue Fall 1996, 46–50.

Kevles, Bettyanne. "Body Imaging." *Newsweek,* Winter 1997–98, 74–76.

Kevles, Bettyanne Holzmann. *Naked to the Bone: Medical Imaging in the Twentieth Century.* New Brunswick, NJ: Rutgers University Press, 1997.

Khafagi, Frederick A., and S. Patrick Butler. "Nuclear Medicine." *The Medical Journal of Australia* 176, no. 1 (2002): 27. http://www.mja.com.au/public/issues/176_01_070102/kha10734_fm.html (accessed August 23, 2006).

Marano, Lou. "Ethics and Mapping the Brain." June 4, 2003. http://www.hawaiireporter.com/story.aspx?03357186-c0f2-4a84-9eb4-0457be143480 (accessed August 23, 2006).

Motluk, Alison. "Cutting Out Stuttering." *New Scientist,* February 1, 1997, 32–35.

"New Device Clearance: Given® Diagnostic Imaging System—K010312." August 1, 2001. http://www.fda.gov/cdrh/mda/docs/k010312.html (accessed August 23, 2006).

"Osteoporosis: A Guide to Prevention and Treatment." Health.harvard.edu, 2006. http://www.health.harvard.edu/special_health_reports/Osteoporosis.htm (accessed December 26, 2007).

"PET Scans Detect Therapy Responses in Esophageal Cancer Patients." April 2003. mskcc.org (accessed April 16, 2003).

"Quantitative Computed Tomography." In *The Encyclopedia of Medical Imaging Volume 1.* http://www.medcyclopaedia.com/library/topics/volume_i/q/quantitative_computed_tomography_qct_.aspx?s=Quantitative+Computed+Tomography&mode=1&syn=&scope= (accessed December 26, 2007).

Raichle, Marcus E. "Visualizing the Mind." *Scientific American,* April 1994, 58–64.

Rajendran, Joseph. "Positron Emission Tomography in Head and Neck Cancer." Abstract, June 6, 2003. http://www.appliedradiology.com/articles/article.asp?Id=855&SubCatID=223&CatID=48&ThreadID=&Search= (accessed August 23, 2006).

Scott, A. M. "Current Status of Positron Emission Tomography in Oncology." Abstract, January–February 2001. http://www.ncbi.nlm.nih.gov/entrez/query.fcgi?cmd=Retrieve&db=PubMed&list_uids=11478353&dopt=Abstract (accessed August 23, 2006).

Susman Ed. "Positron Emission/Computed Tomography Fusion and Magnetic Resonance Imaging Detect Different Cancerous Lesions: Presented at RSNA." *Doctor's Guide,* December 9, 2002. http://www.docguide.com/news/content.nsf/news/85256977005 73E1885256C8A00702AD2?OpenDocument&id=48DDE4A73E09A969852568880078C2 49&c=Diagnostic%20Radiology&count=10 (accessed December 26, 2007).

Wang, Gene-Jack, ed. "Study Reveals Biochemical Signature of Cocaine Craving in Humans." June 13, 2006. http://www.bnl.gov/bnlweb/pubaf/pr/PR_display.asp?prID=06-74 (accessed December 26, 2007).

"What Is DEXA Scanning?" http://www.gorhams.dk/html/what_is_dexa_scanning.html (accessed August 23, 2006).

Wu, D., and S. S. Gambhir. "Positron Emission Tomography in Diagnosis and Management of Invasive Breast Cancer: Current Status and Future Perspectives." Abstract, April 2003. http://www.ncbi.nlm.nih.gov/entrez/query.fcgi?cmd=Retrieve&db=PubMed&list_uids =12756080&dopt=Abstract (accessed August 23, 2006).

"X-Rays Go Digital." October 2003. http://css.sfu.ca/update/vol15/15.3-digital-x-rays (accessed August 23, 2006).

RELATED WEB SITES

http://www.acponline.org/computer/telemedicine/glossary.htm.
http://www.acponline.org/computer/telemedicine/links.htm.

CHAPTER 7

Information Technology in Surgery—the Cutting Edge

CHAPTER OUTLINE

LEARNING OBJECTIVES

After reading this chapter you will be able to

- List some of the uses of computers in surgery.
- Describe the role of computers in surgical planning.

- Define robot, endoscopic surgery, minimally invasive surgery, augmented reality, and telepresence surgery; be aware of the Socrates system, which allows long distance mentoring of surgeons in real time.
- Describe NASA Extreme Environment Mission Operation (NEEMO).
- Describe the Operating Room of the Future.
- List some of the robots used in surgery including ROBODOC, AESOP, ZEUS, and da Vinci.
- Describe some of the advantages and disadvantages of computer-assisted surgery.
- Describe the use of lasers in surgery.

OVERVIEW

Information technology is entering the twenty-first century with profound challenges and extraordinary techniques in the field of surgery. Hardware and software are being developed that help in the planning and carrying out of surgical procedures. Sophisticated simulation software and speech recognition systems, in addition to **robots** equipped with **artificial intelligence**—programmed to "hear," "see," and "respond" to their environments are already helping to perform certain operations. Special system software is used to network all the computerized devices in an operating room.

Health care personnel can use a combination of computer-generated images, virtual and augmented reality, and robotic devices to assist before and during operations. Currently, computer-generated graphics assist in planning surgery, in guiding operations, and in training surgeons and other health care professionals. Enhanced images and precision instruments have made the development of the field of **minimally invasive surgery (MIS)** possible. MIS is surgery performed through small incisions. Most minimally invasive procedures are done using an **endoscope**—a thin tube, which can be connected to a minuscule camera. It projects an image of the surgical site onto a monitor. The surgeon does not look at the patient; instead she or he looks at a monitor on which is projected an *image* of the patient. Thus, much of **computer-assisted surgery** is said to be **image-directed**. **Distance (or telepresence) surgery** performed by robotic devices controlled by surgeons at another site has been successfully performed. It is conceivable that a robot controlled only by a computer program could perform surgery.

COMPUTER-ASSISTED SURGERY

Computer-Assisted Surgical Planning

Computer-assisted surgical planning involves the use of **virtual environment** technology to provide surgeons with realistic accurate models on which to teach surgery and to plan and practice operations. With **virtual reality (VR)** technology, the computer can create an environment that seems real, but is not. VR simulations were first used in the 1940s to train pilots. Currently, these lifelike simulations are used in the health care field. The models created by VR technology can look, sound, and feel real. They can respond to pressure, by changing shape, and to being cut, by leaking. A model such as this, which is interactive, allows surgeons not only to plan surgeries more precisely, but also to practice operations without touching a patient. Some models include a predictive element that shows the results of the doctor's actions. For example, plastic surgeons can practice on a model of a face and see the results of their work. The Netra system allows planning of biopsies, tumor resections, surgical implants, and surgery for motor disorders. The Compass system allows surgeons to plan operations for brain tumors by providing a three-dimensional model from computed tomography (CT) scans and magnetic resonance imaging (MRI). The image is also used as a guide during the operation.

Minimally Invasive Surgery

Minimally invasive surgery (MIS), utilizing an endoscope or a laparoscope, performs procedures through small incisions that involve a minimum of damage to healthy tissue (Figure 7.1 ■).

However, some laparoscopic surgeries involve electronic cutting tools, posing some risk for the patient. Still, there is less bleeding and pain, and a shorter recovery time. This means a shorter hospital stay and lower costs. You will recall that an endoscope projects an image of the surgical field onto a monitor.

Recognizing that a picture on a monitor is not the same as viewing the surgical field, some doctors are attempting to improve the picture by connecting endoscopes to high-definition televisions. Gall bladder disease has been treated with minimally invasive techniques for many years.

One form of minimally invasive robotic surgery is called **endoluminal surgery**. Endoluminal surgery does not require incisions. It is also called natural orifice surgery. For example, devices recently approved by the Food and Drug Administration (FDA) give the surgeon access to the stomach through the patient's mouth.[1,2] "An untethered miniature robot . . . inserted through the mouth would . . . be able to enter the abdominal cavity."[3]

COMPUTER-ASSISTED SURGERY AND ROBOTICS

Computer-assisted surgery makes use of robotics and computer-generated images such as CT scans and MRIs. The robots are under the control of software and the surgeon. Through a combination of hardware and software, a robot may be able to "see" via video devices, and to "hear" through microphones using speech recognition software.

Robots, unlike humans, can hold endoscopes and other instruments without becoming tired or shaky. Robots are also used to scale down the surgeon's motions. Some surgeons report that this makes their hands "rock steady," making surgery on small delicate areas such as the eye safer.

Feedback mechanisms allow the robot to determine the proper pressure and tension needed to manipulate a particular object. Robots are able to compare tissue

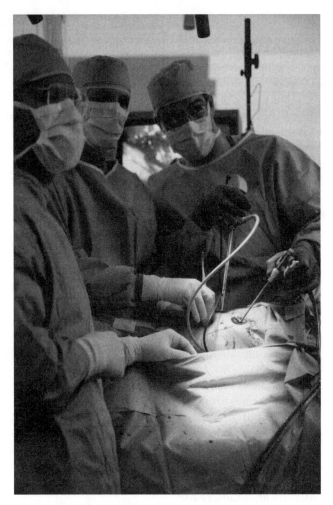

■ **FIGURE 7.1**   Minimally invasive surgery using an endoscope allows procedures to be performed through miniscule incisions. Courtesy of Photodisc/Getty Images.

density and thus "decide" whether tissue is normal or a tumor by remembering its "pressure signature."

Currently, doctors are trying to give robots a delicate sense of touch; the robots will also be able to palpate tissue. To restore the sense of touch to surgeons, a chip containing sixty-four sensors will be inside the patient's body; it will scan the patient. When it encounters a lump, the pressure in a sensor will rise. Outside the patient, the doctor's finger rests on motorized pins that rise or fall according to the sensors. Through the pins, the doctor will feel the object inside the patient's body.

Currently robotics and MIS are being used in complex surgeries. New computer-controlled systems are making it possible to perform trauma surgery (such as femoral fracture fixation) through quarter inch incisions; one such system has received FDA clearance. Minimally invasive knee and hip replacements are also a possibility. FDA-approved hardware and software will make hip replacement through a tiny incision possible; the software allows the surgeon to have more information by keeping track of the implant and the instruments, and their relation to the patient. The information is given to the surgeon in real time.

New instruments are being developed to make surgery even less invasive. Laprotek is developing flexible, computer-controlled catheters; the surgeon can control them inside the patient. The catheters can carry out suturing. European clinical trials began in May 2003.

One program, eXpert Trainer, attempts to teach the special skills that are needed to perform MIS. The skills include working with long instruments, learning "eye-hand disassociation" to work on a patient while looking at a monitor, working in a three-dimensional field while looking at a two-dimensional screen, and to reverse right and left motions and images.

ROBODOC, AESOP, ZEUS, da Vinci, MINERVA, and Other Robotic Devices

The earliest use of a robot in surgery was in hip replacement operations. Integrated Surgical Systems' **ROBODOC** (which is undergoing FDA-approved clinical trials) is a computer-controlled, image-directed robot that performed its first hip replacement in 1992. It can be used only with cementless implants—which constitute about one-third of implants done each year. It has been used in thousands of hip replacement operations worldwide. Because ROBODOC actually cuts into a patient's femur, there have to be strict built-in safeguards. They come from the program that controls the robot and physical limitations on how much ROBODOC can move. Before the operation, the hip navigation system helps surgeons align implants. The surgeon inserts three pins into the patient's hip. ROBODOC will use these as guides for locating the point to start drilling. Currently, some hip replacements are being performed without pins, and studies are being carried out to compare the two methods. ROBODOC works with ORTHODOC, which using CT scans creates a three-dimensional image of the hip. The doctor plans the surgery using the image. The plan is translated into drilling instructions for ROBODOC that drills a perfect opening for the implant. ROBODOC is up to ten times more accurate than a human being.

In a report of U.S. multicenter trials comparing outcomes of hip replacement done with ROBODOC to those performed by hand, it was found that at twenty-four months there were no differences in complications between the two groups; however the group undergoing ROBODOC surgery had no intraoperative fractures. But blood loss and surgical time were greater; the most significant findings were that ROBODOC did "improve implant size, selection, position, and accuracy." One of the advantages of ROBODOC is that it forces surgeons to plan carefully, thus avoiding the wrong-sized implant and reaming defects. The study predicts better long-term performance with ROBODOC. A German study focused on safety. It found that an operation had never had to be stopped for safety reasons with ROBODOC; that the robot itself would stop the surgery if it sensed any errors in data. The surgery could then be completed by hand.

Automated endoscopic system for optimal positioning (AESOP), which was introduced in 1994 by Computer Motion Inc., is the first FDA-cleared surgical robot (Figure 7.2 ■). Originally developed for the space program, AESOP is now used as an assistant in endoscopic procedures. It holds and moves the endoscope under the direction of the surgeon. AESOP was first developed to be controlled by foot pedals. However, currently it responds to voice commands such as "AESOP move left" or "AESOP stop." "AESOP move right" causes a continuous movement for 2.5 seconds. The surgeon can tell AESOP to save a position and later to return to it. Any surgeon who uses AESOP trains the robot to recognize his or her voice. If it fails to recognize the surgeon's voice or command during an operation, a backup system of manual controls can be relied on. Unlike a human assistant, AESOP does not become tired

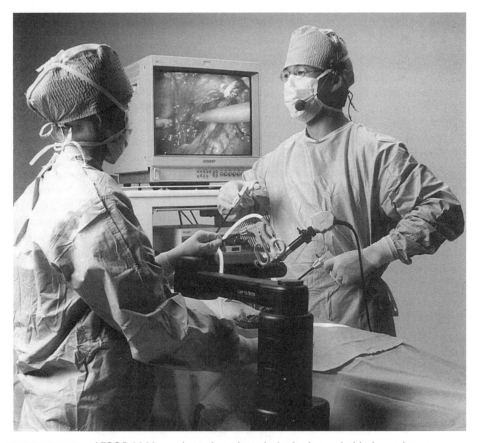

■ **FIGURE 7.2**   AESOP 3000, a voice-activated surgical robotic arm holds the endoscope, providing a steady image. Courtesy of © Intuitive Surgical, Inc.

or shaky. It has been used in a wide variety of procedures including appendectomy, splenectomy, and relief of intestinal obstruction.

In May 1998, in France, heart surgeries were performed on six patients using computers and robots. The incisions were small. The surgeon touched only the console located at a distance of several yards from the patient; she or he could see inside the heart via a three-dimensional camera inside the patient; the robot actually performed the surgery directed by the surgeon. More and more cardiac surgeries are being performed as minimally invasive surgeries.

ZEUS is a robotic surgical system, which will make possible minimally invasive microsurgery. ZEUS has three interactive robotic arms, one of which holds the endoscope, while the other two manipulate the surgical instruments. The surgeon, sitting at a console, controls them. The endoscope is controlled by voice commands. The surgeon manipulates instruments, which resemble surgical tools, while looking at a monitor; the surgeon's manipulations control the robotic arms, which are actually doing the surgery. ZEUS includes a feedback system so that the surgeon "feels" the tissue. The computer-controlled robotic arms also scale down the surgeon's movements, filtering out any hand tremor. This means that a one-inch movement by the surgeon becomes a one-tenth of an inch movement of the robot's surgical instrument. By eliminating the hand's vibrations, ZEUS makes delicate procedures safer. Thus, ZEUS can increase the surgeon's dexterity. Computer Motion Inc., which manufactures ZEUS states that it will be able to perform heart bypass surgery endoscopically, through incisions the diameter of a pencil instead of the traditional thirty-centimeter splitting of the breast bone. ZEUS may be approved for use in coronary bypass, mitral valve replacement, and laparoscopic and thoracic surgery.

Similar to ZEUS, the **da Vinci** robot (Intuitive Surgical, Inc.) was first cleared for assisting in surgery in 1997, for performing some surgeries in 2000, and for performing cardiac surgery such as mitral valve repair in November 2002. A small study in December 2000 found that patients undergoing minimally invasive mitral valve repair have less pain and shorter hospital stays than those who underwent conventional surgery. They returned to work 50 percent faster. Minimally invasive heart surgeries are performed through three tiny incisions: one for the endoscope that projects the surgical field on to a monitor; and the other two for surgical instruments. The instruments are held by a robot. Its wrists can move 180 degrees (a greater range of motion than humans have) and follow the surgeon's hand motions; the surgeon's hands are attached to controls. The surgeon watches the surgery on a screen in three-dimensional, high-resolution images, and can see any part of the surgical field. One advantage of da Vinci is that it mimics the surgeon's hand motions. To control other laparoscopic instruments, the surgeon has to move the opposite way, for instance, to move the instrument right, the surgeon must move left, up is down and so on. On January 17, 2002 the first endoscopic cardiac bypass surgery was performed in the United States. However, the FDA has not yet approved this for widespread use. Da Vinci is also used to repair an inborn condition called atrial septic defect (ASD). Patients born with ASD have an opening between the two upper chambers of the heart, which untreated can result in congestive heart failure, hypertension, and increased risk of stroke. It should be noted that at least one person has died in a robot-aided surgery. Da Vinci was being used to remove a cancerous kidney. However, the patient's aorta was accidentally cut during the surgery and he died two days later. The hospital denied that the robot was to blame.

In 2005, da Vinci was approved for gynecological procedures. It can be used to perform hysterectomies, to remove fibroid tumors, and in all urologic procedures. Cleared for heart surgery in 2004, da Vinci has been used in over two thousand heart and chest surgeries (Figure 7.3 ■).

It can be used in mitral valve repairs and coronary bypass procedures. It is also used in prostate surgery (the most common robotic surgery), gynecological and infertility surgeries. The use of da Vinci has increased from 1500 procedures in 2000 to twenty thousand in 2004.[4–6]

Researchers at Columbia University College of Physicians and Surgeons in New York are currently conducting clinical trials on Evalve® Cardiovascular Valve Repair System. Evalve® is being used for the treatment of mitral valve regurgitation. Untreated, this condition can lead to arrhythmias and congestive heart failure. The valve repair procedure is nonsurgical. Guided by images, a catheter is inserted into the vascular system to the mitral valve where it places a clip to repair the leaky valve.[7]

MINERVA is a robot developed to perform stereotactic neurosurgical procedures. Used to treat some brain tumors, the stereotactic method involves fixing a

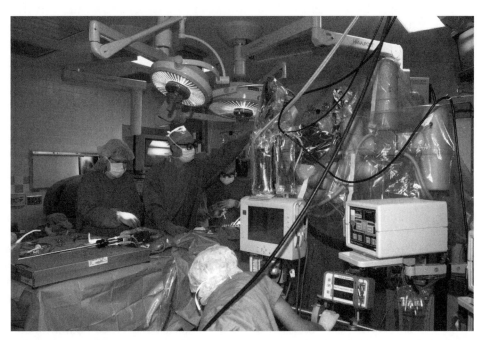

■ **FIGURE 7.3**   The one hundredth mitral valve replacement performed by the da Vinci system. Courtesy of East Carolina University, photo by Cliff Hollis.

metal frame, similar to a cage, on the patient's head. The surgeon uses an MRI or CT scan to calculate how to reach the tumor with a minimum of trauma to surrounding tissue. The surgeon does not see the surgical site and must rely on the CT scan to avoid damaging vital parts of the brain. For successful robot-assisted surgery, the robot must be highly accurate. MINERVA operates inside the CT scan. This enables the surgeon to follow the position of the instruments. The doctor selects the target. MINERVA makes the calculations, and responding to the doctor's commands, performs the procedure. NeuroMate was developed in France for neurosurgical applications and is FDA approved. It has performed over one thousand tumor biopsies. It collects data from images of the patient and with special software plans the path to the tumor. This information is transferred to a control workstation. The surgeon uses all the information including X-rays to command the robot to insert a guide. The guide is then used to introduce a surgical instrument. Less invasive than robot-assisted stereotactic neurosurgery, is stereotactic radiosurgery or gamma knife surgery (see Chapter 6 on Radiology) that does not involve cutting, but uses radiation to shrink certain brain tumors, which then may not need to be surgically removed. The newer cyber knife, because it compensates for patient movement can be used to treat brain and spinal tumors with radiosurgery.

Other robots have been developed. Using **ARTEMIS**, a surgical system that works with the simulation software **KISMET**, a surgeon can perform MIS while viewing three screens, which show the view presented by the endoscope and simulations. ARTEMIS can also perform minimally invasive breast biopsies.

Robots can assist in needle placement in the insertion of nerve blocks for back pain and minimally invasive kidney procedures (percutaneous access of the kidney/remote center of motion (PAKY/RCM)). Acrobat or active constraint robot (ACROBOT) is used for total knee replacement. PROBOT helps in prostate surgery. Steady-hand robot was developed for microsurgery where smaller than human movements of the hand are needed. A robot is being developed in Germany that reduces the risks of extremely delicate spinal surgery; it would make it possible to monitor the surgery in real time, possibly diminishing risks such as paralysis.

System software is required to connect the operating room hardware into a network that a surgeon can control with voice commands. **HERMES** is an FDA-cleared operating system that performs these tasks, allowing the surgeon to use his or her voice to control all the electronic equipment in the operating room, coordinating the endoscope and robotic devices. It also allows the surgeon to adjust lighting with a voice command. The surgeon can use HERMES to take and print pictures and access the patient's electronic medical record including images and other information.

A major problem with surgical robots is their size. In 2006, doctors and engineers at Purdue University were attempting to create "less expensive, portable, and versatile surgical robots . . ." and they planned to include sensors so that surgeons would be able to feel tissue. The sensors would communicate with the computer, which would create a color coded "tactile map." Surgical robots currently cost around $1 million. The portable robot would cost about $250,000.[8]

Augmented Reality

Because much computer-assisted surgery is image-guided, software has been developed that enhances what the surgeon sees. This kind of surgery is called **augmented reality** surgery. It makes use of computer-generated imagery to provide the surgeon with information that otherwise would be unavailable. The computer-generated images may either be fused with the image on the monitor or projected directly onto the patient's body during the operation allowing the doctor to virtually see inside the patient. However, an image on a monitor is two-dimensional. A head mounted display that combines the computer-generated images and the image of the patient allows the surgeon to see a three-dimensional field and see different views by simply turning her or his head instead of adjusting the endoscope, making it more like traditional open surgery. The image and the reality must of course be perfectly aligned (registered) with each other. One use of augmented reality is in using an ultrasound to allow the technician to see an image of the fetus on the abdomen of the patient. Another is in image-guided breast biopsies. It is also used in brain surgery, where an MRI or CT scan may be projected on the patient's head, so that the surgeon can see a tumor, which would otherwise be invisible.

A new four-dimensional model of the human body called CAVEman, has been developed in Canada. It can be used to plan surgery and to educate patients. ". . . the larger-than-life computer image encompasses more than 3,000 distinct body parts, all viewed in a booth that gives the image height, width and depth. . . . It also plots the passage of time [the 4th dimension]." The model looks like it is floating just out of reach. High-resolution computer-generated images can be projected onto CAVEman giving a view of the inside of a particular patient. There is only one finished CAVEman in the world today. Researchers plan to use the model to study the genetic components of several diseases including cancer, diabetes, multiple sclerosis, and Alzheimer's. It will make it possible to "merge patients' diagnostic results . . . internal images and blood tests—in one place." CAVEman can be viewed using three-dimensional glasses and its parts moved by a joystick.[9]

Telepresence Surgery

Telepresence surgery (distance surgery) is at the cutting edge of telemedicine. The National Aeronautics and Space Administration (NASA) first sought to develop telepresence surgery for space flight medical emergencies. Actual surgeries have been performed with the patient and surgeon at a distance and have been successful. Distance surgery thus has the potential of making surgical expertise available on battlefields, space stations, and in remote rural areas. Several research groups are working on telesurgical systems. Some of this work is funded by the Advanced Research Projects Agency (ARPA) of the U.S. Department of Defense, which first conceived of robotic surgery and still sees remote surgery as a way of saving lives on the battlefield and protecting surgeons from dangerous environments. One of the systems that has been developed is the Green Telepresence Surgical System in which surgeons wearing three-dimensional glasses can view the operating room and patient. The system has been used to practice suturing. It has demonstrated its precision by slicing a grape into one-millimeter slices. Distance operations were first performed on animals.

In telepresence surgery, as in MIS, the doctor looks at an image of the patient, not the actual patient. The instruments in the surgeon's hands feel real, but in fact they only direct the robot at a distant site (theoretically hundreds of miles away) that is performing the surgery.

In September 2001, a woman in France had her gall bladder removed by doctors in New York. She spent two days in the hospital. Technically, the surgery made use of high-speed fiber optics, so that time delay was minimal. Much of the system is not yet FDA approved. "It was amazing for the doctors . . . to see the surgical tools suddenly start moving themselves and doing the operation, without any surgeon in the room guiding them," according to one of the doctors on the French team.[10] In this computer-assisted laparoscopic procedure patient and doctor never touch; the surgeon controls the robot through hand signals. Successful prostate cancer surgery was performed in April 2002 between Germany and Virginia. Using the Socrates system, the American doctor was able to see and hear as if he were in the operating room in Berlin; he also controlled AESOP, while the German surgeon performed the surgery. Using Socrates, the remote doctor can teleconnect to the operating room, see and hear, and control devices networked by HERMES. Socrates allows a surgeon in a place to give expert advice in real time to a distant surgeon. **Socrates** is basically a mentoring system, allowing a surgeon in one place to give expert advice in real-time to a distant surgeon. In 2001, the Socrates system was cleared by the FDA, which at the same time created a new classification of device: Robotic Telemedicine Device.

In March 2003, ZEUS was used to perform distance surgery in Canada to correct a patient's acid reflux disease. At one hospital, endoscopic instruments were inserted into the patient's stomach. At another hospital four hundred kilometers away a surgeon used ZEUS to perform the successful surgery. ZEUS's sensors took the information from the surgeon's hand movements and sent it to the distant instruments. The Canadian federal government sees distance surgery as a way of serving its northern population.

NASA Extreme Environment Mission Operation

The NASA Extreme Environment Mission Operation (**NEEMO**) is a series of NASA missions in which groups of scientists live in Aquarius. The major purpose of these projects is to enable astronauts to be operated on in space from earth using wireless technology and robotics. **Aquarius** is the only undersea lab in the world. Aquarius is now sixty-seven feet under the ocean's surface off the Florida Keys. It is thirteen feet wide and forty-five feet long with approximately four hundred square feet of space for living and laboratory activities.[11]

Early NEEMO missions tested living and building in an extreme environment, similar to outer space. NEEMO 7 and 9 included doctors, but no surgeons. One of NEEMO 7's goals was to see whether doctors with no training in surgical techniques could successfully perform surgery with the help of telementoring and telerobotics.

According to one of the family practitioners on board the techniques were "very new for us." The projects used telemedicine techniques to perform gall bladder surgery and suturing on a simulated patient. The project used wireless communications. According to the commander Bob Thirsk, the suturing was not successful. "My perception is that some special skills may be necessary." There were some problems on NEEMO 7 regarding the size of the robotic surgeon (a modified ZEUS) and communication delays. "If a signal is delayed more than 0.7 seconds, a surgeon will begin to have problems controlling the robot."[12,13] NEEMO 9 succeeded in assembling a surgical robot, and completed surgeries controlled by a doctor in Canada.[14]

The NASA NEEMO 12 crew conducted advanced medical experiments using robotic telesurgery (Figure 7.4 ■). Their purpose was to improve future care for astronauts, in part by "overcome[ing] interplanetary lag time." They practiced several emergency procedures on simulated patients. **Raven**, a fifty-pound, mobile surgical robot was used on NEEMO 12 (Figure 7.5 ■).[15,16]

An independent study completed in 2004 that investigated the feasibility of using "real-time or simultaneous surgical consultation and education to students in distant locations, . . . [reported] the successful integration of robotics, video-teleconferencing,

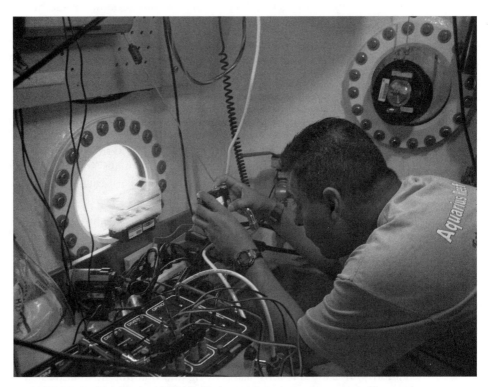

■ **FIGURE 7.4**   Training for NEEMO 12. An astronaut/aquanaut uses a still camera to photograph plants inside the undersea habitat for the twelfth NASA Extreme Environment Mission Operations (NEEMO) mission. Courtesy of NASA.

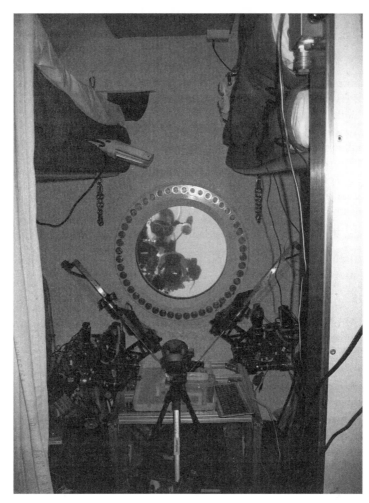

■ **FIGURE 7.5** A two-armed remotely controlled surgical robot from the University of Washington known as Raven is photographed inside the undersea habitat for the twelfth NASA Extreme Environment Mission Operations (NEEMO) mission. Courtesy of NASA.

and intranet transmission using currently available hardware and Internet capabilities." Ninety percent of those viewing anatomical structures telemedically, were able to correctly identify them.[17]

THE OPERATING ROOM OF THE FUTURE

Until very recently picture archiving and communication systems (PACS), the system used to organize and display digital images, could not interact with the operating room. This meant that real-time images were not available to surgeons. Since most computer-assisted surgeries are image directed this was a serious problem. Integration of systems is a current focus of medical informatics.

In the Operating Room of the Future, images from all sources will be integrated and available to surgeons and other personnel. "Multiple image display processors integrate OR video cameras, laparoscopic and endoscopic cameras, MRI, CT, and PET imagery, PACS images, fluoroscopic imaging, ultrasound, patient monitoring data, hemodynamic activity, and patient history on a single, centralized screen for viewing by the surgical team." Information displayed includes a patient's vital statistics, allergies, and the whereabouts of operating room (OR) personnel. Eventually the equipment will be identified and tracked also. The display on four screens (called the wall of knowledge) shows integrated patient information in an easy to understand format, in one location.[18] By 2006, twenty-one operating rooms of the future were in operation in Sloan-Kettering alone. The purpose of this was to enhance patient safety and improve efficiency by providing real-time, integrated information.[19,20]

In some ORs of the future, all personnel including doctors are identified and their movements tracked by **radio frequency identification (RFID) tags**. A list of staff for an operation is displayed and when the doctor or nurse enters the OR, that person's name is brightly lit.[21] RFID-tagged sponges have been created "to help prevent the deadly problem of surgeons accidentally leaving them inside patients." After the surgery, a wand is waved over the patient to check for tags. Because it is so new, no one knows what effect leaving an RFID tag inside a patient would have.[22]

LASERS IN SURGERY

Laser stands for light amplification by the stimulated emission of radiation. Lasers can be used in surgery to cut, vaporize tumors, and seal small blood vessels. A laser beam can be narrowed to the size of a few cells. Lasers are used in gynecology, orthopedics, urology, ear, nose and throat, gastroenterology, and cardiovascular medicine (Figure 7.6 ■).

LASIK is eye surgery that uses lasers to correct vision by changing the shape of the cornea.

DISCUSSION AND FUTURE DIRECTIONS

Computer-assisted surgery encompasses everything from the well-established use of a robotic assistant in an endoscopic procedure to telepresence surgery. It is an evolving field. New robotic devices, nanotechnology, new software, new techniques, and new applications are being developed. Thus, this cannot be an exhaustive survey of the uses of robotics, augmented reality techniques, or minimally invasive surgical procedures. Currently, computer-generated images help make surgery more precise. Making three-dimensional real-time images available in surgery (linking PACS with the operating room) would certainly help. MIS results in smaller incisions, less

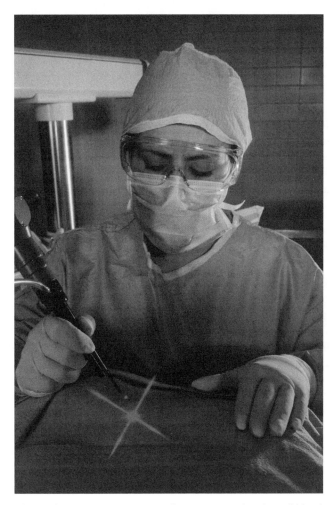

■ **FIGURE 7.6** Lasers in surgery can cut, vaporize tumors, and seal small blood vessels. Courtesy of Corbis RF.

trauma, and therefore less pain and shorter recovery time. This leads to some economic benefits including shorter hospitals stays and less time lost from work. Even though the equipment is quite expensive, it may be less expensive in the long run to use a robot than a human assistant to hold an endoscope in the operating room. However, there are substantial difficulties involved in using MIS. The workspace is small. The doctor is looking at a monitor, not a patient while *indirectly* manipulating surgical instruments. This may cause the surgeon to be less dexterous and have less eye–hand coordination. Research is currently being done to help solve these problems. A glove-like device is being developed to help the surgeon control minimally invasive tools more easily.

Nanotechnology

Nanotechnology is an emerging field of medicine. Nanotechnology works with objects "on the scale of atoms and molecules. . . . A nanometer is one-billionth of a meter." Nanotechnology holds promise in regenerative medicine. Injected into mice with spinal cord injuries, "the nanofibers—thousands of times thinner than a human hair—are the key to not only preventing the formation of harmful scar tissue that inhibits spinal cord healing, but to stimulating the body into regenerating lost or damaged cells." The mice walked![23] Nanotechnology has the potential of helping people with Parkinson's, Alzheimer's, diabetes, and spinal cord injuries. It also regenerated heart cells after a heart attack. The National Research Council warns that along with new possibilities may come new safety hazards.[24]

CONCLUSION

Computer-assisted surgery holds great promise for the future. The use of augmented images to teach surgeons and plan and guide operations can reduce unnecessary cutting and make operations more precise and less invasive. This chapter highlights many of the benefits of minimally invasive procedures and the use of robots. However, it should be remembered that aside from a few established procedures such as cementless hip replacement and gall bladder removal, this field is in its infancy. It is also important to keep in mind the dangers and disadvantages. Looking at a monitor is never quite as good as looking at a live patient; feeling via sensory feedback mechanisms is not the same as actually having one's hands on living tissue. MIS is more difficult to learn and requires more training than traditional surgery. Further, doctors trained in traditional open surgery methods will be understandably reluctant to learn the new methods.

The most experimental area of computer-assisted surgery is telepresence or distance surgery. High-bandwidth channels are required for transmitting endoscopy and networks must be 100 percent reliable because any delay or failure could result in the death of a patient. At the present time, the Canadian federal government is working with doctors to promote the use of distance surgery to treat rural populations. In addition, NASA is conducting experiments in telemedicine in their undersea missions (NEEMO).

Another experimental technology is nanotechnology, which holds promise for the regeneration of cells, tissues, and organs, leading the body to heal itself. It may ultimately relieve the symptoms of diabetes, spinal cord injuries, Parkinson's, heart disease, and cancer among many other conditions.

IN THE NEWS

Excerpt from, "Surgical Device Poses a Rare but Serious Peril"
by Barnaby J. Feder

Kristina A. Fox entered a Portland, Ore., hospital in the fall of 1998 hoping a routine, minimally invasive form of surgery called laparoscopy would relieve a painful gynecological condition.

She went home the same day destined to become part of a simmering debate over whether medical device makers and health care providers have been overlooking—some would say ignoring—an easily preventable, but potentially devastating, laparoscopy hazard.

Severe complications are rare among the 4.4 million Americans who undergo laparoscopic surgery each year . . . But experts say that what happened to Mrs. Fox is a type of injury that occurs far more often than reported.

As in many laparoscopies, Mrs. Fox's surgeon inserted a wand-like electrical tool into her abdomen to cut tissue and seal blood vessels. A miniature video camera let him view his work, but did not show the stray electricity escaping from the wand's shaft. No one suspected when Mrs. Fox was sent home that a wayward spark might have seared a tiny hole in her colon.

Two days later, Mrs. Fox was rushed to the emergency room, perilously ill from the infectious bacteria that had leaked into her abdomen. Mrs. Fox, now 33, ended up with a malfunctioning bladder and disabling pain that despite frequent follow-up treatments—13 operations so far—prevent her from working or bearing children. She has a lawsuit pending against the device makers, the hospital and the doctor involved.

Her lawsuit argues, as do a number of medical experts, that the risk of accidents from laparoscopic surgery could be sharply reduced with the use of fault-detection devices on the market.

"It wouldn't surprise me in the least if it caused more than 100 deaths and 10,000 injuries annually," said Dr. Alan Johns, a Fort Worth gynecologist who frequently teaches courses on the complications of laparoscopy.

Safety advocates say the risk of burns can be reduced by relatively inexpensive scanning devices that can be used before surgery to test electrical wands for insulation cracks. Moreover, the risk can be virtually eliminated by using wands with monitoring systems that shut them down instantly if power is leaking.

The risk of inadvertent burns has been recognized since the invention of the first electrical surgical tools in the late 1920's. But the accident rate soared in the 1980's as laparoscopic versions of the devices became widely used in gynecology, gall bladder removal and gastric bypass surgery.

(continued)

Excerpt from, "Surgical Device Poses a Rare but Serious Peril" *(continued)*

The debate these days is over whether the risks have now been reduced to the point that it is a waste of resources to install safeguard systems or replace the older technology.

The major device makers deny that safer technology is needed. Ethicon Endo-Surgery, a division of Johnson & Johnson, said it had not received any complaints, although it has been named a defendant in a burn lawsuit.

Equipment companies that do acknowledge hearing of electrical mishaps like Mrs. Fox's say they occur in isolated cases where hospitals ignore specified limits on how long or frequently to use wands before replacing them. And many doctors agree.

The InsulScan, the device that scans laparoscopic wands to detect microscopic insulation cracks that can cause burns, was invented by Medicor, a start-up that went bankrupt in 2000 trying to commercialize the device. One of its distributors, privately held Mobile Instrument Service and Repair Inc., took over the business.

Sales are not disclosed but are growing slowly but steadily with backing from Medline Industries, a large medical products distributor, according to Summer L. Babyak, InsulScan's product manager . . . Sales would probably climb if more lawsuits like Mrs. Fox's were filed, but safety advocates say lawyers, like patients, health care providers and insurers, rarely hear of such burns.

CHAPTER SUMMARY

This chapter introduces the student to some of the uses of information technology in surgery.

- Computer-assisted surgery involves the use of computer technology in the planning and/or performance of operations.
- Computer-generated images make planning operations more precise and allow surgeons to practice on realistic models.
- In the operating room, robotic devices, which can "see," "hear," and respond are used as surgical assistants.
  - Robotic devices are used in minimally invasive surgery, much of which involves the use of an endoscope, a viewing device, which can project an image of the surgical site onto a monitor. The image is used to guide the surgeon.
    - ROBODOC, AESOP, ZEUS, da Vinci, and MINERVA are robots used in minimally invasive endoscopic procedures.

- In MIS, three-dimensional, computer-generated images may be fused with the image of the surgical site or actually projected onto the patient to enhance or augment reality.
    - The surgeon's manipulations guide the robotic arms, which operate on the patient. Voice commands control the arm that holds the endoscope.
  - Telepresence surgery, in which the surgeon is at one site and the patient at another site, is being performed. The Socrates system allows a surgeon to mentor another surgeon at a distant location in real time.
    - NEEMO 7 and 9 attempted to demonstrate distance surgery from Canada to the Aquarius off the Florida Keys. NEEMO 12 attempted telesurgery on simulated patients.
  - In the Operating Room of the Future, all information systems will be integrated and available to surgeons.
  - Nanotechnology, using regenerative medicine, may lead to the body healing itself.

KEY TERMS

automated endoscopic
   system for optimal
   positioning (AESOP)
Aquarius
ARTEMIS
artificial intelligence
augmented reality
computer-assisted
   surgery
da Vinci
distance (or telepres-
   ence surgery)

endoluminal surgery
endoscope
HERMES
image-guided
   surgery
KISMET
Laser
MINERVA
minimally invasive
   surgery (MIS)
nanotechnology
NEEMO

radio frequency
   identification
   (RFID) tags
Raven
ROBODOC
robots
telepresence surgery
   (distance surgery)
Socrates
virtual environment
virtual reality (VR)
ZEUS

REVIEW EXERCISES

Multiple Choice

1. A robot _____.
   A. can respond to speech commands
   B. is a programmable machine
   C. A and B
   D. None of the above
2. _____ may be used to help train surgeons and to allow realistic practice operations.
   A. Virtual environment technology
   B. Endoscopes
   C. Robots
   D. ZEUS

3. _____ is a robotic device used in some hip replacement operations.
   A. ROBODOC
   B. AESOP
   C. ZEUS
   D. HERMES

4. An endoscope is _____.
   A. a surgical instrument that cuts into the patient
   B. only used to produce the image the surgeon sees
   C. a thin tube with a light source
   D. B and C

5. Surgery that makes use of computer-generated images to enhance what the surgeon sees is called _____.
   A. virtual reality
   B. augmented reality
   C. telepresence surgery
   D. None of the above

6. Among the benefits of MIS could be _____.
   A. smaller scars
   B. shorter recovery time
   C. less trauma to healthy tissue
   D. All of the above

7. The most frequently done laparoscopic procedure is _____.
   A. gall bladder removal
   B. open heart surgery
   C. brain surgery
   D. knee replacement

8. The first FDA-cleared surgical robot was _____.
   A. ZEUS
   B. HERMES
   C. AESOP
   D. HARRY

9. Computer technology may be involved in _____.
   A. planning operations
   B. assisting in the operating room
   C. training surgeons
   D. All of the above

10. A robot developed to assist in brain surgery is _____.
    A. ZEUS
    B. HERMES
    C. AESOP
    D. MINERVA

True/False Questions

1. The high-bandwidth communications lines needed for distance surgery are in place. _____

2. Computer-generated graphics can give a surgeon virtual X-ray vision. _____

3. One of the advantages of MIS is that the surgeon looks at a monitor not at the patient. _____

4. A robotic device can "decide" whether what it is touching is a tumor or normal tissue. _____

5. Telepresence surgery was first conceived of by the U.S. Department of Defense. _____

6. A disadvantage of MIS is longer hospital stays. _____

7. Virtual reality technology creates environments that seem real but are not. _____

8. Surgeons make use of computer models to plan operations. _____

9. Some surgical robots were originally developed for the space program. _____

10. Hip replacement operations using ROBODOC cannot possibly be as good as those with human surgeons only. _____

Critical Thinking

1. Many challenging issues arise from the innovative uses of computer-assisted surgery and the use of robots in the operating room.
   - Discuss how these developments might affect the patient and the surgeon.
   - What do you consider the responsibilities of the hardware manufacturer?
   - What do you consider the responsibilities of the software publisher?

2. Discuss the advantages and disadvantages of robotic surgery to the patient and the surgeon.

3. Given that computers are playing a more active role in surgery, what steps would you recommend be taken to protect patients from the effects of computer viruses, electrical malfunctions, and software bugs?

4. "Imagine you're having a hip replacement. . . . As you're wheeled into the operating room, you notice the nurses and anesthetist preparing for your surgery. But wait, someone's missing. Your surgeon. You look around the room and finally spot the surgeon, off in the corner keying information into a computer terminal. And there, next to the doctor and computer is a five hundred pound, seven foot-high, jointed steel arm, with a tiny drill attached to one end. It's Robodoc. And it's going to assist in your surgery."[25] How do you feel about being operated on by a robot as opposed to a human being?

NOTES

1. T. Martinez-Serna and C. J. Filipi, "Endoluminal Surgery," *World Journal of Surgery* 23, no. 4 (1999): 368–77, http://www.ncbi.nlm.nih.gov/sites/entrez?db=pubmed&uid=10030860&cmd=showdetailview (accessed December 14, 2007).

2. "FINANCE: Medical Device Company Closes $12 Million Series B Financing," January 19, 2004, http://www.newsrx.com/article.php?articleID=132367 (accessed December 14, 2007).

3. Mark E. Rentschler, Jason Dumpert, Stephen E. Platt, Shane M. Farritor, and Dmitry Oleynikov, "Natural Orifice Surgery with an Endoluminal Mobile Robot" (presented at

the 2006 SAGES Meeting), http://robots.unl.edu/Files/Papers2/Rentschler_Natural_Orifice_Robot_with_figures.pdf (accessed December 14, 2007).

4. Michelle Meadows, "Computer-Assisted Surgery: An Update," July–August 2005, http://www.fda.gov/fdac/features/2005/405_computer.html (accessed December 14, 2007).

5. Carol Marie Cropper, "The Robot Is In—and Ready to Operate," *Business Week*, March 14, 2005.

6. David Samadi, "Prostate Cancer Treatment - da Vinci Robotic Surgery," http://roboticoncology.com/Da-Vinci-Robotic-Prostatectomy.php (accessed December 21, 2007).

7. "Heart Surgery Without the Surgeon: Researchers Test Evalve for Noninvasive Mitral Valve Repair," August 23, 2006, http://www.columbiasurgery.org/pat/cardiac/news_evalve.html (accessed December 14, 2007).

8. Leslie Versweyveld, "Lower Cost, Portable Surgical Robots Could be Smooth Operators," March 2, 2006, http://www.hoise.com/vmw/06/articles/vmw/LV-VM-04-06-13.html (accessed December 14, 2007).

9. Jeffrey Jones, "Virtual Human Puts Doctors Inside Patients," May 23, 2007, http://pune360.com/News/2007/05/27/virtual-human-puts-doctors-inside-patients/ (accessed December 14, 2007).

10. Erica Klarreich, "Is There a Doctor on the Planet?" News@Nature, September 20, 2001.

11. NASA Feature, "About Aquarius," March 28, 2006, http://www.nasa.gov/lb/mission_pages/NEEMO/facilities.html (accessed December 14, 2007).

12. Duncan Graham Rowe, "Scrubbing Up for Robotic Surgery in Space," October 11, 2004, http://www.newscientist.com/article/dn6512-scrubbing-up-for-robotic-surgery-in-space.html (accessed December 14, 2007).

13. Michael Schirber, "NEEMO's Undersea Operations: Making Telemedicine a Long Distance Reality," October 19, 2004, http://www.space.com/scienceastronomy/neemo_surgery_041019.html (accessed December 14, 2007).

14. Tariq Malik, "NASA's NEEMO 9: Remote Surgery and Mock Moonwalks on the Sea Floor," April 19, 2006, http://www.space.com/businesstechnology/060419_neemo9_techwed.html (accessed December 14, 2007).

15. NASA, "NEEMO 12 Mission Journal," May 9, 2007, http://www.nasa.gov/mission_pages/NEEMO/NEEMO12/mission_ journal_3.html (accessed December 14, 2007).

16. "NASA Undersea Mission Planned for May," *Science Daily*, February 27, 2007.

17. Azhar Rafiq, James A. Moore, Xiaoming Zhao, Charles R. Doarn, and Ronald C. Merrell, "Digital Video Capture and Synchronous Consultation in Open Surgery," *Annals of Surgery* 239, no. 4 (2004): 567–73, http://www.pubmedcentral.nih.gov/articlerender.fcgi?artid=1356263 (accessed December 22, 2007).

18. Stefanie Olsen, "Tomorrow's Operating Room to Harness Net, RFID," October 19, 2005, http://www.news.com/Tomorrows-operating-room-to-harness-Net%2C-RFID/2100-1008_3-5900990.html?tag=ne.gall.related (accessed December 21, 2007).

19. "Memorial Sloan-Kettering Cancer Center Using LiveData's OR-Dashboard: 'Wall of Knowledge' Deployed to 21 New Operating Rooms," June 19, 2006, http://www.livedata.com/content/view/83/ (accessed December 14, 2007).

20. "Integrated Operating Room Systems Look to Become OR of the Future," 2006, http://www.medcompare.com/spotlight.asp?spotlightid=123 (accessed December 14, 2007).

21. Olsen, "Tomorrow's Operating Room to Harness Net, RFID."

22. "Tagged Surgical Sponges Help Prevent Deadly Problem," July 18, 2006, http://www.medicalnewstoday.com/articles/47583.php (accessed December 14, 2007).

23. "Nanotechnology Offers Hope for Treating Spinal Cord Injuries, Diabetes, and Parkinson's Disease," *Science Daily*, April 23, 2007, http://www.sciencedaily.com/releases/2007/04/070423080448.htm (accessed December 14, 2007).

24. Barnaby Feder, "Study Says U.S. Has Lead in Nanotechnology," September 26, 2006, http://www.nytimes.com/2006/09/26/technology/26nano.html (accessed December 14, 2007).
25. Kevin L. Ropp, "Robots in the Operating Room," *FDA Consumer,* July/August, 1993, reprinted in 2002, http://www.fda.gov/bbs/topics/CONSUMER/CON00242.html (accessed December 14, 2007).

ADDITIONAL RESOURCES

Ackerman, Jeremy. "Ultrasound Visualization Research." June 15, 2000. http://www.cs.unc.edu/Research/us/ (accessed December 14, 2007).

Argenziano, Michael. "Robotically Assisted, Minimally Invasive Cardiac Surgery." 2002. http://www.nyp.org/masc/davinci.htm (accessed December 14, 2007).

"Artemis Medical Receives 510K Clearance on New Image Guided Biopsy Device." April 22, 2002. http://goliath.ecnext.com/coms2/summary_0199-1664257_ITM (August 23, 2006).

Bargar, W. L., A. Bauer, and M. Borner. "Primary and Revision Total Hip Replacement Using the Robodoc System." September 1998. http://www.ncbi.nlm.nih.gov/entrez/query.fcgi?cmd=Retrieve&db=PubMed&list_uids=9755767&dopt=Abstract (accessed December 14, 2007).

Cleary, Kevin, and Charles Nguyen. "State of the Art in Surgical Robotics: Clinical Applications and Technology Challenges." http://www3.interscience.wiley.com/cgi-bin/abstract/93012897/ABSTRACT (accessed December 14, 2007).

Christensen, Bill. "NEEMO 7: NASA's Undersea Robotic Telemedicine Experiment." October 15, 2004. http://www.technovelgy.com/ct/Science-Fiction-News.asp?NewsNum=227 (accessed December 14, 2007).

Cuellar, Al. "What Is New in Total Hip and Knee Replacement Surgery." August 14, 2006. http://www.ksfortho.com/en/art/?19 (accessed August 23, 2006).

Eisenberg, Anne. "What's Next; Restoring the Human Touch to Remote-Controlled Surgery." May 30, 2002. http://query.nytimes.com/gst/fullpage.html?res=9506EED7113BF933A05756C0A9649C8B63 (accessed December 14, 2007).

Eisenberg, Anne. "What's Next; a Sharper Picture of What Ails the Body." January 24, 2002. http://query.nytimes.com/gst/fullpage.html?res=9E04E7DE113BF937A15752C0A9649C8B63 (accessed December 14, 2007).

"FDA Clearance of da Vinci Surgical System for Intracardiac Surgery Now Encompasses 'ASD' Closure." 2005. http://findarticles.com/p/articles/mi_m0EIN/is_2003_ Jan_30/ai_97073329 (accessed December 21, 2007).

"Florida Man Dies After Surgery Involving Robotic Device." October 31, 2002. http://www.injuryboard.com/national-news/florida-man-dies.aspx? (accessed December 14, 2007).

Hall, Alan. "Surgical Robots Make the Cut." June 14, 2001. http://www.businessweek.com/bwdaily/dnflash/jun2001/nf20010614_799.htm (accessed December 14, 2007).

Hendrickson, Dyke. "EndoVia Sees a Better Surgical Way." *Mass High Tech: The Journal of New England Technology,* September 6, 2002. http://masshightech.bizjournals.com/masshightech/stories/2002/09/09/story14.html (accessed December 14, 2007).

Humphries, Kelly and Delores Beasley. "NASA Prepares for Space Exploration in Undersea Lab." March 28, 2006. http://www.nasa.gov/home/hqnews/2006/mar/HQ_06109_NEEMO_9.html (accessed December 14, 2007).

Lanfranco, Anthony R., Andres E. Castellanos, Jaydev P. Desai, and William C. Meyers "Robotic Surgery. A Current Perspective." January 2004. http://www.pubmedcentral.nih.gov/articlerender.fcgi?artid=1356187 (accessed August 23, 2006).

Livingston, Mark. "UNC Laparoscopic Visualization Research." August 11, 1998. http://www.cs.unc.edu/Research/us/laparo.html (accessed December 14, 2007).

Mack, Michael J. "Minimally Invasive and Robotic Surgery." *JAMA* 285, no. 5 (2001): 568–72.

Matthews, Melissa, Kelly Humphries, Nicole Gignac, and Fred Gorell. "Undersea Habitat Becomes Experimental Hospital for NEEMO 7." August 11, 2004. http://www.nasa.gov/centers/johnson/news/releases/2004/H04-264.html (accessed December 14, 2007).

Meadows, Michelle. "Robots Lend a Helping Hand to Surgeons." *FDA Consumer*, May–June 2002. http://www.fda.gov/Fdac/features/2002/302_bots.html (accessed December 14, 2007).

"Medical Robotics @ UC Berkeley." January 2002. http://robotics.eecs.berkeley.edu/medical/ (accessed December 14, 2007).

"NASA, NEEMO History." March 21, 2006. http://www.nasa.gov/mission_pages/NEEMO/history.html (accessed December 14, 2007).

"New York Weill Cornell Performs Among First Minimally Invasive Kidney Removals in Children and Infants in New York." January 2002. http://www.nycornell.org/news/press/kidney1.html (accessed December 14, 2007).

Peterson, Lynne. "Trends-in-Medicine." April 2004. http://www.crtonline.org/PDF/trends-in-medicine-4-04.pdf (accessed December 14, 2007).

Rafiq, Azhar, James A. Moore, Xiaoming Zhao, Charles R. Doarn, and Ronald C. Merrell. "Digital Video Capture and Synchronous Consultation in Open Surgery." *Annals of Surgery* 239, no. 4 (2004): 567–73. http://www.pubmedcentral.gov/articlerender.fcgi?tool=pmcentrez&rendertype=abstract&artid=1356263 (accessed August 24, 2006).

"Redefining Surgery." August 23, 2006. http://robodoc.com/ (accessed August 23, 2006).

"Remote Control Telemedicine: Sponsored by the National Institutes of Health." http://www.nitrd.gov/ngi/apps/nih/rem.html (accessed December 14, 2007).

"Revolutionizing Trauma Surgery." August 23, 2006. http://ortho.smith-nephew.com/uk/Standard.asp?NodeId=3399 (accessed December 14, 2007).

Dr. Rich. "Robotic Heart Surgery - a Status Report." 2006. http://heartdisease.about.com/library/weekly/aa060401a.htm (accessed August 23, 2006).

"Robot Reduces Spinal Injury Risk." March 12, 2000. http://news.bbc.co.uk/2/hi/health/672815.stm (accessed December 14, 2007).

"Robotic Surgical Assistant for Brain Surgery." NASA Space Telerobotic Program, May 10, 1996. http://ranier.hq.nasa.gov/telerobotics_page/Technologies/0904.html (accessed August 23, 2006).

"Robotic Surgeon to Team Up with Doctors, Astronauts on NASA Mission." April 18, 2007. http://www.physorg.com/news96124114.html (accessed December 14, 2007).

Schaaf, Tracy. "Robotic Surgery: The Future Is Now." Originally published March, 2001. 2006. http://www.devicelink.com/mx/archive/01/03/0103mx024.html (accessed August 23, 2006).

Schurr, M. O., G. Buess, and K. Schwarz. "Robotics in Endoscopic Surgery: Can Mechanical Manipulators Provide a More Simple Solution for the Problem of Limited Degrees of Freedom?" [abstract], November 1, 2001. http://www.informaworld.com/smpp/content~db=all~content=a713750297? (accessed December 14, 2007).

"Simulation Development and Cognitive Science Lab." February 24, 2006. http://www.hmc.psu.edu/simulation/equipment/expert/expert.htm (accessed August 23, 2006).

Stiehl, James. "Computer-assisted Surgery in Adult Reconstruction." 2003. http://64.233.161.104/search?q=cache:gcvMjNmAyyMJ:www.touchbriefings.com/pdf/1680/Steihl.pdf+%E2%80%9CPrimary+and+Revision+Total+Hip+Replacement+Using+Robodoc,%E2%80%9D&hl=en&gl=us&ct=clnk&cd=1/ (accessed August 23, 2006).

Vaze, Ajit. "Robotic Laparoscopic Surgery: A Comparison of the Da Vinci and Zeus Systems." 2002. http://www.bhj.org/journal/2002_4402_apr/endo_208.htm (accessed August 24, 2006).

Versweyveld, Leslie. "Undersea Habitat Becomes Experimental Hospital for Remote Medical Care in NEEMO 7 Project." August 11, 2004. http://www.hoise.com/vmw/04/articles/vmw/LV-VM-09-04-8.html (accessed December 14, 2007).

Versweyveld, Leslie. "Thoroscopic Surgery Robots Now FDA-approved for Use in United States Hospitals." Virtual Medical Worlds, March 6, 2001. http://www.hoise.com/vmw/01/articles/vmw/LV-VM-04-01-12.html (accessed August 24, 2006).

Versweyveld, Leslie. "Socrates Surgical Mentor Allows Surgeon Experts to Provide Remote Guidance in Complex Procedures." Virtual Medical Worlds, March 8, 2001. http://www.hoise.com/vmw/01/articles/vmw/LV-VM-04-01-8.html (accessed August 24, 2006).

Versweyveld, Leslie. "U.S. Food and Drug Administration Kept Busy Approving Surgical Robots from Various Market Competitors." Virtual Medical Worlds, October 17, 2001. http://www.hoise.com/vmw/01/articles/vmw/LV-VM-11-01-20.html (accessed December 14, 2007).

"Virtual Environments for Surgical Training and Augmentation." February 27, 2001. http://robotics.eecs.berkeley.edu/medical/research.html#sim (accessed December 14, 2007).

RELATED WEB SITES

http://www.cts.usc.edu/videos.html

CHAPTER 8

Information Technology in Pharmacy

CHAPTER OUTLINE

LEARNING OBJECTIVES

After reading this chapter, the student will be able to

- Describe the Food and Drug Administration (FDA).
- Discuss uncertified medicines as a safety issue.
- Describe the contributions of information technology to the development and testing of drugs.
- Define biotechnology and rational drug design.
- Discuss the significance of the Human Genome Project (HGP) and its contribution to the understanding of genetic diseases.
- List the uses of computers in clinical drug trials.
- Discuss the relationship of the understanding of the molecular basis of a disease to real breakthroughs in treatment.
- List the uses of computer technology in pharmacies including:
  - The use of computers in the neighborhood drug store, from the printing of drug information for customers, to the full automation of the process of filling prescriptions using robots and barcodes.
  - The use of computers in hospital pharmacies:
    - in centralized dispensing systems using robots and barcodes;
    - in decentralized point-of-use dispensing units;
    - in computerized IVs.
- Discuss telepharmacy—the linking of pharmacists via telecommunications lines to dispensing units in remote locations such as doctors' offices.
- Discuss the impact of information technology on pharmacy, as it affects pharmacists, patients, and hospital administrators.

OVERVIEW

Information technology is transforming all aspects of pharmacy, from the design, testing, and approval of drugs, to the automation of drug stores in the community, to the automation of hospital pharmacies and drug delivery systems. Telepharmacy, or the linking of the prescribing doctor's office with the dispensing pharmacy via telecommunications lines, is expanding.

THE FOOD AND DRUG ADMINISTRATION

In the United States, the **Food and Drug Administration (FDA)** is supposed to oversee the safety and efficacy of new medications:

> The FDA is responsible for protecting the public health by assuring the safety, efficacy, and security of human and veterinary drugs, biological products, medical devices, our nation's food supply, cosmetics, and products that emit radiation. The FDA is also responsible for advancing the public health by helping to speed innovations that make medicines and foods more effective, safer, and more affordable; and helping the public

get the accurate, science-based information they need to use medicines and foods to improve their health.[1]

Just as contributors to *The Journal of the American Medical Association (JAMA)* are required to disclose their financial ties,[2] likewise, we feel, that anyone should be aware of the sources of funding of the FDA. Although much of its budget comes from Congress, since the 1992 passage of **PDUFA (Prescription Drug User Fees Act renewed in 1997, 2002, and 2007)**, which requires drug companies to pay fees to support the drug review process and "companies [to] pay annual fees for each manufacturing establishment and for each prescription drug product marketed," user fees have steadily risen, until in 1992, 51 percent of the FDA's drug review budget came from the companies that the FDA regulates. Between 1996 and 2006, Congressional appropriations to the FDA stayed the same whereas from 1998 to 2005, user fees doubled. In 2004, the $232 million in fees made up 53 percent of the FDA's new drug review budget. In 2006, $380 million came from drug user fees.[3]

> PDUFA authorized FDA to collect fees from companies that produce certain human drug and biological products. Any time a company wants the FDA to approve a new drug or biologic prior to marketing, it must submit an application along with a fee to support the review process. In addition, companies pay annual fees for each manufacturing establishment and for each prescription drug product marketed. Previously, taxpayers alone paid for product reviews through budgets provided by Congress. In the new program, industry provides the funding in exchange for FDA agreement to meet drug-review performance goals, which emphasize timeliness.

In addition to the business funding of FDA, since 1992, Congressional oversight has been sharply curtailed.[4–6]

PDUFA was due to expire in 2007 but was reauthorized by Congress and signed by President Bush on September 27, 2007. User fees to the FDA will rise to $392.8 million, an increase of $87.4 million, by 2008.[7] However, Sean Hennessy and Brian Strom point out in the *New England Journal of Medicine*, "PDUFA Reauthorization—Drug Safety's Golden Moment of Opportunity?" that, "A potentially thorny issue is that the large infusion of cash represented by user fees . . . might result in a conflict of interest for the FDA by creating competing allegiances to pharmaceutical manufacturers and the American People."

The FDA has many advisory panels. Some of their members have financial ties to the drug industry, and the FDA usually follows a panel's recommendations. A study by Public Citizen (a consumer advocacy group) reported in an article by Peter Lurie, et al., in *JAMA*, found that this "did not dramatically sway . . . outcomes." However, both Public Interest and some members of Congress are attempting to eliminate conflicts of interest. Representative Maurice Hinchey (D-NY) stated that "allowing individuals with conflicts of interest to serve on advisory panels endangers the . . . American people . . . [because] pure objectivity is lost." Public Citizen could only study the members who reported conflicts of interest. According to Peter Lurie, ". . . these people . . . are honorable . . ., they would not allow themselves to be influenced. It's the unconscious we need to be afraid of."[8] The Center for Science in the Public Interest points to some FDA actions (or failures to act) including: (i) allowing five companies to market a laser treatment for smoking cessation, which has not been approved by the FDA and (ii) allowing drinks containing nicotine back on the market.[9]

UNCERTIFIED MEDICINES

In June 2006, the FDA released information on drugs that are being sold without FDA review. According to Steven Galson, director of the FDA's Center for Drug Evaluation and Research: "We consider it a significant and serious drug safety issue . . . since these products may pose a risk to consumers." These products include both prescription and over-the-counter drugs. Although these drugs make up less than 2 percent of the market, they include "several thousand prescription medicines including cough remedies, painkillers and sedatives." Most doctors and pharmacists are not aware of this.[10]

Other problems exist besides uncertified medicines. According to the World Health Organization, there is a worldwide epidemic of fake drugs. Fake malaria medicines, tuberculosis and AIDS drugs, and meningitis vaccines are among the most common counterfeits. This epidemic has caused up to 200,000 deaths per year. It could also cause the development of drug-resistant strains of these diseases and others. These new strains could be spread and cause an epidemic or pandemic. Some have gone so far as to call selling fake drugs murder. At the present time, China is thought to be the biggest source for these drugs. People also buy fake drugs over the Internet. There is no effective regulation.[11]

BIOTECHNOLOGY AND THE HUMAN GENOME PROJECT

Rational Drug Design

The technical details of drug design are beyond the scope of this text. However, computers are being used to help design and test new drugs. Genetic tests can be used to determine an individual's response to a specific medication. At St. Jude Hospital in Memphis, children with leukemia are being genetically tested so that medication can be tailored to each patient. This procedure is not covered by medical insurers, and pharmaceutical companies are not interested in manufacturing tailor-made medications.[12] In 2006, computer-aided drug design was being used to help combat human immunodeficiency virus (HIV)/acquired immunodeficiency syndrome (AIDS), tuberculosis, malaria, and hepatitis C.[13] **Biotechnology** sees the human body as a collection of molecules and seeks to understand and treat disease in terms of these molecules. It attempts to identify the molecule causing a problem and then create another to correct it. Specific drugs are aimed at inhibiting the work of specific disease-causing agents. In order to be effective, the drug needs to bind to its target molecule. It needs to fit, something like a key in a lock. To achieve an exact fit, the precise structure of the target must be mapped. Powerful computers allow scientists to create graphical models. Before the availability of computer technology, many drugs were discovered by accident or trial and error. One way of developing drugs with the help of computers is called **rational drug design**. Developing drugs by design requires mapping the structure and creating a three-dimensional graphical model of the target molecule. Because this involves a huge number of mathematical calculations, without computers the process took many years; after the calculations were completed, a wire model of the molecule had to be constructed. Now, supercomputers accurately do the calculations in a small fraction of the time, and graphical software produces the image on a computer screen. This is an example of the field of **scientific visualization**, which is defined by Donna Cox of the National Center for Supercomputing Applications as the process of graphically representing the results of numerical calculations. The model can be manipulated, rotated, and viewed from any angle. Specialized software is used to evaluate a drug's molecular structure, which can then be chemically synthesized. Of course, any compound developed this way still has to be tested in a *real* biological system. The modeling of the target molecule and development of the drug can be repeated several times until a chemical compound is found that satisfactorily inhibits or stimulates the activity of the target site's receptors. Drugs, which are used for Alzheimer's, hypertension, and AIDS, have been developed with the help of computers.

Bioinformatics

The application of information technology to biology is called **bioinformatics**. Although this may be an oversimplification, the field of bioinformatics seeks to organize biological data into databases. The information is then available to researchers who can search through existing data and add new entries of their own. The **Human Genome Project (HGP)** has contributed to making databases of biological information.

The Human Genome Project

The development of new medications is becoming more dependent on knowledge of genes. The HGP, sponsored in the United States by the National Institutes of Health and the Department of Energy, began in 1990 and involved hundreds of scientists all over the world. It was "an . . . effort to understand the hereditary instructions that make each of us unique. The goal is to find the location of the 100,000 or so human genes and to read the entire genetic script, all three billion bits of information, by the year 2005." The project has succeeded in mapping the human genome. One of its goals is an attempt to understand the molecular bases of genetic diseases. This project would be inconceivable without computers and the Internet. Computers are used to keep track of the genes as they are identified; this prevents duplication of effort and ensures that no genes are overlooked. The Internet allows findings to be immediately communicated to scientists working on the project anywhere in the world. Three to four thousand diseases are caused by errors in genes.

Altered genes also contribute to the development of other disorders such as cancer, heart disease, and diabetes. The HGP expects to be able to identify such genes, which might make prevention, early detection, and treatment possible. Once the gene is identified, drugs can be designed. Treatment may include gene therapy to replace the defective gene or the development of drugs. Ultimately, gene therapy may be tailored to specific patients. In 2006, the gene (Runx1) identified with chronic pain was found. It transmits external stimuli to the spinal cord. The finding could lead to the design of more effective pain therapies.[14] The identification of a disease-related gene is simply a starting point for research. For example, one of the genes related to stroke was identified in 2003, but according to Dr. Jonathan Rosand, a stroke specialist at Massachusetts General Hospital, it "is unlikely to yield new treatments any time soon."[15]

In July 2006, scientists made a major breakthrough in understanding the genetic makeup of the *Wolbachia* bacteria that infect mosquitoes and other insects that spread malaria.[16] In August 2006, researchers at the University of Pennsylvania "determined the structure of an important smallpox virus enzyme and how it binds to DNA." This is very important in the creation of a drug to fight smallpox.[17] In August 2006, the genes that increase the risk of heart attack were identified.[18] Hypertension-susceptibility genes were identified in February 2006.[19] It should be noted that although genetic predisposition is important, other factors (such as lifestyle and environment and the extent of public health measures) play a major role in the development of disease.

More than twenty-five million Americans suffer from rare and genetic diseases. The Genetic and Rare Diseases Information Center using information gathered by the HGP provides health care consumers with reliable, immediate, and free information. In one three-month period, the center received one thousand calls and e-mails asking for information.[20]

The HGP is the basis for new databases of biological information. Computers are being used to quickly screen tens of thousands of compounds a day, databases of genes, to find codes that could be useful in drug development. Then a model can be constructed and a drug rationally designed. It is a new form of trial and error, accelerated by computers, producing enormous amounts of information for researchers and computers to analyze.

Developments in Biotechnology

Understanding the molecular basis of a disease can lead to medical advances. In September 1998, the U.S. FDA approved Herceptin as effective against certain types of metastatic breast cancer. Herceptin can work for patients who have too much of a specific gene in their tumor cells. The gene (HER-2/neu) produces a protein that engenders growth in the tumor cells. Herceptin binds to this protein and inhibits its work. According to Dr. Dennis Slamon who directed the research, the development of Herceptin "proves . . . that if we understand what is broken in the malignant cell, we may be able to fix it." Herceptin may also be effective in fighting other cancers including gastric, endometrial, pancreatic, prostate, and colorectal cancers. Many other drugs are in the testing stages.

Lucentis was approved in June 2006 for the treatment of wet macular degeneration. Lucentis is an antibody that binds to a protein that is involved in the formation of blood vessels. In an early study, it was found that patients given Lucentis on the average either maintained or gained vision, whereas the patients who did not take Lucentis, but received traditional treatments, experienced an average loss of vision.

In February 2004, the FDA approved Avastin, an antibody that inhibits the protein that plays a role in the maintenance and metastases of tumors. The protein, called vascular endothelial growth factor (VEGF), helps in the creation of new blood vessels for the tumor. The protein is active in cancers including metastatic, colorectal, kidney, breast, and nonsmall lung cancers. The most extensive trials have been with patients with metastatic colorectal cancer. However, Avastin is also being tested on more than twenty different kinds of tumors.

In November 2004, the FDA approved the use of Tarceva against lung cancer; the following year, Tarceva was approved for use against pancreatic cancer in combination with another drug. It targets a growth pathway in the cell and inhibits its activity, thus slowing or stopping the growth of the tumor in some patients.

In 2003, the FDA approved the use of Xolair as a treatment for asthma. Xolair binds to immunoglobulin E (IgE) antibodies in the blood, which may trigger asthmatic symptoms. This decreases the release of chemicals that lead to the symptoms.

In 2005, several new drugs were approved including:

Arranon	To treat patients with certain cancers
Boostrixa	Booster against tetanus, diphtheria, and pertussis
Byetta	To treat Type II diabetes
Fluarix	A flu vaccine for adults
Fortical nasal spray	For osteoparosis

Source: Approved Biotechnology Drugs (http://www.bio.org/speeches/pubs/er/approveddrugs.asp).

The following drugs have been approved as of 2006:

Amitiza	For the treatment of chronic idiopathic constipation
Dacogen	For the treatment of myelodysplastic syndromes, formerly known as preleukemia
Eraxis	For the treatment of *Candida* fungal infections
Gardasil	For the prevention of cervical cancer caused by the human papillomavirus

Source: Approved Biotechnology Drugs (http://www.bio.org/speeches/pubs/er/approveddrugs.asp).

Antisense technology is one experimental technology used to develop drugs to shut off disease-causing genes. Genasense developed through antisense technology promises to enhance chemotherapy in cancer patients by shutting off the gene producing Bcl-2, which helps cells stay alive. It is given before chemotherapy, radiation, and other cancer treatments to kill cells. Antisense technology is being used to develop treatments for breast cancer and Crohn's disease.[21]

Another new technology aimed at drug development is called **RNA interference** or **RNAi**. RNAi is a natural process for gene silencing. RNA stands for

ribonucleic acid. It is made in the nucleus of a cell but is not restricted to the nucleus. It is a long coiled up molecule whose purpose is to take the blueprint from **deoxyribonucleic acid (DNA)** and build our actual proteins. (DNA is a nucleic acid molecule containing genetic instructions for living things.) RNAi is a process that cells use to turn off genes. The attempt at developing drugs based on RNAi holds the promise of revolutionizing biotechnology.[22] In 2006, RNAi was used to shut off the effects of estrogen in "a specific part of the mouse brain," changing the behavior of the mouse. In another experiment attempting to cure hepatitis B, most of the mice died of liver poisoning. This could introduce a note of caution into the testing of RNAi on humans. This means that although RNAi may be used to help map out genes and neural networks, extreme care should be taken.[23,24]

In 2006, scientists at the University of Illinois "created a synthetic molecule which caused cancer cells to self-destruct." It may lead to new treatments for some cancer patients. However, it has not yet been tested for safety and effectiveness.[25]

Stem cells are cells that can develop into different types of body cells; theoretically, they can repair the body. As a stem cell divides, the new cells can stay a stem cell or become another kind of cell.[26] It is possible that stem cell research may lead to regenerative or rehabilitative medicine. Stem cells are special in a number of ways:

> First, they are unspecialized cells that renew themselves for long periods through cell division. The second is that under certain physiologic or experimental conditions, they can be induced to become cells with special functions such as the beating cells of the heart muscle or the insulin-producing cells of the pancreas.[27]

Many scientists feel that stem cell research may hold the possibility of future cures, preventions, and therapies.[28] In November 2006, scientists succeeded in growing heart valves "using stem cells from the fluid that cushions babies in the womb." These valves might one day be used for babies born with heart defects.[29]

COMPUTER-ASSISTED DRUG TRIALS

Before a drug can be marketed, it has to undergo extensive clinical trials. Some last as long as six years and cost over $100 million. Now, however, software has been developed that allows companies to simulate clinical trials on a computer before the actual trials begin. A simulated drug trial uses information about the drug's effects from earlier trials, animal studies, or trials of similar drugs. By trying out many "what ifs" on computer models, the actual trials can be more precisely designed, making it more likely that they will be definitive. Critics maintain that the models are not precise enough because knowledge of the human body is incomplete. The **Physiome Project** is an international project seeking to create mathematical models of human organs—"digital models of every system and anatomical feature of the human body." It has created a virtual heart using mathematical equations to simulate the processes of the heart. It has been used in studies of irregular heartbeats. A draft of the lungs and skeletal system has been finished. The project is currently working on the digestive system and a database of cellular functions. In the future, the project hopes to model the nervous, endocrine, immune, sensory, skin, kidney–urinary, and reproductive systems. Utilizing these mathematical models, the project hopes to find treatments for conditions such as arthritis and other autoimmune disorders. These mathematical models will not only allow the testing of drugs, but "also enable medical engineers to fashion customized implants . . ." and surgeons to perform "dry runs" of surgeries. The use of these models is still far from reality. Computer-assisted drug trials are not a replacement for actual clinical trials; they are a tool to make the trials more effective.[30] In 2006, the FDA requested that drugs submitted for clinical trials include computer simulations.[31] The purpose of **computer-assisted trial design (CATD)** is to decrease the time and money spent on the trial phase of drug development.

COMPUTER-ASSISTED DRUG REVIEW

After a new drug has been developed, the FDA reviews it. In 1995, the FDA began computerizing the drug review and approval process. This enables them to speed up the process by reviewing data online. According to the *FDA Consumer*, what used to take weeks can now be done in an instant. With FDA computers networked to a drug company's computer, data from clinical trials can be transferred instantly and reviewed more quickly than in the past. It is also easier to do comparisons with other drugs and spot possible problems. According to Roger Williams, associate director of the FDA's Center for Drug Evaluation, the drug review process makes use of giant electronic spreadsheets of perhaps 300 million cells for each review area for each drug. Computers make it possible to organize this massive amount of data.

THE COMPUTERIZED PHARMACY

Computers were introduced in pharmacies more than twenty-five years ago. Initially, drug orders in hospitals could be entered into a computer. The computer system checked for adverse drug interactions and specific patient drug allergies. Today, computers can maintain complete medication profiles of all patients on databases and warn of drug interactions and allergies. This use of the database not only protects patients, but also makes information more easily available for national and international drug studies.

Computers and Drug Errors

Computerizing any aspect of prescription entry, the filling of orders, and dispensing of medications appears to lead to a decrease in medication errors. Today, 61 percent of medication errors in hospitals are caused by transcription errors and illegible handwriting. **Computerized physician order entry system** (CPOE) can lower prescription errors by 66 percent.[32] Currently, computers are utilized in both hospital pharmacies and community drug stores. In any corner drug store, computers provide drug information for patients. According to *Quality Review—a Journal of the USP Practitioners*

Reporting Network, by 1995, almost all pharmacies in the United States used computers to process prescriptions. Although the use of computers makes filling prescriptions faster and easier, and streamlines record-keeping, computers have also been the source of some errors. The errors can be caused by incorrect data entry, an incorrect choice from a computer list, or software error. Incorrect entry of a prescription or an incorrect choice from a list of medications is a human error which can happen whether or not computers are used. However, some errors stem directly from software. In one case, the programmer had used the same abbreviation (DOX100) to designate two different drugs. The incorrect medication lengthened one patient's hospital stay. Another program automatically printed "teaspoonful" when a liquid medication dose did not have a measure entered. This led to an infant being given an overdose of albuterol syrup. Other errors have occurred when software interpreted 1–2 (one to two) as ½.

However, errors in software can be corrected. Generally, all drug errors decline when computers are introduced. Recently, a study was done comparing drug errors before and after the introduction of a computerized physician order entry system in a large hospital. The study looked at errors in drug ordering, administration, and dispensing. Simply introducing a computerized order system cut errors at all three stages. Total errors fell by 55 percent. Errors in ordering fell by 19 percent, in transcription 84 percent, in dispensing 68 percent, and in administering 59 percent. When a menu-driven system was used, dosing errors decreased by 23 percent and allergy errors 56 percent. Another study compared adverse drug events (ADEs) in a 726-bed hospital before and after the introduction of computerized drug ordering. It found 126 errors in the first phase of the study—which had not been caught—and caught 134 errors in the second phase of the study. From the first to the second phase of the study, transcription errors fell to five (84 percent).[33] The reduction in errors is partly due to making orders legible. Second, the computer checks dosage to make sure it is appropriate. It also checks for each patient's drug allergies and any possible drug interaction.

In a study published in the *American Journal of Health-System Pharmacy* in 2006, seven thousand medical errors caused by CPOE were analyzed. Dosing errors were most common. The study traced most errors to "faulty computer interface, miscommunication with other systems, and lack of adequate decision support."[34]

Computer warning systems can be used to prevent ADEs. Serious ADEs occur in about 7 percent of patients admitted to hospitals. Many of these are caused by a physician prescribing either the wrong drug or the wrong dosage, because of lack of knowledge of either the patient or the drug. In 1994, a computerized warning system was designed and put into place in one hospital. The hospital already had in place a database with patient information; the existing system warned of a patient's specific drug allergy and of adverse drug interactions. The new alert system added warnings of other likely ADEs. The warnings were printed out for the pharmacist, who could alert the prescribing physician if he or she believed it was necessary. Physicians reported that the computer-generated alerts made them aware of the potential danger in 44 percent of alerts. "The order changes in these patients were directly attributable to alert notification."[35]

According to the 1999 government report, "To Err is Human," between 44,000 and 98,000 people die in U.S. hospitals each year as a result of medical errors. Seven thousand people die from medication errors both in and out of the hospital. Among the changes the report recommends to reduce medication errors is to "require that all hospitals and health care organizations *implement proven safety practices, such as the use of automated drug ordering systems*" (emphasis added).[36] Four years after the release of the report, one of its authors states, "We've seen pockets of dramatic improvement. Some of the hospitals . . . have had 10-fold reductions in ADEs. But overall, we're a long way from the goal."[37] In 2003, one doctor estimated that 16 percent of physicians scribble illegible prescriptions.[38] The Florida legislature even passed a bill in the spring of 2003 ordering doctors to improve their handwriting.[39]

A Harvard-led study conducted in 2002 and 2003 surveyed several hundred patients in each of the following countries: the United States, Canada, the United Kingdom, Australia, and New Zealand. Twenty-five percent of the people reported that they had experienced either a medical mistake or an error in prescribing. The number of errors grows as the number of doctors seen rises.[40] Several reports in 2003 stressed that the use of computers to write prescriptions and check for errors in dosage is crucial in reducing ADEs. Handheld computers provide immediate access to drug databases and other information. They also make prescriptions legible.

In July 2006, "Preventing Medical Errors" stressed that medication errors are still a serious problem, harming 1.5 million people per year. Several thousand die each year. With the aging population, more medications are prescribed and more errors are made. Like the 1999 Report, "To Err is Human . . .," the 2006 report recommends the use of e-prescribing and electronic health records.[41] One report (October 2006) pointed to the 700,000 Americans who show up in emergency rooms with overdoses or allergic reactions to common prescription drugs including insulin, warfarin, and amoxicillin.[42] Whatever the cause of the error, many doctors would not inform the patient. With an error that the patient was unlikely to notice, 50 percent would tell the patient. Surgeons disclosed errors less frequently.[43]

The Automated Community Pharmacy

Although not yet in common use, fully automated pharmacy systems that can fill prescriptions do exist for community drug stores (Figures 8.1a–f ■). Currently, the use of these systems is expanding with the successful use of robotic systems in Veterans' Administration (VA) pharmacies and hospitals. A fully automated dispensing system involves the employment of a robot. In one such system, a prescription is entered into the pharmacy computer; the pharmacy computer, in turn, activates the pharmacy robot, which first determines what size vial is needed for the prescription—from the three available sizes. A robotic arm grips the correct size. One system has two hundred cells, each containing a different drug. The arm is moved to the correct cell; the tablets or capsules are counted by a sensor and dropped into the vial. The computer prints a label and puts it on the vial, which is delivered via a conveyer belt to the pharmacist. The pharmacist uses a barcode reader to scan the barcode on the label; images of the medication and prescription information appear on the screen. The pharmacist puts the lid on and gives the customer the prescription. One robotic system can fill sixty prescriptions in an hour. Other robotic systems can fill prescriptions for liquid medications as well as tablets and capsules.

Although 49 percent of chain pharmacies used at least two computerized devices, such as barcode scanners or tablet/capsule-counting devices, only 15 percent of independent pharmacies did. Many more chains than independents have

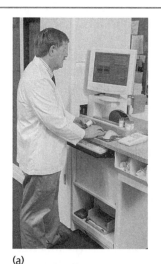

(a)

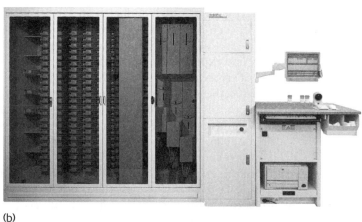

(b)

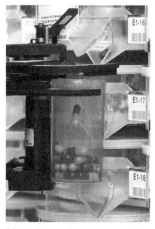

(c)

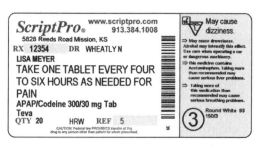

(d)

any computerized devices. Computerization has been hailed as the cure for drug errors. Yet, partly as a result of the increase in new drugs, drug–drug interactions (DDIs) are increasing. A unified computerized system is needed that is linked to databases of DDIs to effectively diminish medication errors. However, some pharmacists feel they are being bombarded with meaningless alerts. It is however possible to design a system which distinguishes between critical and noncritical alerts.[44,45]

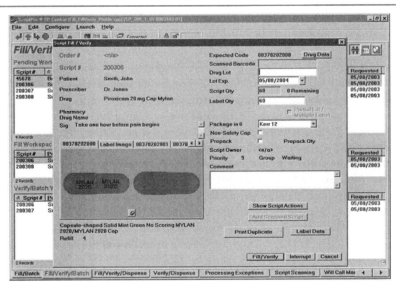

(e)

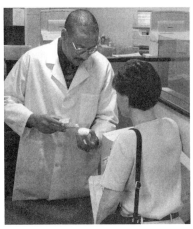

(f)

■ **FIGURE 8.1** ScriptPro SP 200 Robotic Prescription Dispensing System. The ScriptPro fully automated prescription dispensing process begins by (a) entering the prescription into the existing pharmacy computer system. (b) Via the interface, the pharmacy computer sends the fill command to the SP 200. (c) The SP 200 robotic arm then selects a standard vial from one of three vial dispensers in the system. The vial is automatically transported to the correct drug cell, the cell barcode is scanned and the robotic arm engages the cell. The medication is dispensed and counted directly into the vial. The filled vial is automatically delivered to the ScriptPro print/apply labeling unit. At this point, the standard prescription information, (d) barcode and USP auxiliary labels are printed and applied directly to the filled vial. The filled and labeled vial is then delivered on the conveyor to the pharmacist. The pharmacist scans the vial barcode and (e) verifies the prescription with an on-screen image of the medication and script information. (f) The pharmacist then delivers the prescription to the patient, and completes the prescription filling process. Courtesy of ScriptPro.

Automating the Hospital Pharmacy

Hospitals are automating drug distribution systems. An automated hospital pharmacy presupposes the use of barcodes to identify drugs; it involves the use of robots in the hospital pharmacy to fill medication orders, and/or the use of point-of-use dispensing units. A fully automated system may cost as much as $10 million and take several years to install.[46] Drugs are also being administered to patients by computerized infusion pumps. Automated dispensing systems can be centralized or decentralized. In a centralized system, robots are used in the hospital pharmacy to fill prescriptions. In a decentralized point-of-use dispensing system, drug cabinets, similar to ATM machines, are located throughout the hospital. Some hospitals use both robotics and automated point-of-use dispensing.

The Hospital Pharmacy—Robots and Barcodes

In a hospital pharmacy system using a pharmacy robot, medication orders are either faxed to the pharmacy and the information entered into the computer system or entered at a terminal connected with the pharmacy computer. In 2006, only 15 percent of hospitals used a robotic system, up from 4.5 percent in 1999.[47] The information includes the name of the patient, his or her medication, and the dose. **Barcodes** identify each dose of medication, and each dose is kept in a bag. (Any medication that is not identified by a barcode has to be dispensed by hand.) Each patient has a bin into which the robot drops his or her medication. If a barcode is unclear, the robot rejects the dose. The dosages are checked by technicians. In eight hours, one robot can do as much work as six or seven human technicians. The robot, its software, and five years of maintenance are extremely expensive. Hospital administrators maintain that a robot still costs less than hiring six or seven human technicians for eight hours. Hospital managers, like managers in other businesses, see automation as a way to reduce costs, that is, staff, while maintaining service.

Each patient's medications are delivered to the nursing unit on a tray. As an added check on the accuracy of the computer, the barcodes on the patient's wristband and on the medication can be scanned. Dispensing errors are eliminated by using robots in the pharmacy. However, dispensing errors account for only 6 percent of medication errors. More than half occur at the prescribing stage and another third at the distribution stage.

The use of barcodes to identify medications and link them to patients also means that the robot is not only dispensing medication, but also keeping track of inventory. Additionally, it can automatically provide credit for medications, which are not used, and electronically order drugs when the supply is low. The use of barcodes became mandatory in 2004.[48]

Point-of-Use Drug Dispensing

Some computerized hospital pharmacies are using point-of-use dispensing of drugs—a decentralized automated system. Adoption of this technology in healthcare started slowly with only about 50 percent of hospitals using automated dispensing cabinets (ADCs) in 1999; but by 2005, close to 72 percent of acute care facilities had implemented these units.[49] A small computer attached to a large cabinet sits at the nursing unit. It is networked to the hospital pharmacy computer. A nurse types a password, and the unit displays a list of patients. The nurse selects the patient and enters the drug order, and the computer delivers it by opening the drawer containing the medication. The nurse enters the name of the drug and closes the drawer. The computer keeps track of all drug transactions, for billing and inventory purposes. It "counts, dispenses and tracks medications within the hospital." It can generate a variety of reports on patients, drug usage, and nurses. In 2003, the first automated drug dispensing units located in patients' rooms were introduced. Doctors can use them to enter prescriptions. The bedside system will scan the nurse's badge, the patient's wristband, and the medication's barcode. It is linked to databases of information that will help avoid medication errors. It can also keep track of inventory.

Point-of-use dispensing has several advantages over traditional manual dispensing. It shortens the time between the order for a medication and its delivery to the patient. One study found that the waiting time for a first dose of medication went from forty-five minutes to one minute! Automating drug distribution improves patient care in other ways too. Drugs are more likely to be administered on schedule, and significantly fewer doses are missed. Although apparently not reducing dispensing errors to zero like centralized robotic systems claim to do, one study found that a decentralized system decreased dispensing errors by almost one-third. However, many studies disagree on the efficacy of point-of-use dispensing in reducing medical errors.[50]

Decentralized computerized drug delivery has a positive financial impact for the hospital, making it more likely that patients are charged for the medications used. It also decreases the time nurses spend on medication-related activities, such as counting controlled substances, charting, documentation, and billing; a survey of nurses in a surgery unit that had introduced decentralized dispensing found that 80 percent wanted to keep the new system. It also decreased the time that pharmacists spend on problem resolution. Automation (although requiring an initial investment) can save a hospital as much as $1 million over five years in personnel timesavings. About one hundred thousand hospitals are using this system nationwide (2002).

Point-of-use dispensing is also being introduced in clinics and doctors' offices. An automated drug-dispensing unit (something like a vending machine) contains approximately 90 percent of routinely prescribed drugs. A prescription can be entered by a doctor (with a password) and the medication automatically dispensed. However, there are states in which a doctor is not allowed to give a patient prescription drugs without a pharmacist present.

Computerized IVs and Barcodes

Included in the drug errors reported in "To Err is Human" were intravenous (IV) administration errors. In 2005, the "smart pump" was introduced. It "contains several important new safety features including a barcode reader that enables medication verification for IV drugs at the point of care and patient-controlled analgesia (PCA)."[51] Two new safety technologies being introduced in 2006 are barcode medication administration (BCMA) and smart infusion systems with dose error reduction systems (DERS). BCMA uses barcodes to identify each patient and each medication, and according to clinical studies, it might prevent up to 58 percent of

ADEs.[52] Integrating both systems involves barcoding infused medication. IV drugs tend to be higher risk drugs. IV drugs as well as oral drugs can be given to the wrong patient, in the wrong dose; the wrong medication can be given to a patient. The risk is far higher with IV drugs. "A nurse is unlikely to give a patient 10 or 100 pills, but all too easily can commit errors in programming a general-purpose infusion device—e.g., programming 603, instead of 6.3 mg/h—and inadvertently deliver a . . . massive overdose."[53] Using a built-in scanning device, this system links IV drug administration to an adverse drug alert monitor and sounds an alert if a mistake is made. The scanner identifies both the patient and the clinician. This system may avoid many IV medication errors.[54]

Radio Frequency Identification Tags

Radio frequency identification (RFID) tags include an antenna, a decoder to interpret data, and the tag which includes information. The antenna sends signals. When the tag detects the signal, it sends back information.[55] The tags can be used to keep track of anything including medications. Unlike barcodes, RFIDs do not have to be scanned by hand; RFID readers can be embedded anywhere and automatically read the RFID tag. RFID tags are the size of a grain of rice and can contain more information than a barcode.[56] In 2004, the FDA approved implanting RFID tags in people; these tags would include medical information.

▆▆▆ TELEPHARMACY

Telepharmacy involves using a computer, a network connection, and a drug-dispensing unit to allow patients to obtain drugs outside of a traditional pharmacy, at, for example, a doctor's office or a clinic. It should not be confused with the unregulated sale of prescriptions and drugs over the Internet. However, once a patient has a prescription in hand, more and more patients are willing to fill it online "to save time and money," although they did express concerns about safety.[57] Traditional telepharmacy, however, links prescribing physicians with pharmacists via telecommunications lines. It may refer simply to the faxing of prescriptions from the prescribing doctor to the pharmacy for later pickup and to the use of computers to check for adverse drug interaction. However, in a fully computerized telepharmacy system, the physician's and pharmacy's computers are directly linked, and the pharmacist remotely controls a drug cabinet at the physician's office. Once the pharmacist receives the prescription via a telecommunications link, a signal is sent to the remote drug cabinet to open a particular compartment. The dispensing cabinet (at the doctor's office) contains prepackaged drugs, each identified by a barcode. The software prints out a label and patient information and keeps track of inventory. A patient database includes the patient's age, allergies, drug use, diagnosis, and insurance provider. The software checks DDI, drug/allergy interaction, and dosage, and it checks for duplicate prescriptions. Before the patient receives the medication, its barcode is scanned to make sure it is the right drug. The pharmacist and patient could then hold a video teleconsultation. Telepharmacy allows one pharmacist to serve a whole region.

There are several built-in safety checks. The barcode must be correct or the computer will not print a label, and, therefore, the patient will not get the drug. The computer also examines patient allergies, dangerous drug interactions, appropriate dosage, and expiration date; it immediately notifies the prescribing physician if there is a problem. The physician can, however, override the computer's warning. The cabinet in which the drugs are stored is secure and has alarms to guard against theft.

Although not yet in general use, telepharmacy promises to be especially helpful in rural areas and underserved urban neighborhoods where there is no accessible local pharmacy. Using a telepharmacy connection can mean that the patient walks out of the doctor's office with the medication in hand, having already teleconsulted with the pharmacist; neither patient nor pharmacist has to travel. It could prove to be particularly beneficial to populations who cannot travel easily. The elderly, for example, have a poor drug compliance record—due in part to their difficulty traveling. There are several other advantages to telepharmacy. A telepharmacy does not need to fill as many prescriptions as a conventional pharmacy to be cost-effective. Entering prescriptions directly into a computer may cut down on dispensing errors caused by illegible handwriting. Handwritten signatures are no longer necessary. Since the July 2000 law, making the digital signature equivalent to the handwritten signature, the doctor can prescribe without faxes and paper signatures. Dispensing drugs at the doctor's office guarantees that the prescription is filled. Pharmaceutical counseling ensures that the patient understands how to take the medication.

Today, telepharmacy is slowly expanding in part because of a shortage of pharmacists. The expansion is also because of government interest in telepharmacy as a cost-saving device, largely because of the use of generic medications, but also reflecting the higher efficiency of the pharmacist. In 2002, the Department of Health and Human Services (HHS) funded a telepharmacy project designed to serve 13,500 low-income and rural patients. A pharmacist at the central location receives faxes of prescriptions and then sends a signal to a remote "vending machine" where a technician labels the bottle and gives it to the patient. There are five remote locations within a 100-mile radius.[58] The VA, the U.S. Department of Defense (DOD), and the Immigration and Naturalization Service (INS) are also testing telepharmacy systems.[59] The telepharmacy technology can link to the DOD's computerized medical system and can automatically add prescriptions to a medical record.

There are problems with telepharmacy that could slow its expansion. Pharmacy has traditionally been subject to state regulation. Each state has different pharmacy regulations. The National Association of Boards of Pharmacy has model telepharmacy regulations, but only some states have adopted them.

DRUG DELIVERY ON A CHIP

Some medications can currently be delivered on an implanted chip. This is the focus of a great deal of research. The drug is embedded in a chip, which is surgically implanted in the patient. The drug may be released by diffusion. It may be embedded in a biodegradable material that releases as it degrades. One drug, used to treat brain cancer, is a biodegradable implant placed directly on the site from which the tumor was removed. The newest chip to be announced (October 2003) can deliver several medications. It can also deliver specific doses at predetermined times. The chip is in the early stages of development. Medications are embedded in polymers (plastics) that have already been approved by the FDA for other uses in humans. Thus far, the chips have been tested only on animals. Some of its potential uses include delivering an entire course of medication over a period of months, delivering a series of vaccines at the correct time, delivering medication that needs to be taken continuously, including painkillers and medications for chronic conditions. This "pharmacy on a chip" is completely biodegradable. One advantage of using chips to deliver medication is that because they bypass the stomach, they avoid stomach upsets.[60]

In 2006, research continues on a chip that "uses wireless signaling and [a] system of reservoirs that allow precise, efficient delivery of solids, liquids, or gels." It is the size of a stamp, includes one hundred wells that can be filled with drugs, and will deliver substances that are very strong, but have limited stability. Wireless technology can be used to deliver information. It will deliver the correct dose at the correct time. The devices also contain biosensors to deliver information, and the biosensors can be linked to the drug delivery system. The system will not be in human safety trials for a number of years.[61]

THE IMPACT OF INFORMATION TECHNOLOGY ON PHARMACY

Information technology is having a great impact on the field of pharmacy—affecting doctors, patients, pharmacists, and hospital management in different ways. The increasing use of computers requires doctors and pharmacists to be computer literate. The impact of automation on pharmacists is overwhelming. In both the hospital pharmacy and community drug store, robots can do what a human pharmacist has always done, that is, fill prescriptions. This allows pharmacists to be more involved in consulting with patients and physicians. In at least one hospital using a pharmacy robot, pharmacists now accompany doctors on rounds. However, hospitals using robots require fewer pharmacists; managers see this staff reduction as a benefit. It saves money, while maintaining services. It is unlikely that many pharmacists share this view.

The impact on patients appears to be beneficial. The HGP holds the promise of understanding the basis of diseases with a genetic link. This, combined with rational drug design, may lead to the development of effective treatments and cures for many diseases. Automating drug dispensing in hospitals and drug stores has apparently reduced dispensing errors considerably.

Telepharmacy also affects patients, doctors, and pharmacists in different ways. Doctors can send a patient home with medication in hand, after teleconsulting with a pharmacist; patients do not need to travel long distances to fill prescriptions or to consult with a pharmacist. Pharmacists can serve a much wider geographic area, and yet do not need to fill as many prescriptions to stay in business. Pharmacists need to achieve a high degree of computer literacy and familiarity with telecommunications and networks to be involved in telepharmacy.

IN THE NEWS

Excerpt from, "Prevention: Computer Fails Its Drug Test"

by Nicholas Bakalar

According to a study published last week in Archives of Internal Medicine, a computer for hospital physicians reduces errors involving medicines, but it still fails to prevent a large number of "adverse drug events"—defined as overdoses, allergic reactions or other medication-caused problems.

Among 937 randomly selected admissions, researchers at the Salt Lake City Veterans Affairs Medical Center, researchers found 483 drug events that they considered clinically significant.

No evidence suggested that the computerized system was responsible for additional events, but the computer program offered no significant benefits in drug selection, dosage and monitoring, which were largely responsible for the side effects.

Dr. Jonathan R. Nebeker, a V.A. researcher and the lead author, said three-quarters of the adverse drug events were not due to medication error.

"We need to broaden our focus from errors alone," Dr. Nebeker said. "Where computers come in is to help physicians take into account the multiple factors that considered together will make the difference in whether a patient suffers a drug-related injury."

Dr. Steven Rappaport, who oversees computerized systems for the V.A., agrees. "There's a lot more information that a system could provide a doctor," he said. "What's the right dose? What's the right medicine? What's the right kind of lab test to order now that we've started a patient on this medicine?"

May 31, 2005. Copyright © 2005 by The New York Times Company. Reprinted by permission.

CHAPTER SUMMARY

This chapter introduced the reader to the impact of information technology on the field of pharmacy.

- In the United States, the FDA is the agency charged with overseeing the safety and efficacy of drugs and medical devices. Much of its budget comes from drug manufacturers.
- There are a myriad of uncertified medications (prescription and over-the-counter) on the market.

- Computer technology is making a contribution to rational drug design. Because computers can do billions of calculations and then graphically represent the results, it is possible to create graphical models of a target molecule, for which a drug can be specifically designed.
- Bioinformatics is the application of information technology to biology.
- The Human Genome Project is leading to an understanding of the molecular bases of diseases that have a genetic link. This knowledge has led to the development of drugs that are currently in the testing stages.
- Drug trials can be simulated using computers, so that actual trials take less time and cost less and are more likely to be successful.
- Information technology is changing the way pharmacies do business.
  - Computers are used in the corner drug store to provide information for customers and pharmacists. Some drug stores are fully computerized, with robots filling the prescriptions.
  - In hospitals, two computerized pharmacy systems exist (and may co-exist).
    - A centralized system uses robots in the hospital pharmacy to fill drug orders typed in on terminals. The drugs are identified by barcodes. Each patient's medications are then delivered to the unit.
    - In a decentralized point-of-use dispensing system, computers attached to cabinets sit in various places in the hospital. A nurse may enter a password and type in a medication order; the drawer with the medication opens and the nurse can remove it.
    - Both centralized and decentralized systems cut down on drug dispensing errors and on the amount of time personnel spend on medication-related activity.
    - Barcodes can be used to identify medications. RFID tags can also be used.
  - Telepharmacy involves the linking of a pharmacist with a remote drug cabinet in a doctor's office via telecommunications lines.
- Information technology is affecting doctors, patients, pharmacists, and administrators in different ways.

KEY TERMS

antisense technology
barcodes
bioinformatics
biotechnology
computer-assisted trial design (CATD)
computerized physician order entry system
deoxyribonucleic acid (DNA)

Food and Drug Administration (FDA)
Human Genome Project (HGP)
PDUFA (Prescription Drug User Fees Act renewed in 1997, 2002, and 2007)
Physiome Project

radio frequency identification (RFID) tags
rational drug design
ribonucleic acid
RNA interference or RNAi
scientific visualization
stem cells
telepharmacy

REVIEW EXERCISES

Multiple Choice

1. The creation of medications using computers to create a model of the target molecule and design a medication to inhibit or stimulate its work is called _____.
   A. biotechnology
   B. rational drug design
   C. visualization
   D. None of the above

2. The _____ is a project attempting to understand the genetic makeup of the human being.
   A. International Genome Project
   B. National Institute of Health Project
   C. Genetic Script
   D. Human Genome Project

3. A centralized computerized hospital pharmacy system involves the use of _____.
   A. barcodes to identify drugs
   B. robots
   C. A and B
   D. None of the above

4. Which of the following is true of decentralized point-of-use dispensing?
   A. It decreases the waiting time for the first dose of a drug
   B. It increases the likelihood that drugs are administered on schedule
   C. It decreases dispensing errors
   D. All of the above

5. The linking of a drug cabinet in a doctor's office with a pharmacist via telecommunications lines is called _____.
   A. telemedicine
   B. telepharmacy
   C. remote pharmacy
   D. robotic pharmacy

6. Information technology has made the Human Genome Project possible by _____.
   A. enabling scientists to keep track of genes as they are identified, and allowing findings to be immediately communicated via the Internet
   B. making pharmacy robots available internationally
   C. keeping track of new drugs as they enter clinical trials
   D. keeping records of the results of clinical drug trials

7. Telepharmacy raises certain legal problems associated with _____.
   A. the prescribing of drugs that are not FDA approved
   B. interstate licensing of pharmacists
   C. a doctor prescribing medications
   D. None of the above

8. The Human Genome Project may lead to _____.
   A. a more complete understanding of genetics
   B. more accurate predictions of who is likely to develop a disease with a genetic basis
   C. Both A and B
   D. None of the above
9. The use of computers to simulate drug trials _____.
   A. means that we do not need actual clinical trials
   B. means actual clinical trials are more likely to succeed
   C. helps save both time and money
   D. B and C
10. DNA provides a blueprint of genetic information. _____ helps create the proteins.
    A. Biotechnology
    B. RNA
    C. TNA
    D. None of the above

True/False Questions

1. Errors in software can lead to errors in filling prescriptions. _____
2. Understanding the genetic basis of a disease can lead to the development of an effective drug. _____
3. Hospital pharmacy robots can dispense any drug with a barcode. _____
4. Decentralized hospital dispensing units reduce dispensing errors to zero. _____
5. Telepharmacy allows one pharmacist to serve a large geographical area. _____
6. Automation of pharmacy may lead to unemployment among pharmacists. _____
7. Antisense technology attempts to treat cancer by turning off a gene that keeps cells alive. _____
8. Biotechnology sees the human body as a collection of molecules. _____
9. Computers have helped in the development of drugs used to treat AIDS. _____
10. Computer-assisted trial design means that real clinical trials are not needed. _____

Critical Thinking

1. Discuss the advantages and disadvantages of the introduction of computers in a local pharmacy
   (A) from the pharmacist's point-of-view.
   (B) from the customer's point-of-view.
2. As the administrator of a small hospital, discuss the advantages and disadvantages of introducing a centralized computerized hospital pharmacy system using robots.
3. Telepharmacy could prove to be a benefit to elderly patients who have difficulty traveling. However, privacy, security, and legal issues may have to be settled before telepharmacy becomes an established part of health care. Discuss this statement. Consider licensing issues and the lack of security of networked communications in your answer.

4. The same information could be used to deny individuals health insurance or life insurance. What measures would you take to ensure that this did not happen?

NOTES

1. "FDA Mission Statement," http://www.fda.gov (accessed November 21, 2007).
2. "Medical Journal Says It Was Misled Again," Associated Press, July12, 2006, http://www.nytimes.com/2006/07/13/health/13jama.html (accessed November 21, 2007).
3. Diedtra Henderson, "Drug Makers Lobby US to Hike FDA Funds," *The Boston Globe*, July 13, 2006, http://www.boston.com (accessed November 21, 2007).
4. Stanley M. Wolfe, "The 100th Anniversary of the FDA: The Sleeping Watchdog Whose Master is Increasingly the Regulated Industries (HRG Publication #1776), June 27, 2006, http://www.citizen.org (accessed November 21, 2007).
5. Gary W. Lawsen, "Impact of User Fees on Changes Within The Food and Drug Administration," 2005, http://fdastudy.com (accessed November 21, 2007).
6. Larry Thompson, "User Fees for Faster Drug Reviews Are they Helping of Hurting the Public Health?" 2000, http://www.fda.gov (accessed November 21, 2007).
7. "FDA Proposes New Measures to Strengthen Drug Safety under PDUFA Reauthorized User Fee Program," January 11, 2007, http://www.fda.gov (accessed November 21, 2007).
8. Diedtra Henderson, "Study Rebuts Conflict Fears Around FDA Financial Ties of Panels," *The Boston Globe*, April 26, 2006, http://www.mindfully.org (accessed November 21, 2007).
9. "FDA Fails to Protect Americans from Dangerous Drugs and Unsafe Food, Watchdog Groups Say: Agency Captured by Industries It Should be Regulating, According to Rep. Waxman, Public Citizen and CSPI," June 27, 2006, http://www.citizen.org (accessed November 21, 2007).
10. Robert Cohen, "Uncertified Medicines a 'Serious' Safety Issue," July 9, 2006, http://www.nj.com (accessed November 21, 2007).
11. Donald G. McNeil, Jr., "In the World of Life-Saving Drugs, a Growing Epidemic of Deadly Fakes," February 20, 2007, http://www.nytimes.com/ (accessed November 21, 2007).
12. Claudia Dreifus, "Saving Lives With Tailor-Made Medication," August 29, 2006, http://www.nytimes.com/ (accessed November 21, 2007).
13. "Computer-Aided Drug Design," 2006, http://www.medfarm.uu.se/ (December 20, 2007).
14. "Master Genetic Switch Found For Chronic Pain," January 27, 2006, http://www.sciencedaily.com/releases/2006/01/060126195756.htm (accessed December 20, 2007).
15. Nicholas Wade, "Scientists Discover First Gene Tied to Stroke," September 22, 2003, http://www.nytimes.com/ (accessed November 21, 2007).
16. "Gene Breakthrough Heralds Better Prospect For Malaria Solution," July 25, 2006, http://www.sciencedaily.com/releases/2006/07/060725084640.htm (accessed December 20, 2007).
17. "Penn Researchers Determine Structure of Smallpox Virus Protein Bound to DNA," University of Pennsylvania School of Medicine, August 7, 2006, http://www.sciencedaily.com/releases/2006/08/060805131526.htm (accessed December 20, 2007).
18. Robert Langreth, "The Suggestive Gene," August 14, 2006, http://www.forbes.com (accessed November 21, 2007).
19. Binder, A, "Identification of Genes for Complex Trait: Examples from Hypertension," *Current Pharmaceutical Biotechnology* 7, no. 1 (February 2006): 1–13.
20. "Center to Offer Quick, Reliable Source for Genetic Information," National Genome Research Institute, http://genome.gov (accessed November 21, 2007).
21. CenterWatch Clinical Trials Listing Service, 2006, http://www.centerwatch.com (accessed November 21, 2007).

22. "Which Diseases Will RNAi Drugs be Used to Treat and What Barriers Will RNAi Drugs Need to Overcome," July 25, 2006, http://genengnews.com (accessed November 21, 2007).

23. Charles Choi, "RNAi: A New Targeted Silencer?" June 27, 2006, http://the-scientist.com (accessed November 21, 2007).

24. Andrew Pollack, "Mice Deaths are Setback in Gene Tests," May 25, 2006, http://www.nytimes.com/ (accessed November 21, 2007).

25. "Cancer Cell 'Executioner' Found," BBC news, August 27, 2006, http://www.bbc.co.uk (accessed November 21, 2007).

26. "Stem Cell Basics," August 12, 2005, http://www.nih.gov (accessed November 21, 2007).

27. "Stem Cell Information," August 12, 2005, http://www.nih.gov (accessed November 21, 2007).

28. "Stem Cell Research," February 2006, http://www.newsbatch.com (accessed November 21, 2007).

29. "Stem Cell Experiment Yields Heart Valves," Associated Press, November 18, 2006, http://www.nytimes.com/ (accessed November 21, 2007).

30. Michael Behar, "The Doctor Will See Your Prototype Now: How Super-Accurate Sims Can Test the Effects of Drugs on Patients," February 2005, http://www.wired.com/wired/archive/13.02/start.html?pg=9?tw=wn_tophead_4 (accessed December 20, 2007).

31. Andrew Pullan, Nicolas Smith, and Peter Hunter, "Creating the Virtual Human," Health Care and Informatics Review ONLINE, 2006, http://hcro.enigma.co.nz (accessed November 21, 2007).

32. "Computerized Doctors' Orders Reduce Medication Errors," June 27, 2007, http://www.sciencedaily.com/releases/2007/06/070627084702.htm (accessed December 20, 2007).

33. "Study: Computers Cut Mistakes in Doctors' Prescriptions," October 20, 1998, http://www.cnn.com/HEALTH/9810/20/drug.errors.ap./index.html (accessed December 3, 2007).

34. Chunliu Zhan, Rodney Hicks, Christopher Blanchette, et al., "Computerized Prescribing may Reduce Some Harmful Errors, but can Introduce New Errors" [abstract], July 2006, http://ahcpr.gov (accessed November 21, 2007).

35. Robert A. Raschke, MD, MS, Bea Gollihare, MS, RN, Thomas A. Wunderlich, RPh, et al., "A Computer Alert System to Prevent Injury from Adverse Drug Events Development and Evaluation in a Community Teaching Hospital," *JAMA* 280 (1998): 1317–20, http://jama.ama-assn.org/cgi/content/full/15/1317 (accessed February 2, 2008).

36. William C. Richardson, "To Err is Human: Building a Safer Health System," December 1, 1999, http://www8.nationalacademies.org/onpinews/newsitem.aspx?RecordID=9728 (accessed December 20, 2007).

37. Alan Jehlen, "Preventing Medical Errors," *American Teacher*, May/June 2003, http://aft.org (accessed November 21, 2007).

38. Bonnie Darves, "Seven Simple Steps to Prevent Outpatient Drug Errors," *American College of Physicians Observer*, June 2003, http://www.acponline.org/cgi-bin/htsearch (accessed November 21, 2007).

39. John Dorschner, "Study Finds Healthcare Error Prone," May 6, 2003, http://www.vaccinationnews.com/DailyNews/2003/May/06/StudyFinds6.htm (accessed December 3, 2007).

40. John Dorchner, "Study finds healthcare error prone," www.brevardlawyer.com/errorprone.htm (May 6, 2003; August 16, 2006).

41. Gardiner Harris, "Report Finds a Heavy Toll From Medication Errors," July 21, 2006, http://www.nytimes.com/ (accessed November 21, 2007).

42. "Study Finds a Widespread Risk of Reactions to Some Medicines," October 18, 2006, http://www.nytimes.com/ (accessed November 21, 2007).

43. Nicholas Bakalar, "Medical Errors? Patients May Be the Last to Know," August 29, 2006, http://www.nytimes.com/ (accessed November 21, 2007).

44. Nidhi Shah, Andrew C. Seger, and Diane L. Seger, "Computerized Prescribing Alerts can be Designed to be Widely Accepted by Primary" [abstract], May 2006, http://ahcpr.gov (accessed November 21, 2007).

45. Pharmaceutical Research, "National Survey of Community Pharmacies Examines Workload, Available Technology, and Perceptions of Drug Alert Systems," 2006, http://www.ahrq.gov/research/jun06/0606RA2.htm (accessed December 3, 2007).

46. Margie Manning, "Computers to Replace Docs' Scribbles at Barnes-Jewish: $10 Million System will Place Orders for Drugs, Tests; Should be in Place Within Three Years," March 4, 2002, web.uvic.ca/~h351/online_articles.htm (accessed November 21, 2007).

47. Rebecca Logan, "Hospitals Turn to Robots, Bar Codes to Organize Pharmacies," March 3, 2006, http://www.bizjournals.com (accessed November 21, 2007).

48. "Hospitals Turn to Robots, Bar Codes to Organize Pharmacies," June 3, 2006, http://www.bizjournals.com (accessed November 21, 2007).

49. "Guidelines for Safe Use of Automated Dispensing Cabinets," draft document, posted October 16, 2007, Institute for Safe Medicine Practices, http://www.ismp.org/Tools/guidelines/labelFormats/comments/default.asp (accessed February 2, 2008).

50. Michael D. Murray, Pharm.D., M.P.H., "Automated Medication Dispensing Devices," Chapter 11 in *Making Health Care Safer: A Critical Analysis of Patient Safety Practices*, prepared for the Agency for Healthcare Research and Quality, contract no. 290-97-0013, 2001, http://www.ahrq.gov/clinic/ptsafety (accessed February 2, 2008).

51. "Cardinal Health Launches First 'Smart Pump' System to Feature New Bar Code Reader For Safer IV Medication Administration," October 31, 2005, http://www.cardinal.com/content/news/10312005_65252.asp (accessed November 21, 2007).

52. Bryan Houlston, "Integrating RFID Technology into a Drug Administration System, Healthcare and Informatics Review Online," December 1, 2005, http://hcro.enigma.co.nz (accessed November 21, 2007).

53. Tim Vanderveen, "IVs First: A New Barcode Implementation Strategy, Patient Safety and Quality Healthcare," May/June 2006, http://psch.com (accessed November 21, 2007).

54. Harris, "Report Finds a Heavy Toll from Medication Errors."

55. "How RFID Works," http://technovelgy.com (accessed November 21, 2007).

56. "RFIDs: The Pros and Cons Every Consumer Needs to Know About Radio Frequency Tags," June 4, 2005, http://sixwise.com (accessed November 21, 2007).

57. Shelley Freierman, "Most Wanted: Drilling Down/Online Pharmacies; And No Doctor's Scribble," April 11, 2005, http://www.nytimes.com/ (accessed November 21, 2007).

58. Ukens Carol, "Pharmacy Shortage Boosts Telepharmacy," June 3, 2002, http://www.drugtopics.com/drugtopics/Miscellaneous/Pharmacist-shortage-boosts-telepharmacy/ArticleStandard/Article/detail/116637 (accessed December 20, 2007).

59. Ibid.

60. Steve Mitchell, "Scientists Create 'Pharmacy in a Chip'," October 19, 2003, http://web.uvic.ca (accessed November 21, 2007).

61. Special Report: Emerging Technologies, "Implanted Chips That Deliver Your Drugs," June 18, 2002, http://www.businessweek.com/technology/content/jun2002/tc20020618_5119.htm (accessed December 3, 2007).

ADDITIONAL RESOURCES

Ackerman, Kate. "EHR Alerts Prescription Oversights," June 2, 2006, http://www.ihealthbeat.org (accessed November 21, 2007).

Approved Biotechnology Drugs, 2005, http://www.bio.org/speeches/pubs/er/approveddrugs.asp (accessed November 21, 2007).

Baase, Sara. *A Gift of Fire*, Upper Saddle River, NJ: Prentice Hall, 2002: 22–23.

Barker, Kenneth N., Bill G. Felkey, Elizabeth A. Flynn, and Jim L. Carper. "White Paper on Automation in Pharmacy," March 1998, http://www.ascp.com/publications/tcp/1998/mar/ (accessed November 22, 2007).

Borel, Jacques, and Karen L. Rascati, "Effect of an Automated, Nursing Unit-Based Drug-Dispensing Device on Medication Errors," © 1995, American Society of Health System Pharmacists, Inc., originally published in the *American Journal of Health System Pharmacy* 52 (September 1, 1995): 1875–79; Article Review and Commentary, http://www.ajhp.org/cgi/content/abstract/52/17/1875 (accessed November 22, 2007).

Brumson, Bennett. "Consumer Products Produced by Robotics," March 2001, http://www.roboticsonline.com/public/articles/archivedetails.cfm?id=357 (accessed November 22, 2007).

"Cardinal Health Installs New Point-of-Care Technology System in Huron Valley-Sinai Hospital," March 6, 2003, http://www.cardinal.com/us/en/providers/products/pyxis/ (accessed August 17, 2006).

"Cardinal Health Introduces Health Care's First Patient Room Automated Dispensing System For Medications and Supplies," June 2, 2003, http://www.cardinal.com/us/en/providers/products/pyxis/ (accessed August 17, 2006).

Cefalu, William T. and William Weir. "New Technologies in Diabetes Care," September 2003, http://www.patientcareonline.com/ (accessed November 22, 2007).

Chervokas, Jason and Tom Watson. "Doctors Build a Community Online," *CyberTimes*, February 6, 1998, http://www.nytimes.com/library/cyber/nation/020698nation.html (accessed November 22, 2007).

Cobb, Drew. "Improving patient safety—how can information technology help?" *AORN Journal*, August 2004, http://findarticles.com/p/articles/mi_m0FSL/is_2_80/ai_n6159722 (accessed December 3, 2007).

"Computer-Assisted Trial Design," 2003, http://www.pharsight.com/ (accessed November 22, 2007).

"Computers: Errors In—Errors Out," *Quality Review, a Publication of the Practitioners' Reporting Network*, no. 48, revised 8/95, August 1995, http://www.usp.org (accessed November 22, 2007).

Douglass, Kara. "Rx For Speedy Service," September 20, 1997, http://findarticles.com (accessed November 22, 2007).

"FDA Approves Avastin, A Targeted Therapy for First-Line Metastatic Colorectal Cancer Patients," February 26, 2004, http://psa-rising.com/wiredbird/genentech-avastin-feb2004.html (accessed November 22, 2007).

"FDA Approves Xolair, Biotechnology Breakthrough for Asthma," June 20, 2003, http://www.novartis.de/servlet/novartismedia.pdf?id=9793 (accessed November 22, 2007).

"FDA Approves Herceptin For Breast Cancer," September 29, 1998, http://www.newswise.com/articles/view/?id=hercptn2.ucl (accessed November 22, 2007).

Fleiger, Ken. "Getting SMART: Drug Review in the Computer Age," *FDA Consumer*, October 1995, http://www.fda.gov/fdac/features/895_smart.html (accessed November 22, 2007).

"From Maps to Medicine: About the Human Genome Research Project," August 9, 2000, http://whitepapers.zdnet.co.uk/0,39025945,60014727p-39000569q,00.htm (accessed November 22, 2007).

"Genentech Presents Positive Preliminary Six-Month Data from Phase Ib/II Study for Lucentis in Age-Related Macular Degeneration (AMD)," August 18, 2003, http://www.gene.com (accessed November 22, 2007).

"Genentech Receives FDA Fast-Track Designation for Avastin," June 26, 2003, http://www.gene.com/gene/news/press-releases/detail.jsp?detail=6367 (accessed November 22, 2007).

Gump, Michael D. (interview). "Robot Technology Improves VA Pharmacies—U.S. Medicine Interviews . . .," July 2001, web.uvic.ca/~h351/online_articles.htm (accessed November 22, 2007).

Fletcher, Amy. "Hospital Drug Delivery Systems Take High-Tech Route," August 8, 2003, http://denver.bizjournals.com (accessed November 22, 2007).

"Health Plans for Virtual Human," BBC News, May 17, 1999, http://news.bbc.co.uk (accessed November 22, 2007).

Hennessy, Sean and Brian Strom. *New England Journal of Medicine* "PDUFA Reauthorization—Drug Safety's Golden Moment of Opportunity?" April 26, 2007, http://content.nejm.org (accessed November 22, 2007).

HHS. "PDUFA Reauthorization Good for American Patients," 2002, http://hhs.gov (accessed November 22, 2007).

Human Genome Resources Fact Sheet, 2003, http://www.nlm.nih.gov/pubs/factsheets/humangenome.html (accessed November 22, 2007).

Leape, Lucian L. and Donald M. Berwick. "Five Years After To Err Is Human: What Have We Learned?" *Journal of the American Medical Association* 293, no. 19 (May 18, 2005): 2384–90, http://www.cmwf.org/publications/publications_show.htm?doc_id=278113 (accessed November 22, 2007).

Marietti, Charlene. "Robots Hooked on Drugs: Robotic Automation Expands Pharmacy Services," 11/97, *Healthcare Informatics,* November 1997, http://www.ncbi.nlm.nih.gov (accessed November 22, 2007).

"Milestone Demonstrates Pyxis Corporation's Leadership in Development of Automated Medication Technology for Patient Safety," January 10, 2002, http://web.uvic.ca (accessed November 22, 2007).

Neergaard, Lauran. "DNA to Aid in Tailoring Prescription for Patient," *Star-Ledger,* November 3, 2003, 23.

Ouellette, Jennifer. "Biomaterials Facilitate Medical Breakthroughs," American Institute of Physics, October/November 2001, http://www.aip.org (accessed November 22, 2007).

"Physicians Hospital of El Paso Set to Deploy Pyxis Safetynet Technology to Reduce Medical Errors," October 10, 2002, http://www.cardinal.com/us/en/providers/products/pyxis/ (accessed December 3, 2007).

Pollack, Andrew. "Drug Testers Turn to 'Virtual Patients' as Guinea Pigs," November 10, 1998, http://www.nytimes.com/ (accessed November 22, 2007).

Pollack, Andrew. "Merck and Partner Form Alliance to Develop Drugs Based on RNA," September 9, 2003, http://www.nytimes.com/ (accessed November 22, 2007).

Pollack, Andrew. "Mixed Data Leave Doubts on Cancer Drug," September 12, 2003, http://www.nytimes.com/ (accessed November 22, 2007).

"Preventing Death and Injury From Medical Errors Requires Dramatic, System-Wide Changes," *The National Academies,* November 29, 1999, http://www8.nationalacademies.org/onpinews/newsitem.aspx?RecordID=9728 (accessed December 3, 2007).

Raschke, Robert, et al. "A Computer Alert System to Prevent Injury From Adverse Drug Events," *JAMA,* October 21, 1998, 1317–20.

"The RNA Structure Database," September 10, 2003, http://rnabase.org (accessed November 22, 2007).

Sardinha, Carol. "Electronic Prescribing: the Next Revolution in Pharmacy," *Journal of Managed Care Pharmacy,* January–February 1998, http://www.amcp.org/jmcp/vol4/num1/spotlight.html (accessed November 22, 2007).

Schwarz, Harold and Bret Brodowy. "Implementation and Evaluation of an Automated Dispensing System," © 1995 first published in the American Society of Hospital Pharmacists, *American Journal of Health-System Pharmacy,* 52 (April 15, 1995): 823–28 [abstract], 1998, http://www.ncbi.nlm.nih.gov (accessed November 22, 2007).

"Significant Milestones in Biotechnology," Genentech Inc., 2000, http://www.gene.com (accessed November 22, 2007).

Sipkoff, Martin. "Telepharmacy Helps Improve Efficiency," February 2001, http://64.233.169.104/search?q=cache:b5Dr3x35FcoJ:www.qualityindicator.com/common/pdfs/QIP0201.pdf+Sipkoff,+Martin,.+Telepharmacy+Helps+Improve+Efficiency&hl=en&ct=clnk&cd=1&gl=us (accessed December 3, 2007).

"Spokane Pharmacists Test Rx Vending Machine Dispensing," February 2002, http://www.telepharmacysolutions.com/news.html (accessed November 22, 2007).

Stephenson, Joan. "Targeting Medical Errors," *JAMA* 283, no. 3, January 19, 2000, jama.ama-assn.org/cgi/content/full/283/3/325-b (accessed December 3, 2007).

Tamblyn, R., et al. "The Use Of Computers In Health Care Can Reduce Errors, Improve Patient Safety, And Enhance The Quality Of Service—There Is Evidence," March 1, 2005, http://www.informatics.nhs.uk (accessed November 22, 2007).

"Tarceva (erlotnib HCl) Phase II Clinical Trials Initiated in Patients with Malignant Glioma," August 8, 2003, http://www.gene.com (accessed November 22, 2007).

"Thompson Approves Demos to Expand Safety-Net Patients' Access To Prescription Drugs and Pharmacy Services, Lower Drug Prices," HHS News US Department of Health an Human Services, December 18, 2001. http://newsroom.hrsa.gov/releases/2001%20 Releases/vendingmachines.htm (accessed December 3, 2007).

Ukens, Carol. "Manuel the Robot Earns his Long-Term Care Keep," July 10, 2006, http:// www.drugtopics.com/drugtopics/article/articleDetail.jsp?id=353150 (accessed November 22, 2007).

Ukens, Carol. "New Bar-Code Scanner Simplifies Drug Ordering," August 7, 2006, http://www.drugtopics.com/drugtopics/author/authorDetail.jsp?id=6373 (accessed November 22, 2007).

"What is a Helix? And What is RNA and DNA . . .," http://www.chemistry-school.info (accessed November 22, 2007).

"What is RNA?" June 12, 2006, http://www.cancerbackup.org.uk/Aboutcancer/Whatiscancer/ Understandingtermsstatistics/related_faqs/QAs/1080223255 (accessed November 22, 2007).

CHAPTER 9

Information Technology in Dentistry

CHAPTER OUTLINE

LEARNING OBJECTIVES

In this chapter, the student will learn many of the ways that computer technology has impacted the practice of dentistry. The student will be able to

- Describe the use of computers in education.
- Discuss the significance of the electronic patient record in integrating practice management and clinical applications.
- Discuss the impact of changing demographics on dental practice.
- Describe the use of computers in endodontics, periodontics, and cosmetic dentistry.
- Define diagnostic tools including the X-ray, digital X-ray, electronic concordance, and the new tools that use light.
- Define minimally invasive dentistry.
- List the uses of computers in dental surgery.
- Describe the trend toward growing specialization.
- Describe the emerging field of teledentistry.

OVERVIEW

Computers have been transforming dentistry for many years. **Dental informatics** combines computer technology with dentistry to create a basis for research, education, and the solution of real-world problems in oral healthcare using computer applications. Studies are being done on the role of information technology on the dentist–patient relationship.[1]

From the time the patient calls the office for an appointment recorded in an electronic appointment book to the services offered and the instruments in use, even to the pain the patient senses, digital technology plays a role. The earliest application of information technology in the dentist's office, as in so many other offices, was administrative—related to bookkeeping and accounting.

Many dental offices use computers for some aspect of their practice. Computer technology can be utilized in dentistry to help reduce medical errors, to train dentists, to facilitate communication between dentists, to perform administrative, clerical, and managerial functions in the dental office, and not least to enhance patient care.

The practice of dentistry has also been affected by demographic changes in our society over the last century. Younger people (with the significant exceptions of the poor, minorities, and immigrants) have few cavities because of preventive care. Older people are subject to periodontal disease.

EDUCATION

Dentists can surf the Web for online information specific to their professional interests and use e-mail to communicate with each other and their patients. Computer-generated treatment plans are used to help educate patients (Figure 9.1 ■). These plans can be presented on DVDs.

Root Canal

Endodontic
Treatment

Endodontic Treatment

λ Nothing is as good as a natural tooth! And sometimes your natural tooth may need Endodontic (root canal) treatment for it to remain a healthy part of your mouth.

λ Signs to look for include pain, prolonged sensitivity to heat or cold, discoloration of the tooth, and swelling or tenderness in the nearby gums. But sometimes, there are no symptoms.

λ Most patients report that having Endodontic (root canal) treatment today is as unremarkable as having a cavity filled.

Tooth Anatomy

λ A tooth is made up of three main structures :

1. The hard outer covering of ENAMEL.

2. The underlying layer of DENTIN.

3. A soft tissue - the PULP- that is comprised of the blood supply, and the nerve of the tooth, which is housed in the hollow root canal space.

λ The pulp partially nourishes the root from the inside.

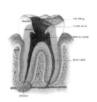

Infection of the Pulp

λ Sometimes the pulp inside your tooth becomes inflamed or infected.

λ This can be caused by deep decay, repeated dental procedures on the tooth, a crack or chip in the tooth, or a blow to the tooth.

λ In any other part of your body, if a similar tissue becomes diseased, the body merely throws it off and forms new tissue. However, a tooth is a unique and different situation. Because the soft tissue within the tooth is totally encased within hard tissue, the body cannot get to it in order to affect repair.

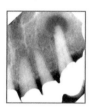

Treatment

It is the role of the dentist to do what the body is unable to do. He must :

- Remove the soft tissue located in the internal spaces (canals).

- Cleanse the area.

- Fill the canals with a special material so that bacteria cannot re-enter the tooth to cause another infection.

Treatment (cont.)

λ The dentist removes the inflamed or infected pulp, carefully cleans and shapes the inside of the tooth, then fills and seals the space.

λ Often it is necessary to place a POST down into the canal space to act as an anchor when large amounts of tooth structure are missing due to disease.

λ While many patients may be in great pain before seeing the dentist, most report that the dentist relieves the pain and that they are comfortable during the procedure.

λ When the endodontic treatment is complete, the tooth is by no means "dead". It receives quite adequate support from the surrounding tissues and may be expected to last as long as any other natural tooth.

Post Op Care

λ For the first few days after treatment, the tooth may feel sensitive - especially if there was pain or infection before the procedure. This discomfort can be relieved with medications.

λ You should not chew or bite on the treated tooth until you have had it restored by your dentist, because it could fracture.

λ Often it is necessary to place a POST down into the canal space to act as an anchor when large amounts of tooth structure are missing due to disease.

■ **FIGURE 9.1** Software is available to help educate patients about dental treatments. This PowerPoint presentation explains Root Canal Therapy. Screen shots are from SOFTDENT Practice Management Software. Courtesy of Eastman Kodak Company.

Although not yet common, virtual reality simulations are beginning to be used in the education of dentists and dental surgeons. Case Western Reserve University that installed virtual dentistry equipment at a cost of $2 million in 2002 is very satisfied with the part virtual reality can play in dental education. The simulators are always available, so students can learn at their own pace. According to faculty members, students learned much faster; they report that students learned drilling techniques in two weeks instead of one full semester. Each station includes a mannequin, drill, syringes, suction, light, cabinets, and a computer monitor—simulating a dentist's office. A camera watches the student's work and sends the student messages. The student is shown what the tooth should look like, and images and evaluations of the student's work via the monitor.[2]

DentSim is a program that uses virtual reality. Its purpose is to teach technical dexterity to dental students. A small pilot study has been completed. The study found that using the program improved technical dexterity. More studies are planned.[3]

ADMINISTRATIVE APPLICATIONS

From the moment a patient calls to arrange an appointment to the electronic submission of the bill to the insurance company, computer technology may be involved. Many dental offices, like other medical offices, use computerized appointment calendars; thus, appointments can be made (and viewed) from any room in the office that has a networked computer (Figure 9.2 ■). Specialized software helps to create treatment plans, to explain plans to patients, and to give postoperative instructions. In offices using fully integrated practice management software, any screen is accessible from any other, simply by clicking the mouse.

The Electronic Dental Chart

Computers were first used by dentists in the 1960s as accounting tools. In the 1980s, computers were used for practice management. The American Dental Association (ADA) began developing guidelines for the fully integrated computerized dental office. The electronic appointment book, electronic accounting software, and electronic record-keeping in which the patient's record includes images, charting, and photos will become more and more common (Figure 9.3 ■). Software that computerizes some clinical procedures (charting, probing, and digital imaging) is beginning to be used. In the future, a patient record that links practice management with all clinical procedures may be developed.

The **electronic dental chart** will be standardized, easy to search, and easy to read (Figure 9.4 ■). It will integrate practice management tasks (administrative applications) with clinical information. It will include all of the patient's conditions and treatments, including images. Although no standards currently exist on what should be in a chart, dental charting software is creating a standard record. The record must include codes for treatment and diagnosis, which will come from the American Dental Association (ADA). The chart should include the following: the ability to

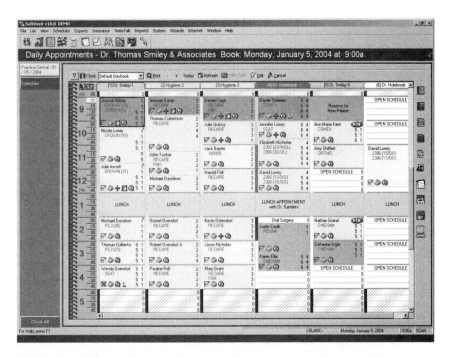

■ **FIGURE 9.2**   An appointment can be made in an electronic appointment book. The screen shot is from SOFTDENT Practice Management Software. Courtesy of Eastman Kodak Company.

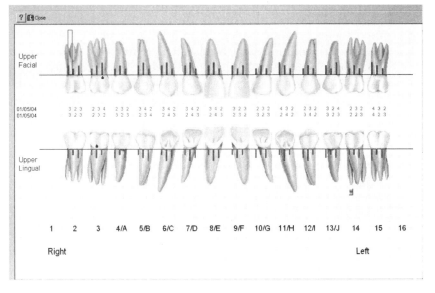

■ **FIGURE 9.3**   Periodontal charting can be done on a computer screen. The screen shot is from SOFTDENT Practice Management Software. Courtesy of Eastman Kodak Company.

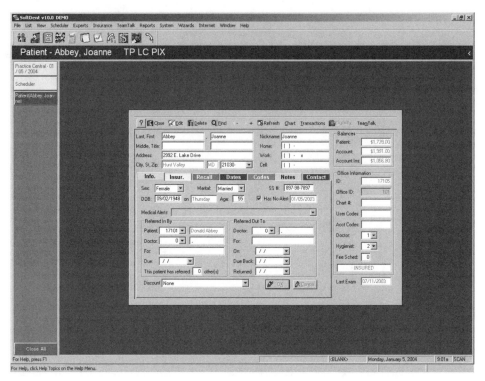

■ **FIGURE 9.4**   All of a patient's information is accessible on any computer on the network. The screen shot is from SOFTDENT Practice Management Software. Courtesy of Eastman Kodak Company.

find patients by name, patient identification numbers, health information such as allergies or conditions that would affect dental care, treatment planning, procedures performed and planned, treatments completed, medical history, and ADA codes. As additions are made they must be dated, and an audit trail of who edited each record must be kept. Files must be password protected. The record includes graphics and text. The chart will be created on a patient's first visit and updated every visit. Not only does it contain clinical information, but transactions can be posted. It also includes the fee schedule and patient's insurance information (including co-payment and deductible). Because much of the chart is made up of images, it is easy for the patient to understand. The patient and dentist can develop treatment plans that take into account medical needs and finances. The chart can be electronically transmitted to specialists.

DEMOGRAPHICS AND THE TRANSFORMATION OF DENTISTRY

In 2000, the surgeon general issued a first report on dental health. The report pointed to changes over the last hundred years. In 1900, most people lost their teeth by middle age. By the middle of the twentieth century, the baby boom generation was taught to take care of their teeth. Bacteria (usually streptococcus) were found to be the cause of tooth decay and periodontal disease in the 1950s and 1960s.

By the late twentieth century, many children were drinking fluoridated water, having their teeth regularly cared for, and thus suffering less decay. This meant that they did not lose their teeth as they aged. However, according to the surgeon general, there is still an "epidemic of oral disease." Victims of this epidemic are low-income, minority, and some immigrant populations. One study traced the high number of cavities in poor children to increased lead levels in the children's blood, plus shortages in calcium and vitamin C.[4] But dental health in general has improved over the last century. These trends—successful preventive treatments in middle-class children and an increasing aging population who have kept their teeth—have changed the conditions dentists are treating and the expectations of patients. Dentists are filling fewer teeth, but increasingly and aggressively treating the more affluent portion of the aging population. This population now seeks dental care to save their teeth. However, this may make the dentist's job more difficult because this population is both old and may be in poor health.

COMPUTERIZED INSTRUMENTS IN DENTISTRY

Computerized instruments have been entering the field of dentistry for several years. From a very expensive machine that creates crowns immediately to fiber optic digital cameras and digital X-rays, computer technology is changing some aspects of dentistry. The **fiber optic camera** is analogous to the endoscope used in surgery. It is used to view an area that is normally difficult to see. The dentist aims a fiber optic wand at the area of the mouth to be examined. The image can be viewed on a monitor by the patient and the dentist. The image can help the dentist see and diagnose problems at a very early stage. An electronic periodontal probe has been developed to replace the sharp steel probe dentists use to measure pockets between teeth and gums. It is more accurate and, one would hope, less painful than its predecessor.

Computer-controlled injections are administered by the WAND™. The **WAND™** includes a microprocessor that measures tissue density; this ensures a steady flow of anesthetic. The microprocessor delivers anesthesia ahead of the needle, numbing the tissue before the needle touches it. It numbs only the injection site—not the tongue, lips or face.

ENDODONTICS

Endodontics is the dental specialty that diagnoses and treats diseases of the pulp. Endoscopes make use of fiber optics to take pictures of the root canal and show them on a screen. Both the dentist and the patient can see and discuss the images, which helps in both diagnosis and educating the patient.

The precision of ultrasonic instruments helps in performing root canal therapy. They are flexible and accurate and allow the dentist to clean out the root without harming the surrounding tissue.

If a patient needs a crown, computers can be used to create a model of the affected tooth. This computer-generated model can be electronically transmitted to another company that uses it to prepare the crown. Too expensive to be common, Computer-Aided Design/Computer-Aided Manufacturing (CAD/CAM) is used by a new machine to create crowns.

PERIODONTICS

Periodontics is concerned with diagnosing and treating diseases of the gums and other structures supporting the teeth. Periodontal disease is caused by bacteria. Untreated, periodontal disease can lead to both tooth and bone loss. The sequence of the genome associated with the pathogen causing gum disease has been identified; this might lead to the development of effective treatments.[5] Tooth loss because of periodontal disease is related to (does not necessarily cause) heart disease.[6] Gum disease is also linked to premature birth.[7] Periodontal disease is more prevalent in older people who have kept their natural teeth. It is also prevalent among African-Americans.[8] Periodontal disease is related to stroke and cancers, especially pancreatic cancer in men.[9] Gum disease, which affects about fifty million Americans, may be a sign of other diseases, for example, diabetes.[10]

The standard method of measuring periodontal pockets (the spaces between teeth and gums) involves probing with a steel-tipped tool, measuring the pockets and noting the depth on a patient's chart. An electronic probe with a flexible tip may be more accurate and less painful. Currently, voice-activated charting is beginning to be used.

Although not widely accepted, lasers are used by some dentists to treat periodontal disease. They apply lasers to soft tissue and root surfaces. This can be added to traditional treatment. However, there is little or no evidence that it is effective.[11]

The change in the conditions for which people seek dental care is related to demographic changes mentioned above. Older adults with their own teeth are more likely to suffer from periodontal disease. Gums recede; roots are exposed and may develop cavities. The more teeth a person keeps, the more these problems develop, and the more visits to the dentist. Further, affluent older adults may seek cosmetic dentistry: "smile makeovers," tooth whitening, and orthodontics.

COSMETIC DENTISTRY

Cosmetic dentistry is becoming more and more widely available: 84 percent of dentists now offer cosmetic treatments.[12] Cosmetic dentistry attempts to create a more attractive smile. To do this, several procedures may be employed. Tooth bleaching may be done at home with bleaching kits or at the dentist's office using lasers. One procedure is called ZOOM. Porcelain veneers may be applied to create a whiter looking tooth. **Bonding** involves the application of a material to the tooth that can be shaped and polished. **Dental implants** can be used to replace missing teeth; computers help plan the exact placement of the implant. Cosmetic dentists and orthodontists employ digital cameras and graphics software.

Some orthodontics is performed via teledentistry. The technician is with the patient, and the clinician directs the technician from afar. Virtual reality three-dimensional images allow the patient to view herself or himself before and after any procedure. Some software even morphs the image—from the face before to the face after—to show the patient how her or his face will be changed by the procedure. Using the virtual reality image, the technician can move individual teeth in virtual reality. The dentist can review the procedure via the Web. When the plan is approved, a real realignment of the teeth can begin.[13]

In other systems, the dental hygienist photographs the patient using a digital camera and simply makes the changes by dragging the mouse on the image of the patient's face on the screen.

DIAGNOSIS AND EXPERT SYSTEMS

Diagnosis is not always clear and simple; dentists need to analyze all sorts of data, such as the clinical presentation of the patient and general medical information. No individual can have all the current information at her or his fingertips. But knowing how to phrase questions and find facts for decision-making is a crucial skill. There are several collections of evidence-based articles and reviews categorized by topic, which dentists can search online. Journals, such as the *Journal of Evidence-Based Dental Practice*, give summaries of articles. Databases, such as MEDLINE, can also be helpful. When doing the search, the dentist needs to be able to frame questions that provide enough information. The question should state the problem clearly and the desired outcome. The computerized search should be of peer-reviewed, evidence-based relevant material.

The dentist then needs to apply the correct factual information to the particular situation to make a diagnosis. In dentistry as in other fields, expert systems or **clinical decision-support systems (CDSS)** can help. Expert systems are a branch of artificial intelligence, which attempts to model computer logic on human behavior. An expert system maintains a large collection of facts relevant to the discipline (dentistry) and rules on how these facts are used in decision-making. The dentist may type in symptoms, and the expert system may respond by asking for more information; finally, diagnoses are suggested. The diagnosis is in the form of an inference: if the patient exhibits swelling, then she or he may have an infection. Expert systems are meant as an aid in diagnosis, not a replacement for the judgment of the dentist. **EXPERTMD** is software that allows the creation of medical and dental expert systems.

Today's CDSS can be tailored to each patient. CDSS "are computer programs that are designed to provide expert support for health professionals making clinical decisions. . . . To help . . . analyze patient data and make decisions regarding diagnosis, prevention, and treatment."[14] Like any expert system, CDSS may remind the practitioner of conditions and diagnoses she or he has not recently encountered.

Patient information is kept in a database. Patients are asked to fill out electronic questionnaires; their answers are automatically sent to the database. The system generates automatic alerts to remind the dentist of any health problems the patient may have. While examining the patient, all charting is done on the computer; cavities and periodontal health are electronically recorded. The CDSS automatically asks the dentist risk assessment questions; the program then classifies the patient's risk assessment. The CDSS then generates a treatment plan for the particular patient. It also informs the patient of specific risk factors, for example, smoking.

DIAGNOSTIC TOOLS

A basic diagnostic tool is a clinical examination using a probe. This method is not completely accurate. More cavities are found by X-rays than by traditional exams.

X-rays

Traditional X-rays have been used for more than one hundred years to diagnose cavities. X-rays are more effective than clinical examination. X-rays can be used because as the mineral content of the tooth decreases, the X-ray shows the cavity as darker. The dentist must then interpret the X-ray correctly. This is not a foolproof method of diagnosis and may not detect cavities at an early stage when minimal intervention is necessary.

Digital Radiography

As an aid in diagnosis, digital X-rays have some advantages. They take less time and expose the patient to 60 to 90 percent less radiation (Figures 9.5 ■ and 9.6 ■). There is a cost savings on film and processing. Dentists will no longer have to store film. The image needs no developing, and the image can be viewed immediately on a monitor, by both the dentist and the patient. The dentist can also enhance the image. The patient can see the digital image more clearly than a small film, and aspects of the digital X-ray can be enhanced to show specific problem areas. Computers can be used to scan X-ray images into a patient's digital file. Like the traditional X-ray, the digital X-ray also needs interpretation. Several studies, however, have found no significant differences in diagnosis between digital and traditional imaging.

Electrical Conductance

Electrical conductance is also currently used to diagnose cavities. An electric current is passed through a tooth, and the tooth's resistance is measured. A decayed tooth

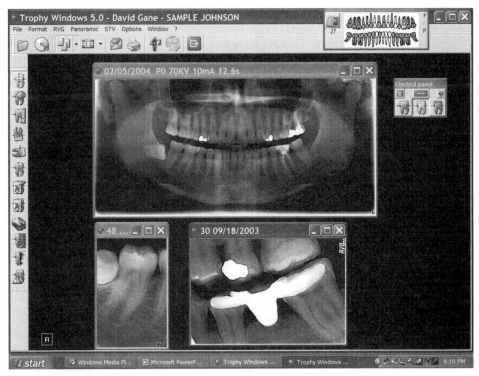

■ **FIGURE 9.5** Digital X-rays expose a patient to less radiation and are immediately displayed on a monitor. The screen shot is from SOFTDENT Practice Management Software. Courtesy of Eastman Kodak Company.

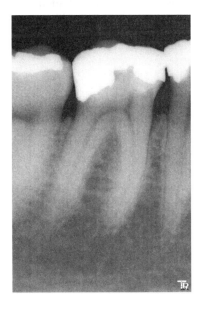

■ **FIGURE 9.6** Digital X-ray. The screen shot is from SOFTDENT Practice Management Software. Courtesy of Eastman Kodak Company.

has a different resistance reading than a healthy tooth. Studies differ on the accuracy of this method, but tend to rate it high in detecting substantial cavities, not early lesions.

Emerging Methods

Traditional clinical exams and X-rays can detect cavities only after they are somewhat advanced. New methods use light to attempt to identify cavities earlier. Studies disagree on their effectiveness. New techniques have also been developed to stop demineralization, which occurs with caries; however, the success of these treatments is not yet known.

Light Illumination

Several methods use light to help diagnose tooth disease. These show promise in diagnosing early lesions. To find decay, a bright light is used to illuminate the tooth, revealing color differences. Decay looks darker because the light is absorbed when a cavity changes the structure of enamel.

Fiber optic transillumination found early lesions (affecting enamel) but was limited in diagnosing advanced caries.

Digital imaging fiber optic transillumination (DIFOTI®) involves using a digital camera to obtain images of teeth illuminated with laser light (Figure 9.7 ■). The images are analyzed using computer algorithms. "They showed a direct correlation . . . between loss of fluorescence and the presence of caries . . . [and] a quantitative correlation of that loss and the amount of caries present."[15] DIFOTI® can find cavities developing behind metal fillings that X-rays would not diagnose.

Intraoral fiber optic cameras allow both patient and dentist to get a close-up tour of the patient's mouth (Figure 9.8 ■). A fiber optic device is aimed at an area of the patient's mouth, and the image appears on the screen. The image can be magnified to show problems, such as small cracks, which might otherwise remain unnoticed until the tooth breaks.

LASERS IN DENTISTRY

Laser stands for **light amplification by stimulated emission of radiation**. Lasers deliver light energy. Depending on the target, the light travels at different wavelengths. Each target absorbs one wavelength and reflects other wavelengths, so each instrument is different. There are several uses of lasers in dentistry. Low-level lasers can find pits in tooth enamel that may become cavities. The Food and Drug Administration (FDA) has approved laser machines for drilling and filling cavities; lasers also reduce the bacteria in the cavity.

Minimally invasive dentistry uses lasers. When surgical lasers are used in place of drills, they burst cells by heating them. One laser works on hard tissue, another on soft tissue. Lasers can quickly harden the material used to fill the tooth, reducing the time a filling takes to complete. Lasers cannot be used where previous fillings or crowns exist.

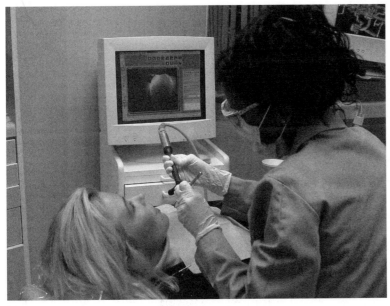

(a)

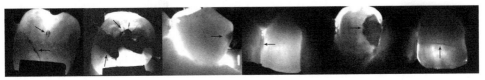

(b)

■ **FIGURE 9.7** (a) Hygienist imaging patient with DIFOTI® system. (b) DIFOTI® images of, from left to right: 1) virgin occlusal caries, 2) recurrent occlusal caries around amalgam, 3) incipient interproximal decay, 4) incipient interproximal decay, 5) recurrent buccal decay around composite, and 6) horizontal anterior fracture. Courtesy of DIFOTI®.

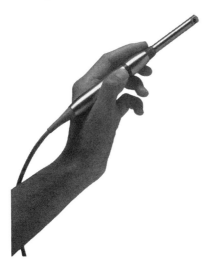

■ **FIGURE 9.8** An intra-oral camera can help reveal problems before they become serious. Courtesy of Eastman Kodak Company.

Lasers are used by periodontists; they can reshape the gums. They can also be used to remove bacteria from periodontal pockets. But their use is limited in root canal therapy. The FDA has approved one laser for treating root canals. Lasers can be used in some instances to help clean out the root canal and to remove bacteria. However, they can only be used in straight canals because the instruments are glass and do not bend. If the temperature is too high, the canal space can be charred and the tooth and surrounding tissue can be damaged.

Lasers also have uses in cosmetic dentistry. Dentists can apply whitening solutions to teeth and activate the solutions using lasers. This can cause the tooth to lighten in a very short time.

MINIMALLY INVASIVE DENTISTRY

Minimally invasive dentistry emphasizes prevention and the least possible intervention. Teeth are constantly affected by acids, which **demineralize** the surfaces. Early lesions beneath the enamel can be treated with calcium, phosphate, and fluoride, which help **remineralize** teeth. Preventive measures include antibacterial rinses and toothpastes, fluoride, diet, sealants, and the use of sugarless gum to increase saliva. The widespread use of fluoride has strengthened tooth enamel but not the dentin. Many cavities, which appear in X-rays, are simply not found by traditional clinical examination. Cavities often appear in hard to see fissures in a tooth. Sealants may be used as a preventative measure. If a cavity is there, minimally invasive techniques may be used to prepare the tooth. Air abrasion can remove small amounts of a tooth; it involves aiming high-speed particles at the tooth. It can be used for the removal of cavities, of defects in the enamel, and to detect cavities in fissures by opening them for inspection. It is relatively painless. It removes less of the tooth than a traditional drill.

Minimally invasive dentistry also makes use of lasers. The laser vaporizes decay by directing a stream of light at the affected area. The lasers are so precise that they affect only the decay, not the tooth. Very few patients require pain medication, and those who do are sensitive to the cold water used, not the laser. The machine is much more expensive than the conventional drill, but it allows fillings to be done so quickly that many more patients can be treated.

SURGERY

Computers play a part in dental surgery, from the delivery of anesthesia to the planning and creation of dental implants. Computerized monitoring devices can keep track of a patient's vital signs. For patients requiring implants, software can create a three-dimensional view of the patient: this allows the dentist to see the exact relationship of the planned implant to the patient's bone. The surgery can be done as a simulation; dental computed tomography (CT) scans allow the surgeon to rotate the implant on the screen so that by the time the patient is operated on, the surgery is planned down to the last detail. The software can measure bone density from the image and predict whether or not bone grafts will be needed. Procedures take less time and are easier for both patient and dentist.

The latest surgical alternative does not use scalpels. It is radiosurgery. According to the Academy of General Dentistry, "radiosurgery is a technique that uses radio waves to produce a pressureless, bloodless incision instead of knives." It is used for the following procedures: cosmetic surgery (to heat bleaching agents), gum surgery, root canal therapy, the removal of a muscle that grows between the two front teeth, and biopsies. There is no bleeding and healing is faster.[16]

THE GROWTH OF SPECIALIZATION

In the last quarter of the twentieth century, only 10 percent of dentists were specialists. This is expected to rise to about 30 percent. This is due in part to the decrease in the number of dentists trained, whereas the number of specialists trained remains constant, so that specialists form a greater proportion. It is also because of changing demographics. As life expectancy increases and dental health improves, more affluent patients who feel they need to be attractive will seek cosmetic dentistry. With the aging population, some dentists will specialize in geriatrics. New technologies that allow dental problems to be diagnosed and treated earlier will result in dentists who specialize in diagnostics. Group practices may increase. In 2000, 108 million people in the United States lacked dental insurance.[17] However, there is the possibility of the inclusion of dental services under health maintenance organizations (HMOs), which will expect preventive care and economical service. Patients may educate themselves via the Internet and expect more from their dentists.

TELEDENTISTRY

Teledentistry programs have been developed to help dentists access specialists, improving patient care. One system uses the Internet and requires a computer and digital camera. The general dentist can e-mail a patient's chart, including images to the specialist who can suggest both diagnosis and treatment. This saves the patient time and travel and gives her or him access to expert advice.

IN THE NEWS

Excerpt from, "Taking Care; The New-Age Dentistry"
by Andrew H. Malcolm

WHEN TODAY'S ADULTS WERE children, it was a popular pastime to portray what the city of the future would be like—air cars gliding serenely between strange-looking buildings towering over clean streets where vehicular traffic moved efficiently. . . . But no one imagined what dentistry would look like in the last decade of the 20th century.

"'It's absolutely amazing what's happened," says Dr. Arthur A. Dugoni, past president of the American Dental Association and dean of the School of Dentistry at the University of the Pacific in Stockton, Calif.

What's happened is that technology has swept through one of the oldest and most maligned professions, revolutionizing its approach, its methods and its capabilities, even the personality of its practitioners. And while the image of the dentist's office as a kind of medieval torture chamber filled with strange smells and muffled moans lingers in the nostrils and ears of many middle-aged patients, the modern-day reality for their children is as different as the city of the future that never was. Dental visits now are usually pain free . . .

For American consumers, who, along with insurance companies, shell out about $42 billion each year to care for their mouths, the dental revolution means, among other things: . . . live video coverage of the mouth by a camera that presents a magnified picture of the teeth, enabling the dentist to locate areas of decay more easily and allows patients to watch what the dentist is doing. Computer-assisted "smile forecasts" that portray on a television screen exactly what a cosmetic procedure, like filling in gaps between teeth, can do to enhance a patient's appearance.

A host of experimental approaches now being studied by researchers . . . include: Lasers that vaporize, in a flash, even the largest pockets of decay. These could eventually eliminate the need for dreaded dental drilling. And "Electronic braces," which can reposition teeth in less than half the time required by conventional orthodontic hardware.

It is all a far cry from the first significant advance in dental work in 1785, when John Greenwood invented a drill run by a foot pedal. With a strong foot a dentist could get that instrument whirling at a speed of 100 revolutions per minute. . . .

In today's jet-age practices, the standard air-driven, water-cooled drill turns a half-million times a minute, although 60 seconds is usually more time than needed to cut through a spot of decay. . . .

Despite the proliferation of new dental treatments, the number of would-be dentists appears to be declining. . . .

Dr. Dugoni sees a shortage of dentists beginning to appear around 1996. . . . He traces the problem to the fact that much dental work is now discretionary, causing some doubts in the minds of would-be dentists about their future financial security. . . . Dr. Dugoni adds, "There has been no glamour in the popular image of dentistry as drilling and filling."

But the current reality of dentistry involves much more than drilling and filling. Dr. Paul Keating, a 34-year-old with a seven-year-old practice in Wilton, Conn., says he now spends only one-third of his time restoring and repairing teeth, primarily replacing old fillings.

Another third of his time goes to preventive work—cleaning teeth and gum lines—and trying to reduce his own tooth repair business by teaching oral hygiene to patients young and old. . . .

The remaining third of Dr. Keating's workday, the growing third, is devoted to cosmetic work, because of more aware dental consumers and the rapidly evolving technology. . . .

And what dentists can now do is tantamount to producing the kind of white-capped brilliance once seen beaming only from the expensive smiles of stars on stage during the annual Oscar presentations. Cosmetic procedures are easier and cheaper than ever before. . . . This has launched an essentially new cosmetic dental business, which may soon make up 40 percent or more of the dentist's workload.

Years ago, Dr. Randolph Shoup's dental practice in Indianapolis involved perhaps 40 percent fillings and 5 percent cosmetic work. Now fillings are a dwindling 15 percent and cosmetic work is surpassing 35 percent, thanks, in part, . . . to a $30,000 video camera. "It lets me communicate with my patients on an entirely different level," says Dr. Shoup.

The video camera is connected to a computer, which presents two images on a television screen: a picture of the patient's existing smile on one half of the screen, and a picture of how the smile will look after Dr. Shoup has completed the cosmetic procedure. With a tap of his foot on a floor pedal, Dr. Shoup can order the machine to take a Polaroid photo of the split image, producing a record of what patient and doctor both agreed to. . . . The camera is also helpful for diagnosing dental problems. . . .

LAST SPRING THE Food and Drug Administration approved the use of a new kind of laser for treating periodontal disease, one of the most common dental problems. With this laser, a dentist can vaporize inflamed or infected gum tissue. . . .

"Dentistry is much closer to medicine now," says Dr. Dugoni. "It involves more science, technology, psychology, business methods. It requires more education. A lot of training time is spent, for instance, on anticipating patient anxieties and stress." New dental students are also trained much more than their predecessors to involve patients in treatment decisions."

CHAPTER SUMMARY

Computers are used in all aspects of dentistry from educating dentists and patients to helping in surgery.

- The electronic patient record may standardize the dental chart and integrate the practice by including all of a patient's information from financial and insurance to clinical information.
- Changing demographics and improved dental health for most children have combined to change the tasks performed by dentists.
- Computer technology is making the tools used by periodontists, endodontists, and surgeons more precise.
- Traditional diagnostic tools are being supplemented by methods based on digital technology and fiber optics.
- Minimally invasive dentistry emphasizes prevention and the least possible intervention.
- Computers play a role in dental surgery, from delivering anesthesia to monitoring a patient's vital signs.
- Lasers are used in many branches of dentistry.
- More and more dentists are specializing in a particular field.
- Teledentistry can deliver expert consults, especially during surgery, at a distance.

KEY TERMS

bonding
clinical decision-support
    systems (CDSS)
cosmetic dentistry
demineralize
dental implants
dental informatics
DentSim
digital imaging fiber
    optic transillumina-
    tion (DIFOTI®)

electrical conductance
electronic dental chart
endodontics
EXPERTMD
fiber optic camera
fiber optic
    transillumination
intraoral fiber optic
    cameras
laser (light amplification
    by stimulated

emission of
    radiation)
minimally invasive
    dentistry
periodontics
remineralize
teledentistry
WAND™

REVIEW EXERCISES

Multiple Choice

1. The _____ is analogous to the endoscope used in surgery.
   A. digital X-ray
   B. laser
   C. fiber optic camera
   D. None of the above

2. _____ is the dental specialty that diagnoses and treats diseases of the pulp.
   A. Periodontics
   B. Endodontics
   C. Cosmetic dentistry
   D. Digital dentistry

3. _____ is the dental specialty that diagnoses and treats diseases of the gums.
   A. Periodontics
   B. Endodontics
   C. Cosmetic dentistry
   D. Digital dentistry

4. _____ is the dental specialty concerned with smile makeovers.
   A. Periodontics
   B. Endodontics
   C. Cosmetic dentistry
   D. Digital dentistry

5. _____ emphasizes prevention and the least possible intervention.
   A. Periodontics
   B. Endodontics
   C. Cosmetic dentistry
   D. Minimally invasive dentistry

6. _____ can find cavities developing behind metal fillings.
   A. Traditional examination
   B. DIFOTI®
   C. Traditional X-rays
   D. Digital X-rays

7. _____ is a software that allows the creation of medical and dental expert systems.
   A. POEMS
   B. MYCIN
   C. INTERNIST
   D. EXPERTMD

8. _____ can remove small amounts of a tooth; it involves high-speed particles aimed at the tooth.
   A. DIFOTI®
   B. Light illumination
   C. Air abrasion
   D. None of the above

9. _____ deliver light energy. Depending on the target, the light travels at different wavelengths.
   A. Lasers
   B. X-rays
   C. Air abrasion
   D. All of the above
10. One study traced the high number of cavities in poor children to _____.
   A. increased lead levels in the children's blood
   B. shortages in calcium
   C. shortages in vitamin C
   D. All of the above

True/False Questions

1. Some orthodontics is performed via teledentistry. The technician is with the patient and the clinician directs the technician from afar._____
2. Dental health in general has improved over the last century._____
3. Teeth are constantly affected by acids, which demineralize the surfaces._____
4. The percentage of dentists who are specialists is not expected to rise._____
5. The change in the conditions for which people seek dental care is related to demographic changes._____
6. The laser vaporizes decay by directing a stream of light at the affected area. _____
7. The earliest application of information technology in the dentist's office was administrative—related to bookkeeping and accounting._____
8. Lasers can always be used in to help clean out the root canal and to remove bacteria._____
9. Lasers are used in cosmetic dentistry._____
10. Traditional clinical exams and X-rays can detect cavities only after they are somewhat advanced._____

Critical Thinking

1. What are the primary functions of computer technology in the dentist's office? In your answer, refer to clinical, administrative, and special-purpose applications.
2. How do you envision dentistry ten years from now?
3. How would you address the need for proper dental care for children who are disadvantaged?
4. What methods would you incorporate to educate people about good oral health care?
5. How would you close the gap between the poor, health care-deficient populace and the affluent, who can afford proper, regular dental care?
6. With an aging population, dentistry will have to reflect the demand for cosmetic surgery. Do you think that insurance should cover this? Why or why not?

NOTES

1. M. Kirshner, "The Role of Information Technology and Informatics Research in the Dentist-Patient Relationship," December 2003, http://adr.iadrjournals.org/cgi/content/full/17/1/77 (accessed December 27, 2007).
2. Susan Griffiths, "Virtual dentistry becomes reality in multimedia lab," *CWRU Campus News,* September 27, 2001, http://www.case.edu/pubs/cnews/2001/9-27/dent-sim.htm (accessed February 2, 2008).
3. Alice Urbankova and Richard Lichtenthal, "DentSim Virtual Reality in Preclinical Operative Dentistry to Improve Psychomotor Skills: A Pilot Study," 2002, http://www.denx.com/research_and_publication_details.asp?id=33 (accessed December 27, 2007).
4. S. Carpenter, "Lead and Bad Diet Give a Kick in the Teeth—Poor Children Are Most Susceptible to Lead Toxicity," June 26, 1999, http://findarticles.com/p/articles/mi_m1200/is_26_155/ai_55165309/pg_1 (accessed January 18, 2008).
5. Joe Hoyle, "Scientists Sequence Genome of Pathogen Associated with Gum Disease," March 3, 2004, http://www.ada.org/prof/resources/pubs/adanews/adanewsarticle.asp?articleid=805 (accessed December 27, 2007).
6. Jennifer Garvin, "Tooth Loss and Cardiovascular Disease," January 4, 2006, http://www.ada.org/prof/resources/pubs/adanews/adanewsarticle.asp?articleid=1735 (accessed December 27, 2007).
7. Nicholas Bakalar, "Gum Disease Is Linked to Rates of Early Birth," nyt.com, October 11, 2005, http://www.nytimes.com/2005/10/11/health/11teet.html (accessed December 27, 2007).
8. Joe Hoyle, "African-Americans Show Higher Prevalence of Periodontitis: Study," June 15, 2004, http://www.ada.org/prof/resources/pubs/adanews/adanewsarticle.asp?articleid=928 (accessed December 27, 2007).
9. "Link Found Between Periodontal Disease and Pancreatic Cancer," January 16, 2007, http://www.hsph.harvard.edu/news/press-releases/2007-releases/press01162007b.html (accessed November 26, 2007).
10. "Gum Disease Can Signal, Even Cause, Other Health Problems," 2005, http://www.dentalplans.com/Dental-Health-Articles/Gum-Disease-Can-Signal,-Even-Cause,-Other-Health-Problems.asp (accessed December 3, 2007).
11. Charles M. Cobb, "Lasers in Periodontics: A Review of the Literature," *Journal of Periodontal* (April 2006), http://www.perio.org/resources-products/pdf/lr-lasers.pdf (accessed December 27, 2007).
12. American Academy of Cosmetic Dentistry, "What Is Cosmetic Dentistry?" 2006, http://www.aacd.com/press/whatis.asp (accessed November 26, 2007).
13. Alton Bishop, Randol Womack, and Mitra Derakhshan, "An Esthetic and Removable Orthodontic Treatment Option for Patients: Invisalign®," *Dental Assistant,* September–October 2002, http://findarticles.com/p/articles/mi_m0MKX/is_5_71/ai_93306390 (accessed December 27, 2007).
14. Eneida Mendonca, "Clinical Decision Support Systems: Perspectives in Dentistry," *Journal of Dental Education* 68, no. 6 (2004): 589–97, http://www.jdentaled.org/cgi/content/full/68/6/589 (accessed December 27, 2007).
15. Kevin E. Smith, "Caries Detection: At Best an Inexact Science: Part II," *Global Dental Newsjournal* (2000), http://cc.msnscache.com/cache.aspx?q=72701680958301&mkt=en-US&lang=en-US&w=259df8d5&FORM=CVRE (accessed January 18, 2008).
16. Academy of General Dentistry, "Blade-Free Radiosurgery Offers New Cosmetic Surgery," 2006, http://www.agd.org (accessed August 10, 2006).
17. Jessica Gorman, "The New Cavity Fighters," *Science News,* August 19, 2000, http://www.sciencenews.org/articles/20000819/bob9.asp (accessed December 27, 2007).

ADDITIONAL RESOURCES

Alipour-Rocca, L., V. Kudryk, and T. Morris. "A Teledentistry Consultation System and Continuing Dental Education via Internet." *Journal of Medical Internet Research* 1 (1999): e110. http://www.jmir.org/1999/suppl1/e110 (accessed December 27, 2007).

American Association of Cosmetic Dentists. "Not Satisfied with Your Smile? You're Not Alone." July 15, 2002. http://www.aacd.com/press/releases/2002_07_15.asp (accessed December 27, 2007).

American Association of Cosmetic Dentists. "Seniors Benefit from Cosmetic Dentistry." June 3, 2002. http://www.aacd.com/press/releases/2003_06d.asp (accessed December 27, 2007).

American Dental Association. "Cosmetic Dentistry." 1995–2003. http://www.ada.org/public/topics/cosmetic.asp (accessed December 27, 2007).

Angier, Natalie. "Dentistry, Far Beyond Drilling and Filling." August 5, 2003. http://www.geocities.com/drkhosla1/News/newsa164.html (accessed August 24, 2006).

Clark, Glenn T. "Teledendistry: Genesis, Actualization, and Caveats." *Journal of the California Dental Association,* CDA (2000). http://www.cda.org/page/Library/cda_member/pubs/journal/jour0200/intro.html (accessed December 27, 2007).

Delrose, Daniel C. and Richard W. Steinberg. "The Clinical Significance of the Digital Patient Record." *JADA* 131 (June 2000): 57s–60s.

Diagnosis and Management of Dental Caries. "Summary." Evidence Report/Technology Assessment: Number 36. AHRQ Publication No. 01-E055. February 2001. http://www.ahrq.gov/clinic/epcsums/dentsumm.htm (accessed August 24, 2006).

Douglas, Chester W. and Cherilyn Sheets. "Patients' Expectations of Oral Health in the 21st Century." *JADA* 131 (June 2000): 3s–7s.

Dove, S. Brent. "Radiographic Diagnosis of Dental Caries." August 29, 2003. http://www.lib.umich.edu/dentlib/nihcdc/abstracts/dove.html (accessed December 27, 2007).

Drisco, Connie H. "Trends in Surgical and Nonsurgical Periodontal Treatment." *JADA.* 131 (June 2000): 31s–38s.

Fonseca, Raymond, Denice Stewart, M. Katie McGee, Noam Arzt, and Jeffery Stewart. "Remote Dental Consultation System." nd. http://64.233.169.104/search?q=cache:auH6oM1HOfkJ:collab.nlm.nih.gov/tutorialspublicationsandmaterials/telesymposiumcd/5A-3.pdf+Remote+Dental+Consultation+Project&hl=en&ct=clnk&cd=1&gl=us (accessed January 6, 2008).

Forrest, J. L. and S. A. Miller. "Evidence-Based Decision Making in Action: Part 1—Finding the Best Clinical Evidence." *Journal of Contemporary Dental Practice* 3, no. 3 (2002): 010–026. http://www.thejcdp.com/issue011/forrest/forrest.pdf (accessed December 27, 2007).

Freydberg, B. K. "Connecting to Success: Practice Management on the Net." *Journal of Contemporary Dental Practice* 2, no. 3 (2001): 050–061. http://www.thejcdp.com/issue007/freydbrg/freyberg.pdf (accessed December 27, 2007).

Glickman, Gerald N. and Kenneth Koch. "21st-Century Endodontics." June 2000. http://jada.ada.org/cgi/content/abstract/131/suppl_1/39S (accessed August 24, 2006).

Goshtasby, A. A. "Intelligent Systems Laboratory." nd. http://www.cs.wright.edu/people/faculty/agoshtas/nih.html (accessed January 6, 2008).

Griffin, Susan. "Virtual Dentistry Becomes Reality in Multimedia Lab." September 27, 2001. http://www.case.edu/pubs/cnews/2001/9-27/dent-sim.htm (accessed August 24, 2006).

Kurtzweil, Paula. "Dental More Gentle with Painless 'Drillings' and Matching Fillings." *FDA Consumer,* May–June, 1999. http://www.fda.gov/fdac/features/1999/399_dent.html (accessed December 27, 2007).

"Laser Dentistry." http://floss.com/ (accessed August 24, 2006).

"NIH Consensus Statement on Dental Caries Management." ADHA Online, 2003. http://www.adha.org/profissues/nih_consensus_statement.htm (accessed December 27, 2007).

Parks, E. T. and G. F. Williamson. "Digital Radiography: An Overview." *Journal of Contemporary Dental Practice* 3, no. 4 (2002): 023–039. http://www.thejcdp.com/issue012/williamson/index.htm (accessed December 27, 2007).

Scanlon, Jessie. "Say Ahhh (and Watch the Monitor)." nyt.com, September 4, 2003. http://query.nytimes.com/gst/fullpage.html?res=9B00E6D71038F937A3575AC0A9659C8B63 (accessed December 27, 2007).

Schneiderman, A., M. Elbaum, T. Shultz, S. Keem, M. Greenebaum, and J. Driller. "Assessment of Dental Caries with Digital Imaging Fiber-Optic Transillumination (DIFOTI): In Vitro Study." Abstract, 1997. http://www.ncbi.nlm.nih.gov/sites/entrez?db=pubmed&uid=9118181&cmd=showdetailview (accessed December 27, 2007).

Stabholz, A., R. Zeltser, M. Sela, et al. "The Use of Lasers in Dentistry: Principles of Operation and Clinical Applications." December 2003. http://www.ncbi.nlm.nih.gov/sites/entrez?cmd=Retrieve&db=PubMed&list_uids=14733160&dopt=AbstractPlus (accessed December 27, 2007).

Stheeman, S. E., P. F. van der Stelt, and P. A. Mileman. "Expert Systems in Dentistry. Past Performance—Future Prospects." April 1992. http://www.ncbi.nlm.nih.gov/sites/entrez?db=pubmed&uid=1564183&cmd=showdetailview (accessed December 27, 2007).

Stookey, George and Gonzalez-Cabezas. "Emerging Methods of Caries Diagnosis." October 2001. http://www.ncbi.nlm.nih.gov/entrez/query.fcgi?cmd=Retrieve&db=PubMed&dopt=Abstract&list_uids=11699969 (accessed August 24, 2006).

Valceanu, Anca. "Ultraconservative and Minimally Invasive Esthetic Restoration of Crown Fractures: Case Study." Summer 2006. https://www.aacd.com/downloads/journal/22-2valceanu.pdf (accessed December 27, 2007).

White, Joel M. and W. Stephen Eakle. "Rationale and Treatment Approach in Minimally Invasive Dentistry." June 2000. http://www.ncbi.nlm.nih.gov/entrez/query.fcgi?cmd=Retrieve&db=PubMed&list_uids=10860340&dopt=Abstract (accessed August 24, 2006).

Informational Resources: Computer-Assisted Instruction, Expert Systems, Health Information Online

CHAPTER OUTLINE

LEARNING OBJECTIVES

After reading this chapter, the student will be able to

- List the many informational resources that computer technology and the Internet have made available and their use in the health care fields.
- Describe the use of computer-assisted instruction (CAI) in health care education.
- Discuss the Visible Human Project; many simulation programs use data from this project.
- Describe simulation programs such as ADAM, which make use of text and graphics.
- Describe simulation programs which make use of virtual reality (VR) to teach surgical procedures, dentistry, and other skills.
- Define patient simulators.
- Be aware of the existence of distance learning programs in health care education.
- Discuss the role of expert systems, such as INTERNIST, MYCIN, and POEMS in health care.
- Describe the resources on the Internet, including medical literature databases, physicians' use of e-mail, general information and misinformation, and support groups, and be able to discuss both the positive and negative consequences of using the Internet as a resource for health information.
- Discuss the availability of self-help software.
- Discuss the uses of computers in psychiatry.

OVERVIEW

Computers and the Internet have made increasing amounts of information available to more people than in the past and have changed the way we teach and learn in many fields. Health care is no exception. Software exists to teach both providers and consumers of health care. The Internet makes vast stores of information available to patients and health care providers and can provide support for people with various illnesses. Self-help programs present information for consumers of health care. Databases, such as MEDLINE, and expert systems, such as MYCIN and INTERNIST, make the latest medical research easily available to health care professionals. The existence of these new informational resources has made it possible for health care professionals to learn in a variety of environments, via distance learning. These same developments have made it necessary for health care providers to be computer literate to take advantage of new and expanding sources of information.

EDUCATION

The Visible Human Project

The **Visible Human Project** is a computerized library of human anatomy at the National Library of Medicine. It began in 1986 and is an ongoing project. It has created "complete, anatomically detailed, three-dimensional representations of the male and female human body." The images are accessible over the Internet. Hundreds of people have used these images on computer screens where they can be rotated and flipped, taken apart and put back together. Structures can be enlarged and highlighted. The images, also available on CD-ROM, have been used by students of anatomy, researchers, surgeons, and dentists who discovered a new face muscle. There is some speculation that the Visible Human's virtual cadavers may replace actual cadavers in medical education. The Visible Human is available for both teaching and research. Some of the projects using data from the Visible Human include several three-dimensional views of the human body and images of magnetic resonance imaging (MRIs) and computed tomography (CT) scans. ADAM, a program, which is used to teach anatomy, uses data from the Visible Human. The data provided by the Visible Human is the source for a virtual colonoscopy.

The National Library of Medicine is moving the project "From Data to Knowledge." Some current aspects of the Visible Human will allow users to see *and feel* anatomic flythroughs on the Web and to see surrounding structures. Students can use a wand to create three-dimensional structures from two-dimensional structures or from segmented slices. Students will be able to build and palpate organs. An **Explorable Virtual Human** is being developed. It will include authoring tools that engineers can use to build anatomical models that will allow students to experience how real anatomical structures feel, appear, and sound.

One goal of the Visible Human was to allow the use of three-dimensional anatomical models in education. The **Vesalius Project** (Columbia University) is creating these models (called maximal models) of anatomical regions and structures to be used in teaching anatomy.[1]

A project called the **Virtual Human Embryo** is digitizing some of the 7000 human embryos lost in miscarriages, which have been kept by the National Museum of Health and Medicine of the Armed Forces Institute of Pathology since the 1880s. An embryo develops in twenty-three stages over the first eight weeks of pregnancy. The project will include at least one embryo from each stage. It will be sectioned and sliced. Each slice will be placed under a microscope, and digital images will be created. Users will be able to access the images on DVDs and CDs and manipulate and study them.

Computer-Assisted Instruction

Computer-assisted instruction (CAI) is used at all stages of the educational process. Drill-and-practice software is used to teach skills that require memorization. **Simulation software** simulates a complex process. The student is presented with a situation and given choices. The student is then shown what effect that choice would have on the situation. Early simulation programs used text and graphics to describe a situation. Later, animation and sound were added. Today, some programs use virtual reality (VR) so that the student actually feels as if he or she were there.

What is the effect of CAI on education for health care professionals? A quantitative analysis was performed of forty-seven studies of the use of CAI in the health science professions in 1992. The studies all compared student performance in CAI with traditional teaching methods. Thirty-two of the studies concluded that CAI is superior. However, the analysis of the studies also concluded that some of the forty-seven studies jumped to conclusions that were unsupported by the data they collected. The statistical analysis concludes that CAI does have a "moderate-sized effect." A later review of literature on CAI found that computers are having "surprisingly . . . a small impact on medical education." However, it was found to be a helpful supplement in some areas of study.

Simulation Software

Simulation programs have been used for many years in nursing education. As early as 1963, computer-based nursing courses were developed using **PLATO (Programmed Logic for Automatic Teaching Operations)**. The student sat before her or his "television screen and . . . electronic keyset similar to . . . a standard typewriter" and was presented with hypothetical patients to evaluate, problems to solve, and questions to answer. The program used both text and graphics. It was judged to be successful in allowing students to progress at their own pace and in their own style of learning. At that time, most schools did not have the computers necessary to use these programs. Now computers are used throughout the educational system, and simulation programs are a taken-for-granted part of health care education. Programs such as **ILIAD** have been used for years and provide hypothetical cases for the student to evaluate. The student's diagnostic abilities are then compared to the computer's. **ADAM** teaches anatomy and physiology. It uses two- and three-dimensional images (some of them created from the Visible Human data) and has versions available for both patients and professionals. It is interactive, allowing the user to click away over one hundred layers of the body and see more than four thousand structures! Using multiple windows, the user can compare different views of one anatomical structure. A program called eXpert Trainer helps students learn the skills needed for minimally invasive surgery (MIS) (see Chapter 7).

Virtual Reality Simulations

During the 1990s, several trends emerged to make VR surgical simulators possible. First, the Visible Human makes three-dimensional models possible. Second, "the rapid adoption of . . . minimally invasive procedures enabled surgeons to perform operations from outside the body and observe their actions on a video monitor." VR simulations can show exactly what the surgeon would see on the monitor. Third, haptic force-feedback systems allow the user to actually feel and manipulate objects in VR.[2]

The newest simulations use VR techniques, requiring the power of supercomputers. Simulations using VR can make medical education safer and more effective. They are particularly useful in teaching procedures, such as colonoscopies, which are guided by *haptic* clues (sense of feel) and where a mistake can seriously harm a patient (Figure 10.1 ■).

Now, before a medical resident operates on a live patient, surgery can be simulated. Students can manipulate surgical instruments while watching a computer

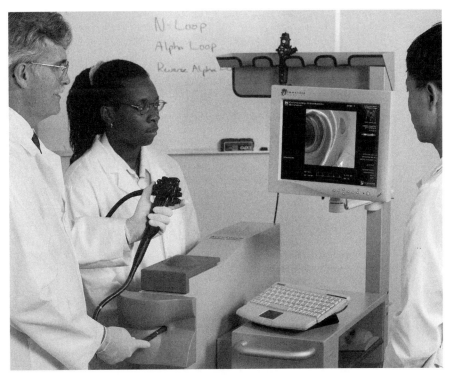

monitor. Motors in the instruments provide resistance so that the student learns how much pressure is required for a particular task (Figure 10.2 ■).

Using a device developed by Dr. Thomas Krummel, of the Penn State College of Medicine, the student can "actually feel . . . [the tissue] . . . as the needle goes through." Dr. Krummel has developed another device using a mannequin and computer imaging, which allows medical students to practice inserting a bronchoscope into a child's trachea. Dr. Krummel has also designed a program to teach surgical skills to new students at Pennsylvania State. The school uses a four-step program, which first teaches skills and then uses a three-dimensional anatomical program. The third step is to perform the tasks learned while monitored by a computer. The last step involves performing the operation on a simulator that mimics the human body and its responses.

VR simulations are also being used to train surgeons to perform minimally invasive operations.[3] Because the surgeon operates in a restricted field which she or he cannot directly see, MIS requires extensive training. One MIS trainer (called **KISMET**) uses "a rough imitation of the . . . abdomen . . . [so] the trainee [can] manipulate the instruments in the usual way. . . . KISMET does all the necessary calculations and generates the virtual endoscopic view."[4] KISMET also allows the student to feel and see how soft tissue reacts to grasping and cutting in real time.

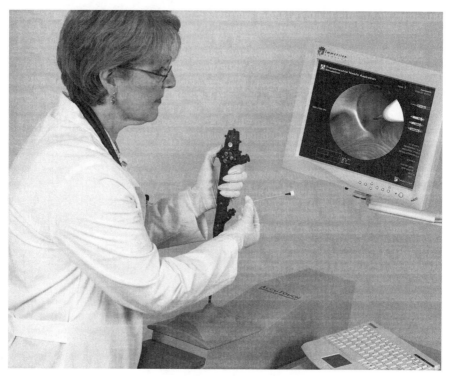

■ **FIGURE 10.2**   Simulation of a bronchoscopy. Reproduced by permission of Immersion Corporation, Copyright © 2007 Immersion Corporation. All rights reserved.

Simulations using VR are currently being developed to teach the administration of an epidural anesthetic, which requires the insertion of a catheter in the epidural space of the spinal column; the only guide is one's sense of feel. A mistake could leave a patient paralyzed. The epidural simulator allows the student to perform the procedure while feeling the resistance of the tissue, but without endangering a live patient. Students can learn to administer an intravenous (IV) from a simulation program instead of practicing on a rubber arm. "The student is able to sense the tactile response of needle and catheter insertion—from the 'pop' as the needle enters the skin through entry into the vein lumen." Simulations are also being used to help teach surgeons to operate on the prostate. As MIS becomes more common, VR simulators that mimic the sights, sounds, and feel of these procedures are being further developed. The Food and Drug Administration (FDA) approved the use of VR simulations to insert a catheter into the carotid artery.[5]

In dentistry, VR simulations make use of mannequins to allow students to practice filling cavities while watching both the mannequin and a monitor. The student feels the tooth via the instruments, learning to distinguish between a healthy and a diseased tooth. The student's work is immediately evaluated. The procedure can be repeated numerous times.

In 2002, researchers created the virtual stomach, a computer simulation. The stomach can be used to study how medications and nutrients decompose and are dispersed. Using the virtual stomach has already led to new knowledge: tablets break down at the bottom of the stomach, and the density of the tablets is important to the speed with which they break down.

Patient Simulators

Human patient simulators (HPS) are programmable mannequins on which students can practice medical procedures (Figures 10.3A–D ■). The simulator has liquids flowing through its blood vessels, inhales oxygen and exhales carbon dioxide, produces heart and lung sounds, has eyes that open and close, pupils that dilate, and a tongue that can swell to simulate an allergic reaction. The student can perform an electrocardiogram, take the pulse, and measure blood pressure and temperature. Medications can be administered intravenously; the mannequin reads the barcode and reacts as it has been programmed to react. Students can practice intubations. They can learn needle decompression of pneumothorax; chest tubes may be inserted. Different kinds of patients can be simulated including a healthy adult, a woman experiencing problems with pregnancy, and a middle-aged man suffering from hypertension. Another mannequin, called **PediaSim**, is a virtual child. It can be programmed also, for instance, to have an allergic reaction to peanuts.

These mannequins can be used in classrooms or in simulated emergency situations. A crowded corner of an emergency room can be simulated, with noise, time limits, and physical constraints for the student. This brings the simulation even closer to reality.

There are many patient simulators that focus on a particular type of patient and specific skills. The first childbirth simulator (not a VR simulator) was created in

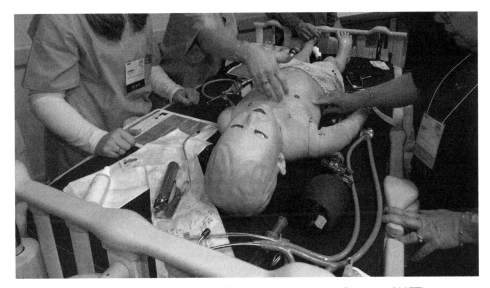

■ **FIGURE 10.3A**   PediaSim: the virtual child. Permission granted, Courtesy of METI.

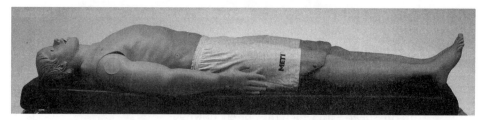

■ **FIGURE 10.3B** Human patient simulator (HPS). Permission granted, Courtesy of METI.

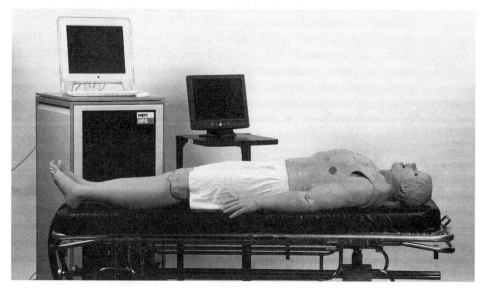

■ **FIGURE 10.3C** HPS System 2. Permission granted, Courtesy of METI.

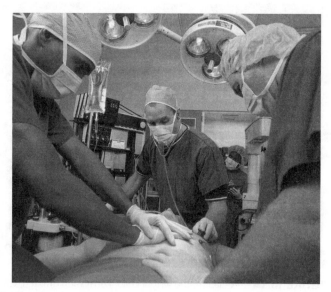

■ **FIGURE 10.3D** HPS in the operating room (OR). Permission granted, Courtesy of METI.

1949; now there are several. There are simulators for teaching laproscopic and endoscopic procedures in interaction with models. There are simulations of "heart attack, drug overdose, vehicular accidents, effects from weapons of mass destruction, bio-terrorism."[6]

Distance Learning

The expansion of information and telecommunications technology has made it possible to learn in a variety of settings—not just the traditional classroom. Distance learning refers to learning in an environment where student and instructor are not physically face-to-face. It may mean anything from simply picking up assignments on the Internet and e-mailing a paper to a professor, to a complete videoconference system where teacher and students see and hear each other via cameras, monitors, and microphones. Distance learning for health care professionals usually falls somewhere in between. A course may use Internet resources, videotapes, and CD-ROMs, along with traditional textbooks and other printed material. Both health science institutions and the government have made educational resources available over the Internet. Through the Learning Center for Interactive Technology, the National Library of Medicine's Cognitive Science Branch provides links to databases, information, and tutorials for health care professionals, making it possible for them to continue learning wherever there is a computer with a link to the Internet. It also is attempting to expand the opportunities for distance learning for health care professionals, and to link existing distance learning sites. Some traditional colleges and universities have degree programs at the graduate and undergraduate level in health sciences that do not require the student to be on campus, but do require self-discipline and access to a computer and the Internet. Public health workers may also learn via distance learning. The **Virtual Hospital** provides online courses for credit for health care professionals.

DECISION SUPPORT: EXPERT SYSTEMS

An expert system (or computerized decision support system) is an attempt to make a computer an expert in one narrow field. Both facts and rules about how the facts are used to make decisions in the field are entered in the computer. Expert systems are a branch of artificial intelligence, which examines how computers behave like human beings, that is, in "intelligent" ways. Expert systems have been used in medicine since the 1950s. They are meant to be decision support systems, which help, but do not replace, medical personnel. They are especially useful when there is a limited, well-defined area of knowledge needed for a decision, which will be based on objective data. The doctor enters symptoms, test results, and medical history. The computer either asks for more information or suggests a diagnosis, and perhaps treatment. Some systems give the diagnosis in the form of a probability.

The computer can suggest conditions that the doctor has not thought of since medical school or has simply not considered. However, it is up to the health care professional to confirm the suggestion by tests. Although these systems are very helpful, they have their drawbacks. Each system is an expert in only one limited area. Expert systems may also spend time eliminating conditions that human experts would not even need to consider. However, with the amount of information available today, a computer's ability to organize is crucial.

Studies of diagnostic software have had mixed results. One study of emergency room patients with chest pain found 97 percent accuracy rate for computers diagnosing heart attacks to 78 percent for doctors. A study of four programs found them to give correct diagnoses 50 to 75 percent of the time. In 1989, a trial using thirty-one undiagnosed cases compared the diagnosis of an expert system in the area of internal medicine called QMR to the best guess of the attending physician and found the following: the accuracy of the physician was 80 percent compared to 85 percent for the expert system and 60 percent for the house staff.

One early medical expert system was developed at Stanford University in 1970. Called **MYCIN**, it aids in the diagnosis and treatment of bacterial infections. The doctor types in data about the patient's symptoms; the computer asks for more information until it has enough to suggest a diagnosis. The computer then asks about any drug sensitivities the patient might have, so that treatment may be suggested. MYCIN's diagnostic accuracy equals or surpasses that of human specialists. **INTERNIST** is another expert system developed at the University of Pittsburgh. It contains information about 500 diseases and their 2900 associated symptoms. A newer expert system developed in England is called **Postoperative Expert Medical System (POEMS)**, which focuses on patients who become sick while recovering from surgery. The **Databank for Cardiovascular Disease** at Duke University is a highly specialized expert system that combines computer monitoring with extensive collections of information on cardiac patients.

In October 1998, a review of decision support systems was published in the *Journal of the American Medical Association (JAMA)*. The review looks at studies of the use of some of the systems during the past quarter century. The quality of expert systems varies. However, in certain areas, specifically, drug use and preventive medicine, "these systems have been shown to improve physician performance and, less frequently, improve patient outcomes."

■ HEALTH INFORMATION ON THE INTERNET

Both doctors and consumers who have access to it use the Internet as a source of health care information. Care should be used when searching for health information; the consumer is required to give personal information. This information is being mined for several purposes, including profiling the person most in need of a product or service. Several groups of health care professionals have created a suggested code of conduct for health-related Web sites: (i) that that they disclose any information that consumers would find useful, including financial ties; (ii) that they distinguish scientific information from advertising; (iii) that they attempt to assure the high quality of information; (iv) and that they disclose privacy risks and take steps to ensure privacy. Any health care professional giving advice or other information over the Web should abide by professional standards. The site needs to make it clear to consumers how they can get in touch with the site manager and should encourage feedback. Owing to the concern over the reliability (or unreliability) of health information, a professor at the University of Minnesota created a site to rate newspaper and magazine health articles.[7]

Some sites, including medical literature databases, are specifically meant for health care professionals. Sixty percent of doctors surveyed said they found Internet information helpful. Many sites are directed to consumers. There are at least 10,000 health-related sites on the Web (excluding support groups). According to the Federal Trade Commission, "consumer online searches for health information are increasing dramatically."[8] Tens of millions of people log on to the Internet looking for information about medication and disease, suggested cures, and support groups. The Internet (with all of its misinformation) has some reliable sites providing good information.

It should be noted that access to health-related information on the Internet is not equally distributed through society, but is restricted to those with access to computers with an Internet connection and the knowledge to make use of them. The digital divide refers to the gap between information haves and have-nots. White and Asian Americans, those with higher incomes, and those with higher education are more likely to have computer and Internet access than low-income, less educated people, and African-Americans and Hispanics. People in rural areas have less access to the Internet than people in urban areas. A February 2002 report from the federal government maintained that the digital divide was disappearing quickly. The Bush administration then lowered funding to government programs that supported community computing centers. However, a 2003 study by sociologist, Dr. Steven Martin at the University of Maryland, concluded that, "Computer ownership and Internet use may actually be spreading less quickly among poorer households than among richer households." Between 1998 and 2001, Internet use grew from 14 to 25 percent among families with annual incomes of less than $15,000; it grew from 59 to 79 percent among families with incomes greater than $75,000. The odds that a poor family would use the Internet grew by a factor of 2.1, whereas the odds for an affluent family grew by 2.6 percent. Dr. Martin predicts that it will be another 20 years before 90 percent of the poorest quarter of the population owns computers.[9]

By 2003, 61.8 percent of U.S. households owned computers, and of those 87.6 percent were linked to the Internet. The percentage of households with broadband connections grew from 9.1 to 19.9 percent from 2001 to 2003. Those with broadband connections are more likely to use the Internet than those with dial-up connections.[10] Although the digital divide is shrinking, it still persists in 2006, according to a federal report. Race and ethnicity, family income, and education all influence Internet use among students. At school, among white students, 67 percent use the Internet; this compares to 58 percent for Asian-Americans, 47 percent for African-American and Native American students, and 44 percent for Hispanic students. At home, 54 percent of white students, 27 percent of Black students, and 26 percent of Hispanic students use the internet. The higher the family income, the more likely a student is to use the Internet (at home or in school). The more education a parent has, the higher the Internet use. Lower use in some ethnic groups is tied to poverty.[11]

In a Pew survey reported in the *New York Times* in March 2006, among adults eighteen and older, "74 percent of whites go online, 61 percent of African-American do and 80 percent of English-speaking Hispanic adults report using the Internet." This compares to the results of a similar study completed in 1998: 42 percent of white adults, 40 percent of Hispanics, and 23 percent of African-American adults reported using the Internet. Among adults as well as among children, higher household income and education are correlated positively with Internet use. Age also correlates negatively with Internet use.[12]

Medical Literature Databases

The capacity of computers to store and organize huge collections of data, to make it accessible, and to transmit it over telecommunications lines forms the basis of online medical literature databases (Figures 10.4 A and B ■). The National Library of Medicine

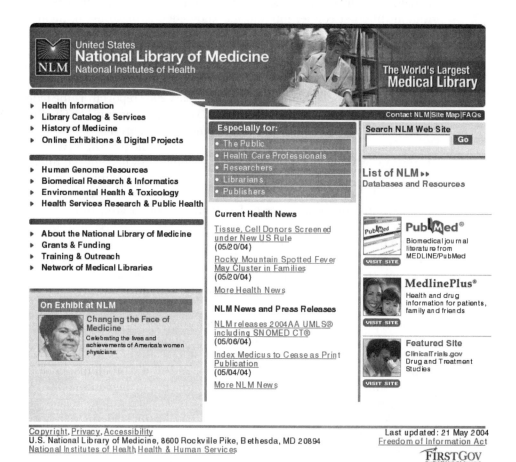

■ **FIGURE 10.4A**   The National Library of Medicine maintains many medical literature databases. Courtesy of National Institutes of Health.

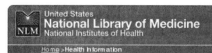

United States
National Library of Medicine
National Institutes of Health

Home >Health Information

Health Information

🖶 Printer-friendly Version

▶ **MedlinePlus - Health Information**
- Over 600 health topics
- A medical encyclopedia with images
- Drug information - Hospitals and physicians
- Latest health news

More about MedlinePlus (Fact Sheet) |Tour |FAQs |MedlinePlus en español

Find a Health Topic by First Letter:
A B C D E F G H I J K L M N O P Q R S T U V W XYZ

▶ **ClinicalTrials.gov**

Provides the public information about clinical trials and opportunities to participate in the evaluation of new treatments and drugs.
More about ClinicalTrials.gov (Fact Sheet) |FAQs
Also see: Clinical Alerts and Advisories

▶ **NIHSeniorHealth**

A web site designed to meet the needs of older adults. Seniors and caregivers can find information on selected topics in an easy-to-read format.

▶ **Tox Town**

An interactive guide about how the environment, chemicals and toxic substances affect human health.
More about ToxTown (Fact Sheet) |Tox Town en español

▶ **Household Products Database**

Information on the health effects of common household products under your sink, in the garage, in the bathroom and on the laundry room shelf.

▶ **Genetics Home Reference (GHR)**

Information about genetic conditions and the genes responsible for those conditions. Includes descriptions of the symptoms, diagnostic process, and treatment options.
More about GHR (Fact Sheet) |Help Me Understand Genetics

▶ **MEDLINE/PubMed - Biomedical Journal Literature**

Provides access to over 12 million references from 4600 biomedical journals. Many of these references link to abstracts and in some cases, the full text of articles.
MEDLINE Fact Sheet |PubMed Fact Sheet|Tutorial |FAQs

▶ **AIDSInfo**

A central resource for current information on clinical trials for AIDS patients, federally approved HIV treatment and prevention guidelines.

Subscribe

Sign up to receive MedlinePlus announcements of new health topics, resources and news headlines.

Related Products/Services

Guide to Healthy Web Surfing
Know what to look for when evaluating the quality of health information on the web.

Health Hotlines
Health-related organizations operating toll-free telephone services

DIRLINE
Directory of health organizations online

■ **FIGURE 10.4B**   The National Library of Medicine *(continued)*.

provides a collection of computerized databases called **MEDLARS (Medical Literature Analysis and Retrieval System)**. The forty databases contain eighteen million references. They are available free via the Internet and can be searched for bibliographical lists or for information.

MEDLINE is a comprehensive online database of current medical research including publications from 1966 to the present containing 8.5 million articles from 3700 journals. Thirty-one thousand citations are added each month. It has been used in hospitals for years. MEDLINE can be used for academic research or to help a doctor identify a patient's problem. Because MEDLINE is updated daily, it gives access to the most up-to-date information to health care personnel (Figure 10.5 ■). Although the information in MEDLINE is meant for professionals, 30 percent of its users are patients. **SDILINE (Selective Dissemination of Information Online)**

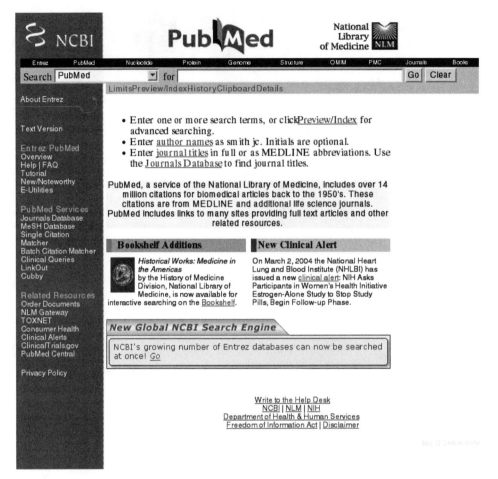

■ **FIGURE 10.5**   PubMed is the search engine used to search Medline. Courtesy of National Institutes of Health.

contains only the latest month's additions to MEDLINE. Other MEDLARS databases include AIDSLINE, AIDSTRIALS, and CANCERLIT. DIRLINE is a guide to online information.

CINAHL (Cumulative Index to Nursing and Allied Health Literature) is a database specifically geared to the needs of nurses and other professionals in seventeen allied health fields. This includes the fields of dental hygiene, occupational therapy, and radiology. CINAHL includes an index of 1000 journals from 1982 to the present, bibliographic citations of books, pamphlets, software, and standards of practice, abstracts or full text of articles where they are available, journals, and descriptions of Web sites.

In 1998, the National Library of Medicine introduced MEDLINEplus, which is meant for the general public (Figure 10.6 ■). In 2001, there were 2.3 hits per month. The information is selected using strict guidelines to guarantee accuracy and objectivity.

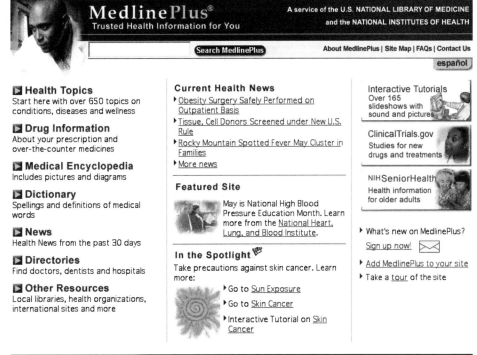

■ FIGURE 10.6   MEDLINEPlus is a database maintained for consumers. Courtesy of National Institutes of Health.

Databases of drug information are also online. **Medi-Span** is a collection of data on drug/drug and drug/food interactions. **Clinical pharmacology** is a database for health care professionals, with the latest information on drugs. It also contains information for doctors to distribute to their patients. **New Medicines in Development** provides information on drugs that have been recently approved and those awaiting approval. **ClinicalTrials.gov** was launched in February 2000; it lists thousands of clinical trials along with their purpose, criteria for participation, location, and contact information (Figure 10.7 ■). **Centerwatch** maintains a Web site that lists 41,000 current clinical trials in the United States. It should be noted, however, that the purpose of drug trials is to test the effectiveness and safety of the medication, not to help those patients participating in the trial. There have been questions raised regarding ethics and adequate safeguards for human subjects who might be drawn in to participating in clinical trials by desperation stemming from illness or poverty. Only one-half of the people who participate in clinical drug trials are actually administered the drug being tested. The other half is given a placebo. Not even the physician knows which patient is receiving which substance. For those interested in the records of drugs that are already on the market, the U.S. FDA's Center for

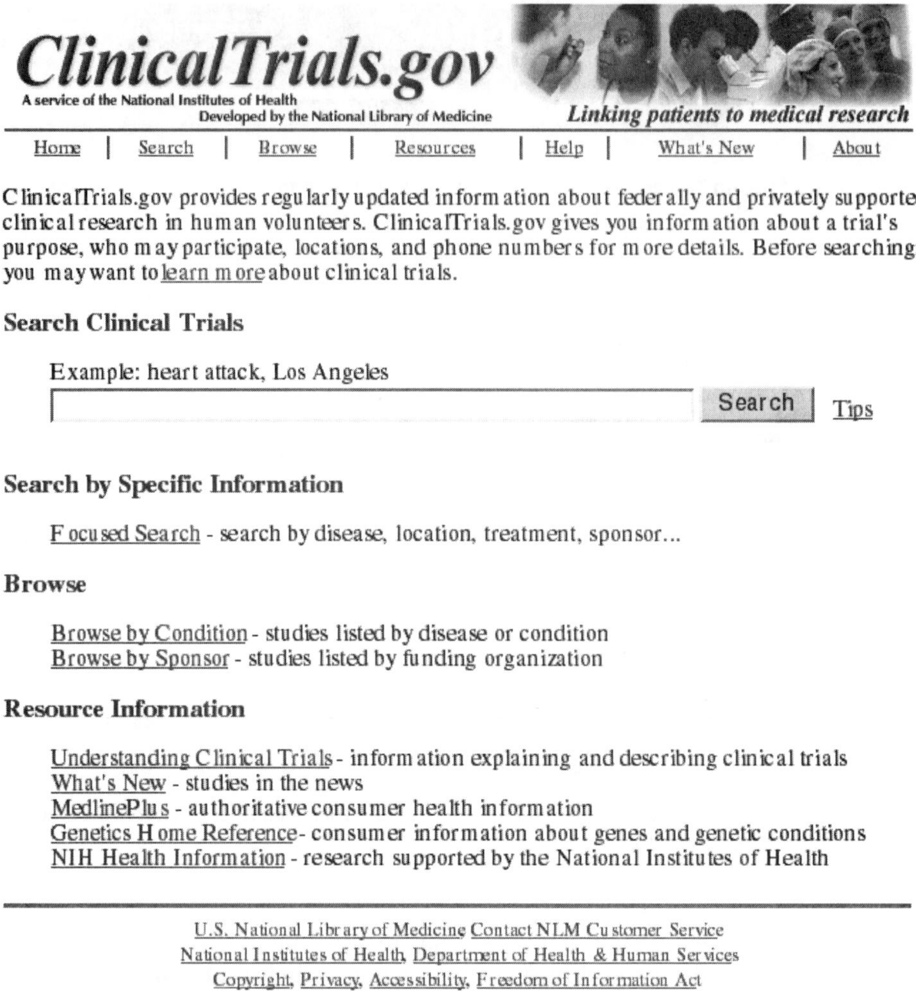

ClinicalTrials.gov

A service of the National Institutes of Health
Developed by the National Library of Medicine

Linking patients to medical research

Home | Search | Browse | Resources | Help | What's New | About

ClinicalTrials.gov provides regularly updated information about federally and privately supported clinical research in human volunteers. ClinicalTrials.gov gives you information about a trial's purpose, who may participate, locations, and phone numbers for more details. Before searching, you may want to learn more about clinical trials.

Search Clinical Trials

Example: heart attack, Los Angeles

| Search | Tips

Search by Specific Information

Focused Search - search by disease, location, treatment, sponsor...

Browse

Browse by Condition - studies listed by disease or condition
Browse by Sponsor - studies listed by funding organization

Resource Information

Understanding Clinical Trials - information explaining and describing clinical trials
What's New - studies in the news
MedlinePlus - authoritative consumer health information
Genetics Home Reference - consumer information about genes and genetic conditions
NIH Health Information - research supported by the National Institutes of Health

U.S. National Library of Medicine Contact NLM Customer Service
National Institutes of Health, Department of Health & Human Services
Copyright, Privacy, Accessibility, Freedom of Information Act

■ **FIGURE 10.7**   ClinicalTrails.gov is a Web site providing information on current clinical trials. Courtesy of National Institutes of Health.

Drug Evaluation and Research maintains a site that provides information on the safety records of drugs and on drug companies and advertisement campaigns. Of course, you should judge information from the FDA as you would information from any other site, bearing in mind that much of the FDA's drug evaluation budget comes from the drug companies it oversees.

Although the existence of these resources is widely known, the effect of their use is not. A review of the literature on the use and effectiveness of electronic information retrieval systems was published in *JAMA* in October 1998. The study found that use is limited: although "physicians have 2 unanswered questions for every 3 patients," they use a computer to search for information only "0.3 to 9 times per physician per month."[13] Further, "most searches retrieve only one fourth to one half of the relevant articles . . ." and how the information retrieved is actually used is not known.

E-mail

A majority of health care consumers who go online to search for advice would prefer information from their own doctors online. Many patients want to establish an e-mail connection with their own physicians. Not only is the information likely to be reliable, but some found an e-mail consultation less intimidating than a face-to-face meeting, enabling them to ask questions that they would not otherwise ask. Yet, few doctors make it available. Doctors express concerns with the time it would take to read and respond to e-mail, problems of liability, and issues of confidentiality and privacy. However, one three-year study of a pediatric practice, which offered free e-mail as an option, found it was an effective way for doctors and patients and their families to communicate. In thirty-three months, a total of 1239 e-mails were received from parents (81 percent) and health care providers (19 percent) alike. Some requested general information (69 percent); others had specific questions (22 percent). Most (87 percent) were answered immediately with suggested treatment and the recommendation to see a doctor. "On average, reading and responding to each e-mail took slightly less than 4 minutes."[14]

Other practices do not deal with e-mail in the same way. In a study of unsolicited e-mail, a fictitious patient sent e-mail to fifty-eight dermatology Web sites around the world. Although the message asked for help with a problem that required attention immediately, only one-half the sites responded. However, of those that responded, more than 90 percent recommended that the patient see a doctor, and 59 percent diagnosed the condition correctly. A questionnaire was sent to the sites that had responded: 28 percent said that they usually do not answer any patient e-mail. Only 24 percent said they answer e-mail communications individually.

In April 2002, a survey was conducted asking doctors and patients for their attitudes towards e-mail. It found that 90 percent of patients would like to exchange e-mail with their physicians, whereas only 15 percent of doctors do exchange e-mail with their patients. Doctors cite concerns with liability (a paper trail), privacy, time, the possibilities of misunderstanding, and the slowness of e-mail compared with conversation. The small percent of doctors who provide e-mail state that patients are calmer when they know there is an open line to their physicians and therefore do not need to communicate as much. Some doctors who provide e-mail for their patients maintain that "no malpractice lawsuits . . . had been filed in which e-mail played a role."[15]

Self-Help on the Web

Tens of millions of adults search the Web for health-related information. Some people visiting health-related web sites may just be doing academic research or seeking to learn. However, many are looking for a diagnosis, treatment, and cure. The numbers of sites either providing advice or linking to sites that provide advice are too numerous to list. Many sites include disclaimers stating in general that, although they attempt to include only accurate information, they are not responsible for the validity of the information presented. The disclaimer may further advise that a medical professional be consulted before any treatment is either started or discontinued. There are sites devoted to almost any disease, condition, treatment, and drug. You can find self-help for depression, stress, addiction, and almost any personal problem you can name. You do not even need to name your problem. One site shows you a human body and invites you to click where it hurts. You are then presented with a list of possible body parts and their possible diseases. If you continue to click, you will be linked to sites that can provide you with information and advice, from "how to treat your own . . ." to where to go for professional help.

Information is not the only online health-related resource. A possibly dangerous development is the availability of both prescription and nonprescription drugs on the Web. The sale of drugs over the Internet is virtually unregulated. A person can log on in one state, find a pharmacy in another state, "consult" (over telecommunications lines) with a doctor, who will then write a prescription, which will be filled through the mail. The prescriptions are signed by physicians whose "examination" of the "patient" may consist of a review of a short questionnaire. Several states are investigating this development, which is (according to several medical boards) either "illegal or does not meet accepted standards of care." In August 2006, two doctors were charged for sending prescription drugs without a face-to-face meeting.[16] Nonprescription drugs are also available.

Support Groups on the Web

The Web provides online support. There are support groups for hospitalized children, people with cancer and other diseases, and for their families and caregivers. Newsgroups, e-mail discussion groups, and live chat groups are available that link people with health- or disease-related interests. **Starbright World** is a network linking 30,000 seriously ill children in one hundred hospitals and many homes in North America. Children in the network can play games, chat, and send and receive e-mail. They can also get medical information.

Support groups exist for virtually every illness. When Dr. Ken Mott, a public health physician, was diagnosed with cancer, he had to travel to receive the treatment he needed. Illness can be isolating. Being in a strange city can compound the isolation. But Dr. Mott, like many other patients, found support and community on the World Wide Web. "Physical disability and pain . . . physical and emotional isolation occur . . . [and] the . . . side effects of treatment . . . leave victims susceptible to depression and withdrawal. But on the Internet and through e-mail I find dimensions of communication for emotional and psychological support that you may not have imagined."[17] It is especially helpful for people with rare diseases. Takayasu arteritis occurs in between 1.2 and 2.6 people per million scattered over the world, making it virtually impossible to form face-to-face support groups. Yet, now the Internet is being used to build a community and disseminate information and give support.

Judging the Reliability of Health Information on the Internet

Anyone can offer information on the Web, with possibly dangerous results. A compliance officer at the FDA related one instance, "A physician was browsing the Web when he came across a site that contained a fraudulent drug offering . . . the person who maintains the site claimed he had a cure for a very serious disease, and advised those with the disease to stop taking their prescription medication. Instead they were told to buy the product he was selling, at a cost of several hundred dollars." Web sites can be run by anyone. More and more sites providing medical information are being operated by unidentified sources, vendors, and manufacturers; many sites are produced by patients. Judging the reliability of a Web site can be difficult. The U.S. Department of Health and Human Services has established a site called http:// healthfinder.gov to help guide people toward reliable sources of information.

In addition, in response to the need to judge the reliability of health information on the Internet, commercial online services have been created. They will research information and clinical trials for you for a fee of between $150 and $500. There are only ten small companies, and no one judges their reliability. Users are advised to look into the qualifications of the searchers and to make sure they do not receive any money from drug companies. Of course, users do not have to hire a service to judge information.

The American Medical Association advises users to judge Web sites as critically as they would judge printed information. The major concern of people using the Web for medical information is privacy. Even though most sites have stated privacy policies, a study found that most do not adhere to them. Users have no way of knowing this. The actual content of the site should be judged on the following criteria: Is there information on the author and is the author reliable? Are the sources of information clear and reliable? Are the sources of funding revealed? Are there any conflicts of interest, for example, does the author or site receive money from any source interested in steering the user toward a particular treatment? Is the information up-to-date? Conflicts of interest bearing on money received from a drug or device company are the most important information to reveal. This does not necessarily make the information invalid. However, you should be very careful using that information and should find backup from another source.

Even reliable sites can provide partial information to doctors as well as to patients. According to one physician, the Web is as attractive to physicians as it is to patients. But even the best sites are incomplete at best. A MEDLINE search produces abstracts of articles, not the articles themselves. The abstract states the conclusion of a study, for example, that a heart drug was found to be effective, but that is not enough information. The abstract leaves out the necessary details: who were the participants and how were they selected, what other medications were they taking, how was the data analyzed, and who designed and financed the study?

Reliable sites do exist. The Virtual Hospital is a comprehensive and authoritative site, which was maintained by the University of Iowa between 1992 and 2006 when its funding was cut. It provides information for patients and health care providers. Its information comes from 350 peer-reviewed sources. Every page displayed contains the author's name, degree, and the peer-review status of the content. Material is presented in a multimedia format and is organized both by type of information (e.g., textbook) and by problem. A health care provider can read a chapter on upper respiratory conditions and view a video clip of the condition. Providers can also complete continuing education credits through the Virtual Hospital by taking an online test. The Virtual Hospital provides information for patients on disease prevention, including immunizations, diet, and cancer screening. Reliable information is also available through **Medscape**, which provides a collection of medical journals online.

SELF-HELP SOFTWARE

For those without an Internet connection, self-help software on CD-ROM provides information, suggests diagnosis and treatment, and may even act as a therapist for people with mild-to-moderate emotional problems, including stress, eating disorders, sexual dysfunction, and depression. Before attempting any self-treatment or taking any medication (even over-the-counter nonprescription medications) and before taking advice on the Internet, you should always check with your physician.

Family health guides on CD-ROM provide more information than a book and are easier to search. According to the president of the Consumer Health Information Research Institute: "They cover a lot of general information very well."

The information you need is on your screen at the click of a mouse. The *Mayo Clinic Family Health Book on CD-ROM* is a comprehensive source of information on health, illness, and medications. The user can quickly learn from text, graphics, and video, how to stop a bleeding cut. The *Doctor's Book of Home Remedies* is a source of information on alternative remedies—such as garlic and salt water for a cold. *Medical HouseCall* allows the user to enter his or her symptoms and responds with possible diagnoses, as well as advice on calling the doctor. Some programs allow the user to enter complete medical histories for each family member. Other guides focus on medications, or fitness, or a specific condition.

COMPUTERS AND PSYCHIATRY

Computers play a part in psychiatry from diagnosis to treatment. **CIDI (Composite International Diagnostic Interview)** is an interview that screens for depression and anxiety. Computers have been used as a tool to screen teenagers for a variety of conditions including suicidal tendencies. A program developed at the Columbia University College of Physicians and Surgeons prompts the interviewer to ask three thousand questions and follow-ups. Anyone flagged by the computer is seen by a psychologist who then makes the diagnosis. Many psychological diagnostic tests, such as **CIDI-Auto**, are self-administered. One company advertises self-administered tests that they claim will help diagnose addiction, thought errors, and even criminal tendencies. They do warn, however, that these diagnoses are meant as suggestions only; they are not conclusive.

The first uses of computers in psychotherapy were in testing; later studies found the online tests comparable to traditional testing. Computers can be better at information gathering than clinicians. Some studies found that some people are more open with a computer-administered interview. More people were willing to participate in a computer-administered interview. A series of studies in 2004 found that computers and the Internet were helpful aids to therapy. "Technological applications . . . include self-help Internet sites, computer-administered therapy, virtual reality therapy . . ." to name a few.[18] The Web-based Depression and Anxiety Test was found effective in diagnosing anxiety disorders and depression. "In computer-guided therapy, the computer itself both determines and provides the feedback to the patient." Several programs that are effective include Fear Fighter for phobias and panic, BTSteps for OCD, Cope and Overcoming Depression Course for depression, and Balance for general anxiety disorder. Two programs have been found helpful for drinking—Behaviorial Self-Control Program for Windows and Drinker's Checkup. Beating the Blues for depression and anxiety was found more effective than live therapy, and computer-aided therapy is cheaper. Although all patients using computer-aided therapies were in telephone contact with live therapists, computers apparently do a good job at some sorts of therapies. There is computer-aided self-help for phobia/panic, nonsuicidal depression, and obsessive-compulsive disorder (OCD). Some patients with OCD and depression were given a self-help book with a telephone number to call a computer-operated interactive voice system. Self-help exposure programs on the Internet or on a PC aided people with panic disorder. Clients can carry palmtops which remind them of techniques to be used in everyday life; this is used as an aid in treating people with generalized anxiety disorder and social phobia. The Web can bring therapy to patients whose conditions may make them unlikely to seek treatment (including those with agoraphobia or OCD).

Later studies tended to confirm the 2004 studies. Online screening programs for anxiety and mood disorders have been "generally equivalent" to assessment by a therapist.[19] Some self-help programs on computers have been shown to be effective; on the Internet users can get feedback, making the programs more helpful. Internet-based treatment was found to be as effective as face-to-face treatment in a number of randomized clinical trials. The use of VR is treating certain phobias and has also been tested in randomized clinical trials and found effective. VR is being used to treat soldiers returning from Iraq with posttraumatic stress disorder.[20] Internet therapy (Interapy) for those suffering from posttraumatic stress disorder was found to be very effective through self-reports. Interapy is also being tried for work-related stress. Interapy was found to be ineffective in treating insomnia. The Internet-based treatment was cognitive behavior therapy in all cases studied. Anxiety disorders have been treated for many years with controlled exposure to whatever provokes the anxiety. Investigations are being performed to see whether the exposure can be done using VR technology.

CONCLUSION

Information technology, specifically the explosive growth of the Internet, has made more information available to more people than ever before. However, the quality of the information varies. Moreover, access is not equally distributed across society, but is restricted to those with computers with Internet connections. Both health care professionals and consumers use these new informational resources. The effects of the use of expert systems and extensive medical literature databases available to health care professionals have not been extensively studied. They apparently do improve physician performance in some areas. There is accurate general information available for health care consumers. However, extreme caution must be exercised in using the Internet or self-help software as a source of health care information.

IN THE NEWS

Excerpt from, "Correcting the Errors of Disclosure"

by Benedict Carey

By now, tales of scientific conflict of interest have become all too familiar. In recent weeks, two top medical journals have been in the news for failing to disclose the financial ties of the academic authors of published papers, one involving antidepressant drugs, the other a medical device approved to treat depression.

But nondisclosure is only part of the story. Companies don't just hire doctors to do research—a practice that in theory ought to help keep businesses scientifically honest—they also trade on the researchers' names. Like producers shopping a new a movie, they go for star power, an A-list cast with names that themselves sell a product, and pull other doctors along, even when the evidence for a treatment is not strong.

Last week, an influential psychiatry journal, Neuropsychopharmacology, said it would print a correction, after revelations that it did not disclose the financial ties of authors of a paper reviewing a new treatment for depression. The treatment, a $15,000 chest implant that sends pulses of electricity to the brain, was approved for depression in 2005 after intense debate over its effectiveness.

At least as important as the failure to disclose financial ties were the authors themselves, and other consultants that the device manufacturer, Cyberonics Inc. of Houston, had hired.

Among them are Dr. Charles Nemeroff, one of the nation's most influential research psychiatrists and the editor of Neuropsychopharmacology; Dr. Dennis S. Charney, of the Mount Sinai School of Medicine, the editor of Biological Psychiatry; and Dr. A. John Rush of the University of Texas Southwestern Medical Center, who led the largest-ever long-term government study on depression.

These are precisely the sorts of experts the field relies on to help evaluate highly disputed data, like those Cyberonics has presented for the treatment.

In a bitter debate over the interpretation of these results, more than 20 experts at the Food and Drug Administration opposed the approval of the device for depression before being overruled by a senior official. . . .

"This is what companies do, try to get top researchers to accept large grants for research, or to consult, because they know those names make them look more legit," said Dr. Daniel Carlat, editor in chief of The Carlat Psychiatry Report . . . who in January reviewed the evidence for the implant and found it unconvincing.

The very presence of those names on papers reviewing the treatment, he said, "is a big part of the salesmanship that comes after getting approval."

One of the company's primary consultants, Harold Sackeim, a professor of psychiatry and radiology at Columbia, said that if device makers could not hire the field's top experts, effective new devices would never be approved. . . .

He added that he and other academic doctors advising the company "are a pretty small group, we all know each other, and the gestalt in the group carries a lot of weight."

The company has focused on promotion, as have some of its consultants. At an American Psychiatry Association meeting . . . Dr. Rush sat in the Cyberonics booth, describing the benefits of the therapy to curious psychiatrists. . . .

And the recent review article that appeared without full disclosure was not focused on whether the device worked for depression, or for whom. It was a speculative essay about its mechanism of action—about how it worked.

One of the supposed strengths of American science is that it is decentralized and diverse: there are dozens of top researchers who are competitive and critical, enforcing a high standard. But when many or most of the leading figures are playing for the same team—an all-star team—that lineup itself may carry the day, regardless of the science.

CHAPTER SUMMARY

Chapter 10 introduces the reader to the vast informational resources made available by computer technology and the Internet.

- Computer-assisted instruction has been used in the education of health care professionals since the 1960s.
  - Drill-and-practice software teaches facts that require memorization.
  - Simulations teach students to evaluate situations and solve problems, as well as teaching skills. Some simulation programs use data from the Visible Human, an ongoing project that contains thousands of images of one male and one female cadaver.
  - Currently, simulation programs are making use of virtual reality techniques, so that the student actually feels as if he or she were performing a procedure. Simulations using virtual reality are used to teach many skills including surgical procedures, administration of epidural anesthesia, and dentistry.

- Patient simulators provide realistic programmable mannequins on which students can practice procedures.
- Computers and telecommunications have made distance learning possible.
- Expert systems such as INTERNIST, MYCIN, and POEMS are used as decision support systems to help in diagnosis.
- The Internet makes a huge amount of information (and misinformation) available to both health care providers and patients. The effects of its use have not yet been evaluated.
  - Medical literature databases such as MEDLINE provide access to the latest research.
  - The Internet provides opportunities for lifelong, distance learning for health care professionals.
  - Health-related information on the Web can be accurate (such as that provided by the Virtual Hospital) or of dubious value. The user must use caution and common sense. The Internet also has online support groups for people with illnesses and for their families.
- Self-help software is available on CD-ROM and, if used with caution, may provide useful information.
- Some computer programs appear to help those with various conditions, such as OCD, panic disorders, and posttraumatic stress disorder.
- Information should be carefully and critically scrutinized. Always look at the credentials of authors and who is paying for the research. Look for any ties between researchers and the devices and medications they are investigating. Be aware of conflicts of interest.

KEY TERMS

ADAM
Centerwatch
CIDI (Composite International Diagnostic Interview)
CIDI-Auto
CINAHL (Cumulative Index to Nursing and Allied Health Literature)
clinical pharmacology
ClinicalTrials.gov
Databank for Cardiovascular Disease

Explorable Virtual Human
human patient simulators
ILIAD
INTERNIST
KISMET
Medi-Span
MEDLARS (Medical Literature Analysis and Retrieval System)
MEDLINE
Medscape
MYCIN
New Medicines in Development
PediaSim

PLATO (Programmed Logic for Automatic Teaching Operations)
Postoperative Expert Medical System (POEMS)
SDILINE (Selective Dissemination of Information Online)
simulation software
Starbright World
Vesalius Project
Virtual Hospital
Virtual Human Embryo
Visible Human Project

REVIEW EXERCISES

Multiple Choice

1. The most comprehensive medical literature database is _____.
   A. SDILINE
   B. AIDSLINE
   C. MEDLINE
   D. None of the above

2. _____ is a programmable mannequin of a child on which students can practice procedures.
   A. Childsim
   B. PediaSim
   C. The Small Virtual Patient
   D. None of the above

3. _____ is an expert system that helps in diagnosis.
   A. MYCIN
   B. INTERNIST
   C. None of the above
   D. A and B are both expert systems

4. _____ is a computerized library of human anatomy.
   A. The Visible Human
   B. The Virtual Hospital
   C. The Databank of Cardiovascular Disease
   D. None of the above

5. The best place to look for *authoritative* general health care information online for consumers would be _____.
   A. Medlineplus
   B. Centerwatch
   C. Any search will find authoritative information
   D. There is no reliable information on the Internet.

6. Which of the following is likely to be a source of reliable health care information on the Internet?
   A. A site maintained by a drug company
   B. A site maintained by a patient
   C. A site maintained by a university
   D. None of the above is likely to provide reliable information.

7. _____ is a database of the most recent additions to MEDLINE.
   A. MEDLARS
   B. AIDSLINE
   C. NEWLINE
   D. SDILINE

8. Which of the following is currently being taught with the aid of simulations using virtual reality?
    A. Minimally invasive surgical techniques
    B. The administration of epidural anesthesia
    C. Some aspects of dentistry
    D. All of the above
9. _____ is a program which teaches anatomy by allowing the student to use a mouse to click away layers of the body.
    A. ILIAD
    B. ADAM
    C. KISMET
    D. None of the above
10. It is not difficult to find support groups on the Web. Starbright World _____.
    A. attempts to link seriously ill children in hospitals in the United States
    B. is a network of AIDS patients
    C. is a network of people with cancer
    D. is a network of families of people with cancer.

True/False Questions

1. Expert systems will eventually replace doctors. _____
2. All the information on the Internet is reliable and accurate. _____
3. MEDLARS is a collection of medical literature databases. _____
4. The Visible Human provides anatomically detailed, three-dimensional representations of the male and female human body. _____
5. The Virtual Hospital was a service of the University of Iowa that provided up-to-date, accurate health-related information on the Web. _____
6. In order to post health-related information on the Internet, a person needs to pass a rigorous exam. _____
7. Information on current clinical drug trials is available on the Internet. _____
8. Some studies have contended that there are programs which are helpful in treating mild clinical depression. _____
9. ADAM is a program that teaches anatomy. _____
10. Simulation programs were used in health care education as far back as 1949. _____

Critical Thinking

1. Discuss the advantages and disadvantages of using virtual reality simulations in health care education.
2. It is possible to become a physician assistant in a distance learning program without being physically present on a campus or setting foot in a classroom. How do you think this might affect education?
3. Given the many uses of information technology in health care today, anyone entering a health care field must be computer literate and computer competent. Discuss this statement.
4. The Internet provides unparalleled informational resources for both consumers and providers of health care. This may be helpful. However, it may be quite

dangerous. Comment on the positive and negative aspects of the availability of health-related information on the Internet.

5. One of the characteristics of the Internet is anonymity—you can hide our identity, and so can anyone else. Discuss the possible effects of this on Internet support groups.

NOTES

1. Celina Imielinska and Pat Molholt, "Incorporating 3D Virtual Anatomy into the Medical Curriculum, Communications of the ACM," *CACM* 48, no. 2 (2005): 49–54.
2. Mark Scerbo, "Medical Reality Simulators: Have We Missed an Opportunity?" 2005, http://www.hfes.org/web/BulletinPdf/bulletin0505.pdf (accessed August 9, 2006).
3. Anthony G. Gallagher, E. Matt Ritter, Howard Champion, Gerald Higgins, Marvin P. Fried, Gerald Moses, C. Daniel Smith, and Richard Satava, "Virtual Reality Simulation in the Operating Room," 2005, http://www.pubmedcentral.nih.gov/articlerender. fcgi?&pubmedid=15650649 (accessed January 18, 2008).
4. "The 'Karlsruhe Endoscopic Surgery Trainer': A 'Virtual Reality' based Training System for Minimally Invasive Surgery," http://www-kismet.iai.fzk.de/TRAINER/mic_trainer1. html (accessed February 2, 2008).
5. "Virtual Reality Simulation Technology Improves Carotid Angiography Skills," Medical Studies/Trials, May 3, 2006, http://www.news-medical.net/?id=17717 (accessed December 29, 2007).
6. AIMS Industry Council, "What Is Medical Simulation?" 2006, http://www.medsim.org/what_medsim.asp (accessed December 28, 2007).
7. "Web Site to Rate Content of Health Care News," *Star-Ledger,* April 17, 2006.
8. "2001 Report to Congress on Telemedicine," February 2001, http://www.hrsa.gov/telehealth/pubs/report2001.htm (accessed December 29, 2007).
9. Lisa Guernsey, "A Dissent on the Digital Divide," nyt.com, September 18, 2003, http://query.nytimes.com/gst/fullpage.html?res=9F0DE7D6153AF93BA2575AC0A9659C8B63 (accessed December 28, 2007).
10. U.S. Department of Commerce, "A Nation Online: Entering the Broadband Age," September, 2004, http://www.ntia.doc.gov/reports/anol/index.html (accessed November 13, 2006).
11. "Digital Divide Still Separates Students," eschoolnews.com, September 6, 2006, http://www.eschoolnews.com/news/top-news/index.cfm?i=41296&CFID=2272416&CFTOKEN= 83744007 (accessed December 28, 2007).
12. Michel Marriott, "Digital Divide Closing as Blacks Turn to Internet," nyt.com, March 31, 2006, http://www.nytimes.com/2006/03/31/us/31divide.html (accessed November 13, 2006).
13. Robert Trowbridge, M.D. and Scott Weingarten, M.D., M.P.H., "Clinical Decision Support Systems," chapter 53 in *Making Health Care Safer: A Critical Analysis of Patient Safety Practices,* prepared for the Agency for Healthcare Research and Quality, contract no. 290-97-0013, 2001, http://www.ahrq.gov/clinic/ptsafety (accessed February 2, 2008).
14. Stephen Borowitz and Jeffrey Wyatt. "The Origin, Content, and Workload of E-mail Consultations." *JAMA* 280 (1998): 1321–24.
15. Katie Hafner, "'Dear Doctor' Meets 'Return to Sender,'" nyt.com, June 6, 2002, http://query.nytimes.com/gst/fullpage.html?res=9C0CE1DC1F3AF935A35755C0A9649C8B63 (accessed December 28, 2007).
16. "Internet Pharmacy Doctors Charged," nyt.com, August 2, 2006 (accessed August 6, 2006).

17. Ken Mott, "Cancer and the Internet." *Newsweek,* August 19, 1996, 19.
18. Michelle G. Newman, "Technology in Psychotherapy: An Introduction," *JCLP* 60, no. 20 (2004): 141–45, http://www3.interscience.wiley.com/cgi-bin/abstract/106570982/ABSTRACT?CRETRY=1&SRETRY=0 (accessed December 28, 2007).
19. Paul M. G. Emmelkamp, "Technological Innovations in Clinical Assessment and Psychotherapy," *Psychotherapy and Psychosomatics,* 2005, http://content.karger.com/ProdukteDB/produkte.asp?Doi=87780 (accessed December 28, 2007).
20. Carlos Bergfeld, "A Dose of Virtual Reality," businessweek.com, July 26, 2006, http://www.businessweek.com/technology/content/jul2006/tc20060725_012342.htm?chan=top+news_top+news (accessed December 28, 2007).

ADDITIONAL RESOURCES

ADAM. 2006. http://www.adam.com (accessed August 24, 2006).

Aschoff, Susan. "A Diehard Patient." sptimes.com, April 30, 2002. http://www.sptimes.com/2002/04/30/Floridian/A_diehard_patient.shtml (accessed December 28, 2007).

Association of Schools of Public Health Distance Programs. 2003. asph.org (accessed August 24, 2006).

Beamish, Rita. "Computers Now Helping to Screen for Troubled Teen-Agers." *New York Times,* December 17, 1998, G9.

Bitzer, Maryann D., and Martha C. Boudreaux. "Using a Computer to Teach Nursing." In *Computers in Nursing.* Edited by Rita D. Zielstorff, 171–85. Rockville, MD: Aspen, 1982.

"Chapter 2. Review of the Literature." 2003. http://herkules.oulu.fi/isbn9514270215/html/c216.html (accessed January 6, 2008).

Choi, James J. "Viewing Virtual Hospital Content on a Personal Digital Assistant." March 2004. http://lib.cpums.edu.cn/jiepou/tupu/atlas/www.vh.org/welcome/help/vhpdausers.html (accessed August 24, 2006).

"CIDI Composite International Diagnostic Interview." 1999. http://www.hcp.med.harvard.edu/wmhcidi/ (accessed January 18, 2008).

Classen, D. C. "Clinical Decision Support Systems to Improve Clinical Practice and Quality of Care." *JAMA* 280, (1998): 1360–1.

Eisenberg, Anne. "The Virtual Stomach (No, It's Not a Diet Aid)." nyt.com, October 31, 2002. http://query.nytimes.com/gst/fullpage.html?res=9807EFDC103FF932A05753C1A9649C8B63 (accessed December 28, 2007).

Eng, Thomas R., et al., "Access to Health Information and Support: A Public Highway or a Private Road?" *JAMA* 280 (1998): 1371–5.

Epstein, Randi Hutter. "Sifting Through the Online Medical Jumble." nyt.com, January 28, 2003. http://query.nytimes.com/gst/fullpage.html?res=9901EED81239F93BA15752C0A9659C8B63 (accessed December 28, 2007).

"Evaluating Medical Information on the Web." November 17, 2003. http://www.ornl.gov/sci/techresources/Human_Genome/posters/chromosome/evaluate.shtml (accessed August 24, 2006).

"eXpert Laparoscopic Trainer." February 24, 2006. http://www.hmc.psu.edu/simulation/equipment/expert/expert.htm (accessed August 24, 2006).

"Fact Sheet." The Visible Human Project, February 16, 2001. http://www.nlm.nih.gov/research/visible/visible_human.html (accessed December 28, 2007).

Ferguson, Tom. "Digital Doctoring—Opportunities and Challenges in Electronic Patient-Physician Communication." *JAMA* 280 (1998): 1361–2.

Fisk, Sandra. "Doc in a Box a Home Health Software Guide." *Better Homes and Gardens,* August 1995, 44–52.

Griffith, Susan. "Virtual Dentistry Becomes Reality in Multimedia Lab." 2001. http://www.cwru.edu/pubs/cnews/2001/9-27/dent-sim.htm (accessed August 24, 2006).

Hamilton, Robert A. "FDA Examining Computer Diagnosis." *FDA Consumer Magazine,* September 1995. http://www.fda.gov/fdac/features/795_compdiag.html (accessed August 24, 2006).

"Health Information On-Line." *FDA Consumer Magazine,* June 1996, revised January 1998. http://www.fda.gov/fdac/features/596_info.html (accessed August 24, 2006).

Hersh, William, and David Hickam. "How Well Do Physicians Use Electronic Information Retrieval Systems? A Framework for Investigation and Systematic Review." *JAMA* 280 (1998): 1347–52.

"How to Evaluate Health Information on the Internet: Questions and Answers." August 28, 2002. http://www.cancer.gov/cancertopics/factsheet/Information/internet (accessed December 28, 2007).

"KISMET Medical Applications," 2001, http://iregt1.iai.fzk.de/KISMET/kis_apps_med.html (accessed December 3, 2007).

Kolata, Gina. "Web Research Transforms Visit to the Doctor." nyt.com, March 6, 2000. http://query.nytimes.com/gst/fullpage.html?res=9D03E1D61538F935A35750C0A9669C8B63 (accessed December 28, 2007).

Le, Tao. "Medical Education and the Internet: This Changes Everything." *JAMA* 285, no. 6 (2001): 809.

Lindberg, Donald A. B. "The National Library of Medicine's Web Site for Physicians and Patients." *JAMA* 285, no. 6 (2001): 806.

Maddox, Peggy Jo. "Ethics and the Brave New World of E-Health." November 21, 2002. http://www.nursingworld.org/MainMenuCategories/ANAMarketplace/ANAPeriodicals/OJIN/Columns/Ethics/Ethicsandehealth.aspx (accessed December 28, 2007).

"Medical Databases." 2003. medic8.com (accessed August 24, 2006).

"Medical Databases." March 19, 2002. allhealthnet.com (accessed August 24, 2006).

Morrow, David J. "Safety Data from F.D.A." nyt.com, September 10, 1998. http://query.nytimes.com/gst/fullpage.html?res=9B0DEED7103EF933A2575AC0A96E958260 (accessed December 28, 2007).

The National Library of Medicine. "The Visible Human Project®." September 11, 2003. http://www.nlm.nih.gov/research/visible/visible_human.html (accessed August 24, 2006).

O'Connor, Anahad. "Images of Preserved Embryos to Become a Learning Tool." nyt.com, March 25, 2003. http://query.nytimes.com/gst/fullpage.html?res=9C07E6DF1730F936A15750C0A9659C8B63 (accessed December 28, 2007).

"Patient Simulator Program: HPS Capabilities." http://www.cscc.edu/nursing/pspcapabilities.htm (accessed December 28, 2007).

Patsos, Mary. "The Internet and Medicine: Building a Community for Patients with Rare Diseases." *JAMA* 285, no. 6 (2001): 805.

"PediaSim Capabilities." http://www.cscc.edu/nursing/pspedsimcap.htm (accessed August 24, 2006).

Prutkin, Jordan. "Cybermedical Skills for the Internet Age." *JAMA* 285, no. 6 (2001): 808.

"Psych Screen, Inc." psychscreen.com (accessed August 24, 2006).

"Public Health Workforce Development." May 12, 2003. http://www.phf.org/phworkforce.htm (accessed December 28, 2007).

Rajendran, Pam R. "The Internet: Ushering in a New Era of Medicine." *JAMA* 285, no. 6 (2001): 804–5.

"Robertson Janice Guidelines for Physician-Patient Electronic Communications." December 6, 2004. http://www.ama-assn.org/ama/pub/category/2386.html (accessed August 24, 2006).

Rubin, Rita. "Prescribing On Line . . . Industry's Rapid Growth, Change Defy Regulation." *USA Today,* October 2, 1998, 1, 2.

Speilberg, Alissa. "On Call and Online, Sociohistorical, Legal and Ethical Implications of E-mail for the Patient-Physician Relationship." *JAMA* 280, no. 15 (1998): 1353–9.

"Starbright World." starbright.org (accessed August 24, 2006).

Termen, Amanda. "Closing the Digital Divide with Solar Wi-Fi." News.com, August 2, 2006. http://news.zdnet.com/2100-1035_22-6101071.html (accessed December 28, 2007).

Terry, Nicolas. "Access vs Quality Assurance: The e-Health Conundrum." February 14, 2001. http://jama.ama-assn.org/cgi/content/full/285/6/807 (accessed August 24, 2006).

"Virtual Hospital." 2008. http://www.uihealthcare.com/vh/ (accessed January 12, 2008).

"The Visible Human Project: From Data to Knowledge." May 3, 2001. nlm.nih.gov/research/visible/data2knowledge.html (accessed August 24, 2006).

Urbankova, Alice, and Richard Lichtenthal. "DentSim Virtual Reality in Preclinical Operative Dentistry to Improve Psychomotor Skills: A Pilot Study." 2002. http://www.denx.com/research_and_publication_details.asp?id=33 (accessed December 29, 2007).

"What's New on Virtual Hospital?" 2004. http://lib.cpums.edu.cn/jiepou/tupu/atlas/www.vh.org/welcome/whatsnew/index.html (accessed August 24, 2006).

Winker, Margaret A., Annette Flanagin, Bonnie Chi-Lum et al. "Guidelines for Medical and Health Information on the Internet." August 7, 2001. http://www.ama-assn.org/ama/pub/category/1905.html (accessed August 24, 2006).

Zuger, Abigail. "HEALTH: Hospital, Clinic, Practice: 3 Views of Doctors and the Web; Reams of Information, Some of It Even Useful." nyt.com, October 25, 2000. http://query.nytimes.com/gst/fullpage.html?res=9D04E2DF1E3CF936A15753C1A966 9C8B63&sec=&spon=&pagewanted=all (accessed December 29, 2007).

RELATED WEB SITES

The Federal Trade Commission (FTC) looks into complaints about false health claims on the Internet. Their Web page can help consumers evaluate claims. http://www.ftc.gov/bcp/conline/edcams/cureall is the Federal Trade Commission's *Operation Cure-all* page.

The Food and Drug Administration (FDA) regulates drugs and medical devices. *Buying Medicines and Medical Products Online* is at http://www.fda.gov/oc/buyonline.

The National Cancer Institute is located at http://cancer.gov.

The Harvard School of Public Health provides consumers with *Ten Questions to Help Make Sense of Health Headlines* at http://www.health-insight.com.

The Journal of the American Medical Association is available at http://jama.ama-assn.org.

The National Library of Medicine provides access to Medline and Medline*plus* at http://www.nlm.nih.gov.

CHAPTER

11

Information Technology in Rehabilitative Therapies: Computerized Medical Devices, Assistive Technology, and Prosthetic Devices

CHAPTER OUTLINE

LEARNING OBJECTIVES

After reading this chapter, you will be able to

- Describe the contribution made to the design of medical devices by information technology and be able to discuss the advantages of computerized medical monitoring systems over their predecessors.
- Describe the use of computerized devices in delivering medications.

- Discuss the Americans with Disabilities Act of 1990 and be able to discuss the impact digital technology has had on assistive devices for people with physical challenges.
  - List assistive devices for those with impaired vision, speech, hearing, and mobility.
  - Discuss speech recognition devices, speech synthesizers, and screen readers.
- Describe the contributions computer technology has made to the development of prosthetics.
  - Discuss the contribution of computer technology to the improvement of myoelectric limbs.
  - Discuss the contributions computer technology has made to improving sight for the blind and hearing for the deaf.
- Define functional electrical stimulation.
  - List its uses in implanted devices such as pacemakers.
  - Discuss its use in simulating physical workouts for paralyzed muscles and restoring movement to paralyzed limbs.
- Discuss the risks posed by implants.
- Discuss the uses of computers in rehabilitative therapies.

OVERVIEW

Digital technology, particularly the microprocessor, has had an enormous impact on the creation, design, and manufacture of medical devices, adaptive devices, and prosthetics. Computers have improved the design of some devices with health care applications and made possible a whole range of new ones. In hospitals and medical offices, **computerized medical instruments** with embedded microprocessors are more accurate than their predecessors. In the work place and the home, the impact of information technology on people who are physically challenged is tremendous. Assistive, or adaptive, technology allows some people with disabilities to work and/or live independently.

    Prosthetic devices (replacement limbs and organs) that contain motors and respond to electrical signals existed prior to computers. However, prosthetic devices designed and manufactured with the help of computers and containing microprocessors are more sensitive, lighter, and more flexible and can work almost as well as natural limbs. **Computerized functional electrical stimulation (CFES or FES)** is a technology that involves delivering low-level electrical stimulation to muscles. Used for many years in pacemakers, CFES is now being used to strengthen muscles paralyzed by spinal cord injury or stroke. CFES is being used experimentally to restore the ability to stand and walk to paraplegics.

COMPUTERIZED MEDICAL INSTRUMENTS AND DEVICES

Computerized medical instruments are "electronic devices equipped with microprocessors [which] provide direct patient services such as monitoring ... [and]

administering medication or treatment."[1] Computerized drug delivery systems are used to give medications. Insulin pumps include a battery-operated pump and a computer chip. The pump is not automatic. However, the chip allows the user to control the amount of insulin administered. Insulin is administered via a plastic tube inserted under the skin; the tube is changed every two or three days. The pump is worn externally and continually delivers insulin according to the user's program. In March 2001, the Food and Drug Administration (FDA) approved a new device for glucose testing. It is worn like a watch and takes fluid through the skin using electric currents; electrodes measure the glucose. The measurements are taken every twenty minutes, and an alarm goes off if the levels are too low. Tests showed that this method was not as accurate as the finger prick and is not meant to replace it, but to reveal trends. Electronic intravenous (IV) units not only are programmable, but also can detect incorrect flow and sound an alarm. Some units can be programmed to administer several drugs through several channels. IV anesthesia can be administered via a mechanical syringe infusion pump, controlled by complex and sophisticated software.

Computerized monitoring systems that collect data directly from patients via sensors have been used for many years. These devices can provide continuous oversight of a patient's condition and can be programmed to sound an alarm under certain conditions to notify human personnel of a change. Computerized **physiological monitoring systems** that analyze blood, **arrhythmia monitors** that monitor heart rates, **pulmonary monitors** that measure blood flow through the heart and respiratory rate, **fetal monitors** that measure the heart rate of the fetus, and **neonatal monitors** that monitor infant heart and breathing rates are devices that are standard and accepted.

Computerized instruments are both more accurate and more reliable than their predecessors. For example, an infusion pump can be set at the desired rate and that rate will be maintained. Its predecessor, whose flow had to be estimated, could have its rate changed by the patient's movements. Computerized cardiac monitors are able, unlike their predecessors, to distinguish between cardiac arrest and a wire coming loose.

Monitoring devices may or may not be linked to a network. Stand-alone devices include IV pumps, electrocardiograms (ECG) (Figure 11.1 ■) and cardiac monitors, defibrillators, temperature pulse respiration (TPR), and blood pressure monitors. When devices are networked, patients can be monitored from a central location within the hospital such as a nurses' station, or even from a physician's home. Networked devices can interact with each other; for example, a cardiac monitor can communicate with a medication delivery device. Networked equipment is most common in emergency rooms, operating rooms, and critical and intensive care units. Because a network makes patient information immediately available anywhere in the hospital and allows a specialist to consult with the emergency room online, it can reduce response time in emergencies.

Computerized Devices in Optometry/Ophthalmology

An ophthalmologist is a doctor who treats eye diseases. An optometrist examines the eye and prescribes glasses. Computerized devices help make eye care, from preliminary vision testing to surgery, more precise. Computerized instruments are used

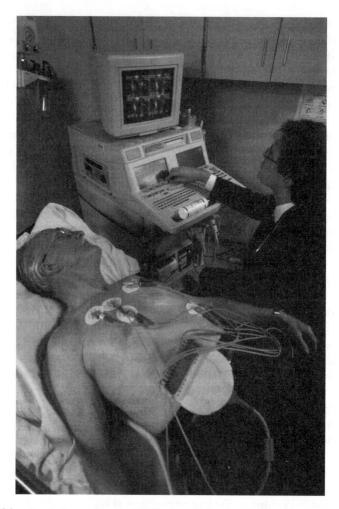

■ **FIGURE 11.1** An electrocardiogram (ECG) records the electrical activity of a heart. Courtesy of Brand X Pictures/Jupiter Images.

to measure refractive error and the shape of the cornea. The **Optomap Panoramic200** examines the retina without dilation using low-powered red and green lasers. The image can be reviewed right away and is larger than that produced by conventional examination. It can help in the early detection of retinal tears, macular degeneration, and diabetic retinopathy. Tools called **biomicroscopes** are used for diagnosis of cataracts. **Tonometers** measure eye pressure. **Corneal topography** uses a computer to create an accurate three-dimensional map of the cornea so that the health care professional can see the shape and power of the cornea. The **Heidelberg retinal tomograph (HRT)** uses lasers to scan the retina, resulting in a three-dimensional description. This technique can detect glaucoma before any loss of vision. **GDx Access** uses an infrared laser to measure the thickness of the retinal nerve fiber. It is used for the early detection of glaucoma. Computers help to make cataract surgery more precise. In such surgery, the eye's lens is replaced by an intraocular lens (IOL). The most precise measurements are needed to determine which IOL to implant. **Optical biometry** refers to the IOL calculations. Traditionally, ultrasound was used for the measurement; it required anesthesia. The IOLmaster takes precise measures in a shorter time and requires no anesthesia. The **Tracey visual function analyzer** measures how well you can see by measuring how your eye focuses light. This data helps in surgical or laser vision correction. Computers are also used to custom design contact lenses.

A newly developed type of glasses may improve the vision of people with tunnel vision, which can be the result of retinitis pigmentosa or glaucoma. The device "combines a camera, computer and transparent computer display on a pair of glasses." People using them would be able to see through the transparent part of the lens, but would also see a tiny version of a wider (peripheral) field superimposed on the lens.[2]

The FDA has approved the testing of retinal implants, but they have not yet been approved as of 2006. In a healthy eye, the retina changes light into electrical signals. The retinal implant contains thousands of light detectors; it also changes light into electric signals. Currently, scientists around the world are studying computer chips that will replace the retina. One major disagreement is where the chip should be implanted: under the retina close to light-detecting cells or near the retinal layer that sends nerve impulses to the brain. The way light is sent to the implant also differs—through a camera or via infrared signals that come from a device mounted on lens frames. The chip will (if successful) treat retinitis pigmentosa and macular degeneration. A chip developed in Germany in 2006 is in clinical trials. Two successful implants in previously blind people were performed in 2005.[3]

Currently, computer software helps restore some sight to the legally blind. Software developed in France calculates the dimensions for glasses that will maximize the amount of light transmitted to any part of the retina that is still functioning. The program calculates the location and size of the portion of the retina that is still working and the level of magnification necessary to restore sight. Using the program has led to a 50 percent improvement in vision. This improvement means that someone who was blind can walk without the aid of a cane or dog.

A prototype of **smart glasses**, developed at the University of Arizona, will soon be able to automatically change focus. The lenses are two flat pieces of glass; between them in a 5-micron space is liquid crystal. The liquid crystal is coated with a transparent electrode that transmits light. At present, the prototype glasses need to be switched on and off before they will change focus. Soon they will automatically adjust (like a camera lens). In the future, you will not need prescriptions for new glasses, just a new program.[4]

In 2007, P2, an integrated system which will automate the examination and treatment of the eye, will be introduced to the U.S. market. It will take the ordinary eye exam and computerize it. It "combines capabilities for three-dimensional imaging, analysis, and treatment and picture archiving and communications system (PACS)-like data archiving." (Figure 11.2 ■).[5]

In ophthalmic surgical training programs, virtual reality simulations are beginning to be used. The **EYESI surgical simulator** allows doctors to learn new surgical

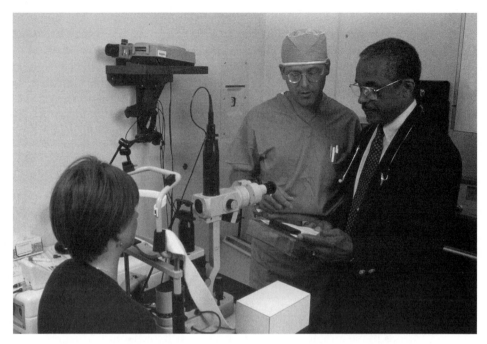

■ **FIGURE 11.2**   A computerized eye exam. Courtesy of Brand X Pictures/Jupiter Images.

skills and techniques "in preparation for surgery on the human eye." In 2006, the program was being evaluated by New York University to test its effectiveness.[6]

ASSISTIVE DEVICES

The **Americans with Disabilities Act of 1990** prohibits discrimination against people with disabilities and requires that businesses with more than fifteen employees provide "reasonable accommodation" to allow the disabled to perform their jobs. Thus, employers are required to provide not only entrance ramps for people in wheelchairs, but hardware and software that make computers usable by people with disabilities. Many assistive devices have been developed. **Adaptive technology** makes it possible for people with disabilities to exercise control over their home and work environments. Some assistive devices allow people with physical challenges to work with computers and other office equipment. Others simply improve the quality of life. For example, at Boston University, scientists are developing a system based on computer-generated noise that helps elderly people keep their balance. It sends random vibrations to the feet, which automatically adjust their balance.

Wheelchairs are being developed that not only help move people around, but climb stairs and allow them to reach a high shelf. The iBOT wheelchair stands up on its back wheels if the user needs to climb stairs and raises the seat to allow reaching. An even smarter wheelchair is being developed. It includes sensors and a computer, and the user can simply tell it where to go or use a touch panel. The wheelchair finds its way, using laser radar to find objects in its way; a computer calculates a new path if necessary.

Sensors can also be embedded in fabrics and clothing. The sensors detect motion and send signals to a computer that displays the activity. Smart clothing can help to monitor chronically ill patients, such as those with heart conditions.[7]

Computer technology can help those with impaired vision, hearing, speech, and mobility. People with low or no vision can use speech recognition systems as input and speech synthesizers for output. Brain input systems are being developed for people who lack the muscle control to use alternative input devices.

Hearing impairment is not a barrier to computer use. However, computers do expand the means of communication that hearing-impaired people can access. Computers can be used as text telephones and can send and receive e-mail. Special modems can communicate with both **text telephones** and computers. Computer-aided transcription makes use of a typist entering verbal communications at a meeting. The communications are then displayed as text on a monitor.

Assistive technology encompasses many areas. People with low vision can use a large type display on a monitor. Braille keyboards allow the blind to type. Blind users can use keyboard alternatives to mouse clicks as commands (for example, [ALT]-F-O, instead of clicking on the open icon). In 2003, a Braille telephone organizer was developed. It combines the functions of the cell phone, note taker, and wireless Internet connector. It can receive information and either read it to the user or allow the user to read it in Braille. Text can be entered using its Braille keyboards.

Speech recognition is useful for people who do not have the use of their hands and for the vision impaired. It promises that you can give computer commands or dictate text. Speech recognition hardware includes a microphone and a chip inside the computer that converts the spoken word to digital data that the computer can process. The digitized word is compared to a database of words in the computer's memory; if a match is found, the word is recognized. Speech recognition systems enable the user to give voice commands to their computers instead of clicking with a mouse, and to write, edit, and format text documents by dictating instead of typing. Great progress has been made in recent years, until speech recognition is almost perfect. Speech recognition systems which may not be able to distinguish between some English words and phrases—"hyphenate" sounds exactly like "–8" (hyphen 8); "the right or left" sounds like "the writer left"—can now be corrected by voice. The newest systems do not require training, and their error rates are close to zero.

Using **page scanners**, speech synthesizers, and screen reader software, printed text can be digitized and input and then read aloud by the computer. A scanner converts printed text into a form the computer can accept as input, that is, it digitizes it. Speech synthesis refers to the ability of a computer to talk; voice output devices turn digital data into speech-like sounds, allowing the computer to talk or read *to* a vision-impaired user or speak *for* a speech-impaired user. Speech synthesis requires both hardware and software. The **speech synthesizer** is really a computer in itself with a processor, memory, and an output device. The software is loaded into the synthesizer's memory. The microprocessor generates speech output and translates binary code to speech. A speaker and amplifier are also necessary. **Screen reader software** tells the speech synthesizer what to say, for example, to read the text description of an icon.

Ray Kurzweil (2006) invented a new portable speech-synthesizing device that uses a digital camera and a hand-held organizer called the Kurzweil–National Federation of the Blind Reader. The device takes a picture of the written text, scans, and reads it. You do not have to be near a computer to use it. It also contains a memory that can save pages.[8]

People with impaired vision are not the only users of speech recognition software. People who have lost the use of their hands also find it useful; instead of typing, they can talk to the computer. Other input devices include the **head mouse**, which moves the cursor according to the user's head motions. **Puff straws** allow people to control the mouse with their mouths.[9] Some computers allow input through eye movement. The newest eye input system does not require the user to stare at letter after letter, but allows the eye to move down a column of letters and stop on one. The chosen letter floats on the screen, and the software predicts the next most likely letters. For example, if the user selected a q, u would be the next most likely letter. After the u, the next letter would be an a, e, i, or o. Users of this system can type at twenty-five words per minute, compared with fifteen words per minute using an onscreen keyboard.[10]

Perhaps, most amazing are programs that attempt to translate electrical impulses from the brain into a mouse click. A quadriplegic can, after a period of training, click a mouse by contracting facial muscles or simply thinking. In 2003, a system that enabled a user to give a command by furrowing his or her brow on which a sensor was taped was demonstrated. Robotic arms and computer mice could be controlled using the sensor. Paralyzed stroke patients could speak on the telephone.

Augmentative Communication Devices

An **augmentative communication device** is any device that helps a person communicate. Medicare began covering these devices in 2002. Those who lack the ability to speak or whose speech is impaired can have a computer speak for them. The device should allow the user to communicate basic needs, carry on conversations, work with a computer, and complete assignments for work or school. It should work with environmental controls at home, but travel with the user. It should enable the user to communicate with anyone, and say anything. It should be easy to use. There are devices which allow the user to type a message on a traditional keyboard and the computer speaks aloud. Some keyboards can be easily operated by one finger. Other devices, as you recall, allow the user to select letters by gazing at an area on the screen, which displays the characters. For people whose speech is impaired, there are devices that enhance speech—making the unintelligible comprehensible—and allow normal communication. Many of these devices are user friendly, that is, easy for people with no computer background to use. Some are specifically designed for children—allowing the user to move an electric pointer to select a picture symbol. Some devices for children have the words organized by part of speech, the English word appearing above the symbol. These devices include synthesized voices. More sophisticated devices included spelling, word prediction, and preprogrammed messages. Portable devices allow the user to communicate anywhere. A device, which the user wears on a belt, allows a user to communicate by pressing buttons to play prerecorded messages and carry on simple conversations.

Environmental Control Systems

Environmental control systems (ECS) help physically challenged people control their environments. Speech recognition technology can be used in the home to control appliances. Butler-in-a-Box has been made by Mastervoice since 1986. It not only understands and obeys voice commands, but also responds in a human voice. Using this system, one can control home appliances with voice commands. It also acts as a speaker phone which will dial or answer calls on command. Other ECS allow the installation of a single switch to control the operation of several appliances (including other controllers). A device even exists that holds the book the user is reading and turns the pages.

ECS can be used to control any electrical appliance in the home. This would include lights, telephones, computers, appliances, infrared devices, security systems, sprinklers, doors, curtains, and electric beds. Voice, joysticks, or switches may control the system. This may enable physically challenged people to live independently at home. One small study reported that twenty-seven of the twenty-nine people with spinal injuries who used an ECS for one year "reported that it increased their independence."[11] Other studies found similar results. Several telephones have been developed. It should be noted that all of these systems required that the user be trained and comfortable with the technology and that the technology be reliable.

Another newer use of environmental controls is to help in language development in children. Many environmental controls include infrared capability. One possibility is using an action toy that moves back and forth to teach the concepts of backwards and forwards or fast/slow. In toys that require children to take turns, words such as My turn/Your turn could be taught.[12] Research is also being done into the possibility of using augmentative communication devices for patients who are only voiceless for a short time, because of illness or surgery.

▨ PROSTHETIC DEVICES

Prostheses are attempts to replace natural body parts or organs with artificial devices. **Myoelectric limbs**—artificial limbs containing motors and responding to the electrical signals transmitted by the residual limb to electrodes mounted in the socket—predate computers. However, computer-related research has improved myoelectric limbs and had an immense impact on prosthetics in general. Developments related to computers include the tiny circuitry used by the sensors that receive the electrical signals and the motors which move the limb, the use of computers in the design and manufacture of limbs, and the improvement of the sensors used in prostheses.

Today, microprocessors can be embedded in a prosthetic limb and make the limb more useful and flexible. Sensors are attached to muscles in the residual limb. The patient must be able to control these muscles. Contracting the muscles generates electrical impulses. A microprocessor processes and amplifies the electrical impulses, sending them as control signals to the prosthesis. The microprocessor controls the tiny motor that moves the artificial limb. Combined with natural-looking prostheses, the results can be a life-like limb (Figure 11.3 ■).

Computer-aided design and manufacturing (CAD/CAM) systems also improve prostheses by making the fit better. The artificial limb must be fitted to the natural limb. CAD/CAM systems have been developed to design both the socket and limb. With CAD/CAM, thousands of measurements can be taken and a three-dimensional model created on the computer screen to create a perfect custom fit for each patient. CAD/CAM is also used in dentistry to help create individually fitted prostheses.

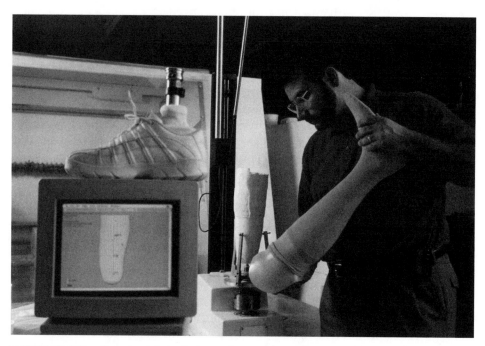

■ **FIGURE 11.3**   Computers help design and manufacture life-like limbs. Courtesy of Brand X Pictures/Jupiter Images.

Computers have made other advances possible. A knee socket has been developed which includes a computer chip that allows patients to walk naturally. Energy-storing feet contain plastic springs or carbon fibers, which are designed to help move the prosthesis. A relatively new lower leg prosthesis is called the C-leg or computerized leg. It includes a prosthetic knee and shin system controlled by a microprocessor. It is made of lightweight carbon fiber and gets its power from a rechargeable battery. With a traditional prosthesis, the user has to think about each step. But the C-leg analyzes gait fifty times per second; it anticipates movement, and thus thinks for the patient. It is supposed to adjust to uneven ground by itself, but results from studies are mixed. It requires less energy for walking at speeds slower or faster than usual, but not at the walker's usual speed; the user does not have to think about changing walking speed. In small studies, patient satisfaction is found to be high. Most study participants chose to keep the C-leg as opposed to a conventional prosthesis. However, in water, the C-leg has been known to short out in at least one instance.[13]

People with computerized prosthetic limbs not only walk but can play sports, run, climb mountains, and—using a prosthetic hand developed at Rutgers University in 1998 with fingers that can be controlled separately—even play the piano! Soon prosthetic limbs will include sensors that allow a person to feel hot and cold. Temperature sensors in the prosthesis would send signals to electrodes on the natural limb. The information is sent to the brain, which registers sensation. Sense-of-feel systems are also being developed so that breakable objects can be manipulated. Today (2007), the Veteran's Administration and the Defense Advanced Research Projects Agency are investing in better and better prosthetic limbs—including a thought-controlled arm—for the many amputees returning from war.[14]

Osseointegration is a technology that allows the integration of living bone with titanium implants. The bone actually grows around the implant, which is thus integrated into the body. It has been used in dentistry, in cranial and maxillofacial reconstruction since 1952. In 1990, its use was expanded to other prostheses. It has many benefits over traditional prostheses, including more control, and less pain. Among the disadvantages are the necessity for two surgeries, long rehabilitation, and risk of infection which can lead to reamputation.[15]

Computer technology is also helping people who are hearing impaired. A digital hearing aid (essentially a tiny computer), which can be programmed to meet individual needs and adjust to background noise, became available in 1996. Although it cannot help the profoundly deaf, many people found it better at picking up faint sounds than older models. Digital technology has also made possible the development of the cochlear implant (cleared by the FDA in 1996), a device, which has been shown to be of some benefit to hearing-impaired people with intact auditory nerves. The device consists of an internal element surgically implanted behind the ear and a small computer that can be carried. The computer, which is a speech processor, digitizes sound. It is attached to the implant by a cord. The computer sends the digitized code to the implant and then to the inner ear where it is interpreted as sound. Although called an implant, because of its size, most of it is not actually implanted. The size is needed to accommodate the power needs of translating analog to digital signals. However, in 2003, a researcher from the Massachusetts Institute of Technology began working on a low-power analog device that would be fully implanted.

One of the problems of hearing aids is that they may amplify sound, but do not indicate where the sound is coming from. Researchers in Sweden are creating a system, which includes microphones in eyeglasses; when the sound is heard, it is analyzed by a computer. Pads in the frames of the glasses will vibrate, telling the user where the sound originated.

In 2006, the newest hearing aids include "digital processing and directional microphones." Sound is more natural. Speech is clearer. Background noise is minimized. They are worn behind the ear; only a small tube enters the ear. If you wear hearing aids in each ear, the wireless e2e (ear-to-ear) system coordinates the hearing aids for better sound. Hybrid implants "combine a traditional hearing aid with a modified electrode similar to . . . a cochlear implant." They provide the best sound.[16]

A new development is Acceleglove. It uses sensors that detect hand and finger movement and sends signals to the computer. The computer associates the hand movements with a particular word. It then translates the sign language into text and speech.[17]

COMPUTERIZED FUNCTIONAL ELECTRICAL STIMULATION TECHNOLOGY

Myoelectrically controlled prostheses, you recall, use the electrical impulses transmitted by muscles to stimulate movement in artificial limbs. CFES (or FES) directly applies low-level electrical stimulation to muscles that cannot receive these signals from the brain. CFES technology was originally developed by NASA. FES has been used for many years in pacemakers and other implanted devices. It is now used to strengthen paralyzed muscles with exercise. It can be used to simulate a full cardiovascular workout for people who are paralyzed, reducing the secondary effects of paralysis. FES even makes it possible to restore movement to some limbs paralyzed by stroke and spinal injury. By stimulating the correct muscles, people who are paralyzed can walk. The amount of electricity is controlled by a microprocessor, which uses feedback from the body to adjust itself.

A normal arm or leg moves because a specific muscle contracts in response to an electrical signal from the brain. A spinal cord injury can prevent these signals from traveling between the brain and any muscle below the injury. Although the muscles still have the ability to move, they do not receive the necessary signals. FES stimulates the muscles directly, sending the electrical signals using electrodes on the skin's surface. On April 1, 2003, Medicare began covering the Parastep system, one system using FES (called functional neuromuscular stimulation) that allows paraplegics to walk. In 2003, in a seventeen-year follow-up study of two patients using FES, it was found that "Although the FES system was devised as a temporary means of achieving functional activation . . . it was found to be effective and relatively safe for more than 17 years."[18] In 2002, the National Institutes of Health gave a 3.1 million dollar grant to the University of Delaware's Center for Biomedical Engineering to develop a system using FES and robots that will assist paralyzed stroke patients. The robot will help move the patient's legs to teach him or her to walk. They hope to develop an FES device that is small and wearable.

FES is used in many implanted medical devices, some of which we have come to take for granted. Computers delivering electrical stimulation to the heart are permanently embedded in the human body as pacemakers. A more advanced pacemaker, based on two-way communications technology developed by NASA, allows the doctor to regulate the pacemaker from outside the patient's body, even via the Internet. More complicated than a pacemaker, an implantable cardioverter defibrillator monitors heart rate and gives a jolt of electricity when needed. According to the U.S. FDA, in a clinical study, it restored normal heart rate in 91 percent of the patients. Devices are being tested and approved constantly. In 2006, the FDA planned to have outside experts monitor devices (such as defibrillators) once they were on the market.[19] In September 1997, the FDA approved an implanted neural prosthesis that restores some hand movement to quadriplegics. The device includes a tiny battery and microprocessor "implanted in the chest and connected to electrodes wired under the skin to eight thumb and finger muscles of the dominant hand. Jerking an externally mounted device on the opposite shoulder signals the implant to move the thumb and fingers." After a period of training, the device enabled quadriplegics to feed themselves and hold a pen. An implantable defibrillator can monitor the heart, and, when it detects an arrhythmia, it converts it to a normal heart rhythm. In March 1998, the FDA approved a breathing pacemaker. It controls breathing by sending electrical impulses to the phrenic nerve.

In July 1997, the FDA approved an implanted device that reduces seizures in people with epilepsy by delivering electrical signals to the brain. Implanted pacemakers (Activa) for the brain are also used to help control the tremors of Parkinson's. This device has wires that connect to the electrodes in the brain. Pacemakers for the brain are being tested for the treatment of bipolar disorder and depression. Research is being done on the use of implanted computerized devices to predict and prevent seizures. Bluetooth technology makes it possible for computerized devices to be linked, so that when a pacemaker senses a heart attack, a cell phone will dial 911.

Electronic stimulation is also being used to prevent chronic pain. Electronic devices are implanted and send low levels of electrical energy to nerves. This does not allow the pain signals to reach the brain.[20]

In 2006, a new implantable device using FES—a **neuroprosthesis**—was developed. It uses "low levels of electricity in order to activate nerves and muscles in order to restore movement." The electrodes are implanted. They are powered by a switch outside the body. When it is turned on, the patient can move limbs that had been paralyzed.[21]

In 2004 and 2005, the FDA approved two devices (**Neuromove** and **Biomove 3000**) for stroke patients. Both devices help to stimulate the muscles to avoid atrophy and increase both the range of motion and blood circulation. The devices help to communicate with paralyzed muscles through electrical stimulation of the brain. The devices work as follows: "When you think about moving a muscle and the device detects the . . . signal in the muscle, the Biomove then sends a stimulation signal to that muscle to cause it to contract providing positive reinforcement by active biofeedback. In most cases, repetitive use causes the brain to assign new brain cells to control that muscle."[22-24]

In 2005, the FDA approved a pilot clinical study of the **BrainGate Neural Interface System** for ALS (Lou Gehrig's disease). The system involves implanting a chip in the brain that will convert brain cell impulses to computer signals.[25] In 2006, in the pilot clinical trial, "A man with paralysis of all four limbs could directly control objects around him . . . using only his thoughts." The device, called BrainGate, is surgically implanted. It includes a sensor that records brainwaves and interprets them. Two patients with the implants who suffered from spinal cord injuries can now hold a conversation and control a cursor at the same time. One of them was able to control a robotic arm. From the first, the patients were able to move limbs by thinking about the motion and ". . . activity was evoked by imagined actions." The Braingate sensor is implanted in the brain.[26]

Neuromodulation is a new field that may help treat disorders of the central nervous system including chronic pain. It ". . . involves implanting an electrode within the nervous system, such as on or below the surface (cortex) of the brain, the spinal cord or the peripheral nerve. A pacemaker-like device called a neurostimulator is implanted in the upper chest and connected under the skin to the electrode. The device is programmed to deliver an electrical current to stimulate targeted nerve cells and nerve fibers in the brain, spinal cord and peripheral nerve."[27]

RISKS POSED BY IMPLANTS

Many of the developments we have mentioned in this chapter involve surgically implanting chips or mechanical devices in human beings. These include heart pacemakers, neural implants, drug delivery systems, and some devices under development, such as the retinal implant. Although millions of people are walking around with implants, we should remember that implants pose some risks including rejection of the implant and infection at the site. Some implants can cause blood clots and require the user to take anticlotting medications. Research is currently being done to lower the risks of implants. Some scientists are focusing on creating more user-friendly materials that the human body will accept. Research is beginning at Rensselaer Polytechnic Institute in New York. Using a technique called **microdialysis**, the project will attempt to look at the body's response to an implant at the cellular level. A tiny probe would take a sample of fluid at the point where the implant and body meet. The analysis of this fluid can show early signs of rejection or infection.

■■■■ COMPUTERS IN REHABILITATIVE THERAPIES

A computerized program called **HELEN (HELp Neuropsychology)** contains diagnostic analyses that keep track of specific tests and tasks performed by the stroke patient. The tasks and methods of solving them are kept in a database. HELEN also contains a rehabilitative module. Tasks are provided for the patient. The methods used to solve the task becomes information for the neuropsychologist. Interactive procedures allow the patient to try different solutions to the problem. "The system contains tasks that relate to perception, memory and attention, including writing, reading, and counting." Deficits can be pinpointed, and problems that engage the intact portion of the brain can be presented. The patient can control the pace of rehabilitation. HELEN hopes to supplement the program with virtual reality to make it more interesting for the patients. Some of the tasks are used with the Internet, for example, the patient is asked: How many pictures do you see? How many black and white? Patients are also asked to put sentences in order.[28]

Motion monitor is a "computer-based system [which] gives physical therapists real-time, objective measures of the motion of each joint in the patient's body." It involves the placing of electrodes on the patient; they are read by magnetic trackers. This information becomes an animation that both the physical therapist and patient can see in real time.[29] It results in objective measures of how a limb is moving for the therapist. It is also used to educate patients to avoid harmful movements.

FES has been used for many years in several forms of rehabilitation. Electrical stimulation can help to simulate a workout for muscles that are not being used because of injury. This may prevent the atrophy of the muscles. It can be used for strengthening the muscles and helping in voluntary activity. A physical therapist must place the electrodes correctly and adjust the amount of electricity.

Virtual reality is being used experimentally to help people with amputations control phantom pain. The system gives the illusion that the amputated limb is still there. Using a headset, the patient sees himself or herself with two arms or legs. They are able to use the physical limb to control the virtual limb. Five patients have tried the system. "Four out of the five patients report[ed] improvement in their phantom limb pain."[30]

Many people lose their eyesight because of a neurological condition or disease. Magnetic resonance imaging (MRIs) and computed tomography (CT) scans can be used to diagnose these conditions. Some stroke victims lose their vision following a stroke. However, new therapies have emerged. "The approach is predicated on a revolution sweeping the field of neurobiology: the discovery that the adult brain isn't fixed . . ., but rather has the ability to 'rewire' itself." **Vision replacement therapy** (VRT) retrains the brain. Using dots on a computer screen, the aim is to stimulate peripheral vision. This therapy can be effective years after the stroke occurred. The therapy may be used to treat other conditions such as obsessive-compulsive disorder (OCD).[31]

■■■■■ CONCLUSION

Information technology has made possible major improvements in medical devices. This chapter could not be an exhaustive survey because new devices are being developed and approved every year. Computerized monitors (whether stand-alone or networked) can continuously collect data from patients, notifying hospital personnel of a change. Adaptive technology will continue to improve the quality of life of people with disabilities. Assistive devices make it possible for people who are physically challenged to work and live independently. Computerized prostheses have been developed that work almost as well as natural limbs. FES is used in implanted devices, such as pacemakers, and to restore movement to paralyzed limbs. Computer programs are now being used in the rehabilitation of stroke patients.

IN THE NEWS

Excerpt from, "Paralyzed Man Uses Thoughts to Move a Cursor"

by Andrew Pollack

A paralyzed man with a small sensor implanted in his brain was able to control a computer, a television set and a robot using only his thoughts, scientists reported yesterday.

Those results offer hope that in the future, people with spinal cord injuries, Lou Gehrig's disease or other conditions that impair movement may be able to communicate or better control their world.

"If your brain can do it, we can tap into it," said John P. Donoghue, a professor of neuroscience at Brown University who has led development of the system and was the senior author of a report on it being published in today's issue of the journal Nature.

In a variety of experiments, the first person to receive the implant, Matthew Nagle, moved a cursor, opened e-mail, played a simple video game called Pong and drew a crude circle on the screen. He could change the channel or volume on a television set, move a robot arm somewhat, and open and close a prosthetic hand. . . .

Mr. Nagle, a former high school football star in Weymouth, Mass., was paralyzed below the shoulders after being stabbed in the neck during a melee at a beach in July 2001. . . .

Implants like the one he received had previously worked in monkeys. . . .

[B]ut the paper in Nature is the first peer-reviewed publication of an experiment in people with a more sophisticated implant . . . The paper helps "shift the notion of such 'implantable neuromotor prosthetics' from science fiction towards reality," Stephen H. Scott, professor of anatomy and cell biology at Queen's University in Ontario, wrote in a commentary in the journal.

The sensor measures 4 millimeters by 4 millimeters—less than a fifth of an inch long and wide—and contains 100 tiny electrodes . . . and was connected to a pedestal that protruded from the top of his skull.

When the device was to be used, technicians plugged a cable connected to a computer into the pedestal. So Mr. Nagle was directly wired to a computer, somewhat like a character in the "Matrix" movies.

Mr. Nagle would then imagine moving his arm to hit various targets. The implanted sensor eavesdropped on the electrical signals emitted by neurons in his motor cortex as they controlled the imaginary arm movement.

Obstacles must be overcome, before brain implants become practical. For one thing, the electrodes' ability to detect brain signals begins to deteriorate after several months, for reasons not fully understood . . . Further, the testing involving Mr. Nagle required recalibration of the system each day, a task that took technicians about half an hour.

Still, scientists said the study was particularly important because it showed that the neurons in Mr. Nagle's motor cortex were still active years after they had last had a role to play in moving his arms.

The implant system, known as the BrainGate, is being developed by Cyberkinetics Neurotechnology Systems Inc. of Foxborough, Mass. The company is now testing the system in three other people, who remain anonymous: one with a spinal cord injury, one with Lou Gehrig's disease and one who had a brain stem stroke . . .

Dr. Jonathan R. Wolpaw, a researcher at the New York State Department of Health, said the BrainGate performance did not appear to be substantially better than that of a noninvasive system he is developing using electroencephalography, in which electrodes are placed outside the scalp.

"If you are going to have something implanted into your brain," Dr. Wolpaw said, "you'd probably want it to be a lot better."

Dr. Donoghue and other proponents of the implants say they have the potential to be a lot better, because they are much closer to the relevant neurons . . . which get signals from millions of neurons all over the brain. . . .

After more than a year, Mr. Nagle had his implant removed so he could undergo another operation, which allowed him to breathe without a ventilator. He can control a computer by voice, so he does not really need the implant. But he said he was happy he had volunteered for the experiment.

"It gave a lot of people hope," he said.

CHAPTER SUMMARY

Chapter 11 introduces the reader to the uses of digital technology in medical instruments, adaptive and assistive devices, and prostheses, and to the use of FES technology.

- Computerized medical instruments with embedded microprocessors are used to monitor patients and administer medication.
  - Computerized drug delivery systems are programmable and can detect incorrect flow.
  - Computerized monitoring devices include physiological monitoring systems, arrhythmia monitors, pulmonary monitors, fetal monitors, and neonatal monitoring systems. They continuously monitor a patient's condition and can be programmed to sound an alarm and notify personnel of a dangerous change.
  - Some monitors are part of a network; this makes it possible to check the patient's condition from a central location and can decrease response time in emergencies.
  - Information technology has had a tremendous impact on people with disabilities.
  - The Americans with Disabilities Act of 1990 requires employers to provide "reasonable accommodation" for people with disabilities on the job. Digital technology has made this possible.
    - Speech recognition technology allows people without sight or without the use of their hands to interact with computers. Other special input devices include head mice and puff straws.
    - Page scanners, speech synthesizers, and screen readers enable the computer to speak to you if you cannot see the screen, and for you if you cannot speak.
    - Speech recognition can also be used to control appliances in the home, allowing disabled people to live independently.
- Prostheses are artificial replacement limbs and organs.
  - Myoelectric limbs contain a microchip and motor and respond to contractions of the muscle of the natural limb. They work almost as well as natural limbs.
  - CAD/CAM is used in the design and manufacture of prosthetic limbs.
  - Computer technology has contributed to the development of a prosthetic hand whose fingers can be separately controlled and prostheses, which can sense hot and cold.
  - Computer technology is also contributing to developments, which help restore hearing and sight, and movement to paralyzed limbs.
  - Computer technology with neural interfaces is allowing stroke victims and people with spinal cord injuries to control their bodily movements and to some degree their environments.
- Computerized functional electrical stimulation delivers low-level electrical stimulation to muscles.
  - It is used in implanted devices such as pacemakers and to stimulate paralyzed muscles, even enabling the paralyzed to walk.
- Implants pose the risk of infection and rejection.
- Computer programs that recognize that the brain is not a fixed entity are now being used in the rehabilitation of stroke patients, even years after the stroke occurred.

KEY TERMS

adaptive technology
Americans with
    Disabilities Act of
    1990
arrhythmia monitors
assistive technology
augmentative communi-
    cation device
biomicroscopes
Biomove 3000
BrainGate Neural
    Interface System
computerized functional
    electrical stimula-
    tion (CFES or FES)
computerized medical
    instrument
corneal topography

environmental control
    systems
EYESI surgical
    simulator
fetal monitors
GDx Access
head mouse
Heidelberg retinal
    tomograph (HRT)
HELEN (HELp
    Neuropsychology)
microdialysis
motion monitor
myoelectric limbs
neonatal monitors
Neuromove
neuroprosthesis
optical biometry

Optomap Panoramic200
osseointegration
page scanners
physiological monitor-
    ing systems
prosthetic devices
puff straws
pulmonary monitors
screen reader software
smart glasses
speech recognition
speech synthesizer
text telephones
tonometers
Tracey visual function
    analyzer
vision replacement
    therapy

REVIEW EXERCISES

Multiple Choice

1. Computerized medical devices have some advantages over their predecessors. Among them are: _____.
    A. they require no human intervention
    B. they do not have to be programmed
    C. they can be programmed to detect values outside of a certain range and sound an alarm
    D. None of the above
2. Networked devices _____.
    A. can reduce response time in emergencies
    B. are most often found in ERs, CCUs, and ICUs
    C. cannot display findings in a central location
    D. All of the above
3. Puff straws, head mice, and speech recognition software could be characterized as _____.
    A. prosthetic devices
    B. assistive devices
    C. adaptive devices
    D. B or C

4. Glasses in which the lenses are two flat pieces of glass; between them in a 5-micron space is liquid crystal coated with a transparent electrodes which transmits light are called _____.
   A. spy glasses
   B. smart glasses
   C. crystal glasses
   D. All of the above

5. _____ is an alternate input device that a blind person could use.
   A. Braille keyboard
   B. joystick
   C. A or B
   D. screen reader

6. The system that involves implanting a chip in the brain that will convert brain cell impulses to computer signals is called _____.
   A. Verichip
   B. Brainchip
   C. Thinkgate
   D. Braingate

7. CFES delivers low-level electrical stimulation and is used _____.
   A. in pacemakers
   B. to simulate workouts for paralyzed muscles
   C. to restore movement to paralyzed muscles
   D. All of the above

8. The _____ restores some measure of hearing to deaf people with intact auditory nerves.
   A. artificial ear
   B. cochlear implant
   C. hearing pacemaker
   D. prosthetic ear

9. Prosthetic limbs, which contain motors and respond to signals transmitted by the muscles in the residual limb, are called _____.
   A. energy-storing limbs
   B. myoelectric limbs
   C. computerized limbs
   D. motorized limbs

10. Discrimination against people with disabilities is prohibited by the _____.
    A. Civil Rights Act
    B. Fourteenth Amendment to the U.S. Constitution
    C. Americans with Disabilities Act
    D. None of the above

True/False Questions

1. It is possible to control the mouse pointer with thought waves. _____
2. Computer software can help restore some sight to people who are legally blind. _____

3. Hardware and software exist that will allow you to control your home environment by giving voice commands. _____
4. Myoelectric limbs are made possible by computers. _____
5. A computerized program called HELEN (HELp Neuropsychology) contains diagnostic analyses that keep track of specific tests and tasks performed by the stroke patient. _____
6. Electronic stimulation is being used to prevent chronic pain. _____
7. Implanted pacemakers for the brain are used to help control the tremors of Parkinson's. _____
8. Networked devices can interact with each other. _____
9. Computerized cardiac monitors cannot distinguish between cardiac arrest and a wire coming loose. _____
10. Speech recognition software can understand whatever you say. _____

Critical Thinking

1. Evaluate your work space at home, school, or work. How would you design an adaptive environment for people who are mobility impaired?
2. How would you design an adaptive environment for people with speech impairments?
3. How would you design an adaptive environment for people who are blind?
4. The quality of life can be greatly enhanced with the extraordinary CFES technology and advances in prosthetic devices. However, the present cost to the patient can be prohibitive. How would you make this technology available to anyone who needs it?
5. How will the health care professions be affected by all the computerized and technical advances concerning disabilities?

NOTES

1. Lawrence Krieg. "Introduction to Computerized Medical Instrumentation." February 2004. http://courses.wccnet.edu/computer/mod/mod-m.htm (accessed December 27, 2007).
2. "Computer Display on Glasses Helps to Overcome Tunnel Vision," September 11, 2006, http://www.mtbeurope.info/news/2006/609009.htm (accessed January 6, 2008).
3. Dan Roberts, "Microchip Implantation," February 10, 2007, http://www.mdsupport.org/library/chip.html (accessed December 27, 2007).
4. "UA Optical Scientists Develop Switchable Focus Eyeglass Lenses," innovations-report.com, April 4, 2004, http://www.innovations-report.com/html/reports/medical_technology/report-57456.html (accessed December 27, 2007).
5. "Clarity Medical Systems Announces Major Move into Adult Eye Care Market," Pleasanton, July 2, 2006, http://www.hoise.com/vmw/06/articles/vmw/LV-VM-07-06-39.html (accessed December 3, 2007).
6. "Virtual Reality Gaining Acceptance in Ophthalmic Surgical Training Programs," August 1, 2006, http://www.med.nyu.edu/communications/news/pr_190.html (accessed December 27, 2007).

7. "Smart Pants: Computer Engineers Develop Clothes that Sense and Interpret Movements," April 1, 2006, http://www.sciencedaily.com/ (accessed November 27, 2007).

8. J. D. Biersdorfer, "A Scanner-Reader to Take Along Anywhere," nyt.com, July 13, 2006, http://www.nytimes.com/2006/07/13/technology/13blind.html?ex=1310443200&en=a9 311e255a6b8d11&ei=5090&partner=rssuserland&emc=rss (accessed December 27, 2007).

9. "The Dasher Project," August 2, 2006, http://www.inference.phy.cam.ac.uk/dasher/ (accessed August 2, 2006).

10. Ibid.

11. *Environmental Control Systems for People With Spinal Cord Injuries: A Report on Research Undertaken by the Ability Research Center,* September 1999, Ability Research Centre, http://www.abilitycorp.com.au/ftp/research/environmental_controls_systems_report.pdf (accessed February 16, 2008).

12. Annalee Anderson, "Language Learning Using Infrared Toys," 2003 Conference Proceedings, www.csun.edu/cod/conf/2003/proceedings/68.htm (accessed August 24, 2006).

13. Steven Rainwater, "Heroic Cyborg to Receive Medal," February 2006, http://robots.net/article/1826.html (accessed December 27, 2007).

14. David Dishneau, "Veterans in the Line of New Technology," *Star-Ledger,* July 17, 2007, 1, 51.

15. Miki Fairley, "Osseointegration: In the Wave of the Future?" September 2006, http://www.oandp.com/edge/issues/articles/2006-09_03.asp (accessed December 14, 2007).

16. Dianne Hales, "New Help for Hearing Loss," May 14, 2006, http://www.parade.com/articles/editions/2006/edition_05-14-2006/Hearing_Loss (accessed December 27, 2007).

17. "Breaking Sound Barriers," sciencedaily.com, March 1, 2006 (accessed November 27, 2007).

18. S. Agarwal, R. Kobetic, S. Nandurkar, and E. B. Marsolais, "Functional Electrical Stimulation for Walking in Paraplegia: 17-Year Follow-up of 2 Cases," Abstract, Spring 2003, http://www.ncbi.nlm.nih.gov/sites/entrez?db=pubmed&uid=12830975&cmd=showdetailview (accessed December 27, 2007).

19. Barry Meier, "FDA Plans to Intensify Oversight of Heart Devices," nyt.com, April 7, 2006, http://www.nytimes.com/2006/04/07/business/07device.html (accessed December 27, 2007).

20. "Rechargeable Spinal Cord Stimulators for Chronic Pain," spine-health.com, 2006, http://www.spine-health.com/research/stim/stim01.html (accessed December 27, 2007).

21. Cynthia Bowers, "New Device Gives Hope to Paralyzed," cbsnews.com, July 17, 2006, http://www.cbsnews.com/stories/2006/07/17/earlyshow/health/main1808040.shtml (accessed December 27, 2007).

22. "Some Biomove 3000 Questions," http://biomoveusa.com/FAQ-Biomove-3000.htm (accessed August 8, 2006).

23. "Zynex Medical's NeuroMove™ System Cited in New Clinical Study of Stroke Recovery Therapies," *Business Wire,* October 26, 2005, http://findarticles.com/p/articles/mi_m0EIN/is_2005_Oct_26/ai_n15736093 (accessed January 6, 2008).

24. "Biomove 3000 System," January 27, 2005, http://www.fda.gov/cdrh/pdf4/k042650.pdf (accessed December 27, 2007).

25. Catherine Calacanis, "FDA Approves Research to Study Brain Chip for ALS," August 3, 2005, www.telemedicineinsider.com (accessed August 3, 2005).

26. Leigh Hochberg, Mijail D. Serruya, Gerhard M. Friehs et al., "Neuronal Ensemble Control of Prosthetic Devices by a Human with Tetraplegia," *Nature* 442 (2006): 164–71, http://www.nature.com/nature/journal/v442/n7099/abs/nature04970.html (accessed December 27, 2007).

27. "The Neurostimulator: Pacemaker for the Brain," September 2006, http://www.froedtert.com/HealthResources/ReadingRoom/FroedtertToday/September2006Issue/PacemakerfortheBrain.htm (accessed December 27, 2007).

28. Cecilia Sik Lányi, Julianna Szabó, Attila Páll, and Ilona Pataky, "Computer Controlled Cognitive Diagnostics and Rehabilitation Method for Stroke Patients," ERCIM News No. 61, April 2005, http://ercim.org/ (accessed November 27, 2007).

29. "Sports Injury Prevention & Performance: 3D Imaging System Helps Athletes Recover from Injuries," December 1, 2006, http://sciencedaily.com/ (accessed November 27, 2007).

30. "Virtual Reality Lets Amputees 'Control' Missing Limbs," sciencedaily.com, November 15, 2006, http://www.sciencedaily.com/releases/2006/11/061115093227.htm (accessed December 27, 2007).

31. Sharon Begley, "Wall Street Journal Feature: NovaVision™ VRT™ Research & Improvements for Stroke Vision Loss Patient," novavision.com, February 1, 2005, http://www.novavision.com/wall-street-journal-feature-novavision-vrt-research-improvements-for-stroke-vision-loss-patient-nid-61.html (accessed December 27, 2007).

ADDITIONAL RESOURCES

"$3.1 Million NIH Grant Funds Research to Help Stroke Patients." October 17, 2002. http://www.udel.edu/PR/UDaily/01-02/NIHgrant101702.html (accessed August 24, 2006).

ALS Association, Patient & Family Services >> Assistive Technology, 2004. http://www.alsinfo.org/psprogat.html (accessed November 20, 2006).

Anderson, Sandra. *Computer Literacy for Health Care Professionals.* New York: Delmar, 1992.

Berck, Judith. "Tools for Blind Students." nyt.com, August 6, 1995. http://query.nytimes.com/gst/fullpage.html?res=990CE7D9143DF935A3575BC0A963958260 (accessed December 27, 2007).

Bhattacharjee, Yudhijit. "Smart Wheelchairs Will Ease Many Paths." nyt.com, May 10, 2001. http://www.nytimes.com/2001/05/10/technology/10NEXT.html?ex=1198904400&en=49d403d1d3597ed8&ei=5070 (accessed December 27, 2007).

Bhattacharjee, Yudhijit. "So That's Who's Talking: A Hearing Aid Points to the Sound." nyt.com, September 27, 2001. http://query.nytimes.com/gst/fullpage.html?res=9D03E1D6133AF934A1575AC0A9679C8B63 (accessed December 27, 2007).

Boch, Otto. "C-Leg: New Generation Leg System Revolutionizes Lower Limb Prostheses." http://www.ottobockus.com/products/lower_limb_prosthetics/c-leg_article.asp (accessed December 27, 2007).

Carroll, Linda. "Doctors Look Ahead to 'Pacemakers for the Brain.'" February 18, 2003. http://www.mindcontrolforums.com/news/pacemakers-for-brain.htm (accessed August 24, 2006).

"Cochlear Implants." August 16, 2006. http://www.nidcd.nih.gov/health/hearing/coch.asp (accessed December 27, 2007).

"Early Infection and Rejection Detection: Microdialysis Technique May Help Implants Stay Put Longer." July 28, 2003. http://www.rpi.edu/web/Campus.News/july_03/july_28/stenken.htm (accessed December 27, 2007).

Eisenberg, Anne. "Analog over Digital? For a Better Ear Implant, Yes." nyt.com, May 29, 2003. http://query.nytimes.com/gst/fullpage.html?res=9901E7DE1F31F93AA15756C0A9659C8B63 (accessed December 27, 2007).

———. "Beyond Voice Recognition, to a Computer That Reads Lips." nyt.com, September 11, 2003. http://query.nytimes.com/gst/fullpage.html?res=9401E3DC133BF932A2575AC0A9659C8B63 (accessed December 27, 2007).

———. "A Chip That Mimics a Retina but Strains for Light." nyt.com, August 9, 2001. http://query.nytimes.com/gst/fullpage.html?res=9F0DE3D7163FF93AA3575BC0A9679C8B63 (accessed December 27, 2007).

———. "A Gaze That Dictates, with Intuitive Software as the Scribe." nyt.com, September 12, 2002. http://query.nytimes.com/gst/fullpage.html?res=9B0CEED81531F931A2575AC0A9649C8B63 (accessed December 27, 2007).

———. "The Kind of Noise That Keeps a Body on Balance." nyt.com, November 14, 2002. http://query.nytimes.com/gst/fullpage.html?res=9F01E6D61F31F937A25752C1A9649C8B63 (accessed December 27, 2007).

————. "What's Next: A Chip That Mimics Neurons, Firing Up the Memory." nyt.com, June 2, 2002. http://query.nytimes.com/gst/fullpage.html?res=9906E3D9173FF933A157 55C0A9649C8B63 (accessed December 27, 2007).

————. "What's Next: Glasses So Smart They Know What You're Looking At." nyt.com, June 28, 2001. http://www.nytimes.com/2001/06/28/technology/28NEXT.html?ex= 1198904400&en=1d794cee7a240466&ei=5070 (accessed December 27, 2007).

————. "When the Athlete's Heart Falters, a Monitor Dials for Help." nyt.com, January 9, 2003. http://query.nytimes.com/gst/fullpage.html?res=9B03E0DE113EF93AA3575 2C0A9659C8B63 (accessed December 27, 2007).

"Environmental Control Systems for People with Spinal Cord Injuries." 1999. http://www. abilitycorp.com.au/ftp/research/environmental_controls_systems_report.pdf (accessed January 18, 2008).

"FDA Approves Electronic Capsule for Stomach Disorder." ihealthbeat.org, July 21, 2006. http://www.ihealthbeat.org/articles/2006/7/21/FDA-Approves-Electronic-Capsule-for-Stomach-Disorder.aspx?topicID=53 (accessed December 27, 2007).

"FDA Approves New Glucose Test for Adult Diabetics." FDA News, March 22, 2001. http:// www.fda.gov/bbs/topics/NEWS/2001/NEW00758.html (accessed December 27, 2007).

Felton, Bruce. "Technologies That Enable the Disabled." nyt.com, September 14, 1997. http:// query.nytimes.com/gst/fullpage.html?res=9A0CE3D81139F937A2575AC0A961958260 (accessed December 27, 2007).

Gallagher, David. "For the Errant Heart, a Chip That Packs a Wallop." nyt.com, August 16, 2001 (accessed August 24, 2006).

Garibaldi, Matthew. "Myoelectric Prostheses Offer Advantages." Winter 2006. http://www. ucsfhealth.org/common/pubs/ortho/winter2006/myoelectric/index.html (accessed December 27, 2007).

Glassman, Mark. "A Braille Phone Organizer Connects the Dots and the User." nyt.com, April 17, 2003. http://query.nytimes.com/gst/fullpage.html?res=9C0DEFDD163AF9 34A25757C0A9659C8B63 (accessed December 27, 2007).

Grady, Denise. "Digital Hearing Aids Hold New Promise." nyt.com, June 4, 1997. http:// query.nytimes.com/gst/fullpage.html?res=9C07E2D6123DF937A35755C0A961958260 (accessed December 27, 2007).

Happ, Mary, Kathryn Garrett, and Tricia Roesch. "Feasibility of an Augmentative Device for Head and Neck Cancer Patients." May 15, 2002. http://www.ons.org/research/ funding/SummaryReports/summaryReportsSm.shtml (accessed January 18, 2008).

Henkel, John. "Parkinson's Disease: New Treatments Slow Onslaught of Symptoms," US FDA, 1998. http://www.fda.gov/Fdac/features/1998/498_pd.html (accessed December 27, 2007).

Junker, Andrew H. "A Revolutionary Approach to Computer Access: Coherent Detected Periodic Brainwave Computer Control." 2003. http://brainfingers.com/ (accessed November 20, 2006).

Klonoff, David C. "Diabetes and Telemedicine: Is the Technology Sound, Effective, Cost-effective, and Practical?" 2003. http://care.diabetesjournals.org/cgi/content/ full/26/5/1626 (accessed January 6, 2008).

Krcmar, Stephen. "The Stuff of Dreams." April 2006. http://www.rehabpub.com/features/ 42006/7.asp (accessed August 24, 2006).

Lazzaro, John. *Adaptive Technologies for Learning and Work Environments.* Chicago, IL: American Library Association, 1993.

Marriott, Michel. "Wired by a Kindred Spirit, the Disabled Gain Control." nyt.com, April 24, 2003. http://query.nytimes.com/gst/fullpage.html?res=9A01E3D71F3AF937A1575 7C0A9659C8B63 (accessed December 27, 2007).

Mathur, Ruchi and William C. Shiel. "Insulin Pump for Diabetes Mellitus." http://www. medicinenet.com/insulin_pump_for_diabetes_mellitus/article.htm (accessed December 3, 2007).

"Medicare to Pay for FES Walking System." 2002. http://sci.rutgers.edu/forum/archive/index.php/t-47354.html (accessed December 27, 2007).

"New Device Approval: GlucoWatch® Automatic Glucose Biographer—P990026." March 22, 2001. http://www.fda.gov/cdrh/pdf/P990026.html (accessed December 27, 2007).

"New Device Approvals: Medtronic Model 7250 Jewel®AF Implantable Cardioverter Defibrillator System—P980050/S1." April 1, 2001. http://www.fda.gov/cdrh/mda/docs/p980050s001.pdf (accessed December 27, 2007).

"New, Light Prosthetics Helping Amputees Function Better: Computerized Prosthetics Offer Better Fit." March 2005. http://www.wnbc.com/print/2267223/detail.html (accessed January 6, 2008).

Norwood, Robert. "NASA Technologies Contribute to Medical Breakthroughs." *Advanced Technologies,* March–April, 1998.

Nussbaum, Debra. "Bringing the Visual World of the Web to the Blind." *New York Times,* March 26, 1998, G8.

Ouellette, Jennifer. "Biomaterials Facilitate Medical Breakthroughs." American Institute of Physics, October/November 2001. http://www.aip.org/tip/INPHFA/vol-7/iss-5/p18.pdf (accessed December 27, 2007).

"A Pacemaker for the Brain." 2005. http://www.clevelandclinic.org/health/health-info/docs/1900/1937.asp?index=8782&src=news&ref=1900/1937.asp?index=8782 (accessed December 27, 2007).

"Pacemaker for the Brain May Offer Hope for Parkinson's Disease." 2006. http://mentalhealth.about.com/library/sci/0102/blparkins0102.htm (accessed December 27, 2007).

Rachkesperger, Tracy. "Growing Up with AAC." 2006. http://www.asha.org/public/speech/disorders/GrowingUpAAC.htm (accessed December 27, 2007).

Senn, Jim. *Information Technology in Business: Principles, Practices, and Opportunities.* 2nd ed. Upper Saddle River, NJ: Prentice Hall, 1998.

Skillings, Jonathan. "Prosthetics Go High Tech." cnetnews.com, August 3, 2005. http://www.news.com/Prosthetics-go-high-tech/2008-1082_3-5816267.html (accessed December 27, 2007).

Taub, Eric. "Typing with Two Hands, No Fingers." nyt.com, May 1, 2003. http://query.nytimes.com/gst/fullpage.html?res=9C0CE5D81F3DF932A35756C0A9659C8B63 (accessed December 27, 2007).

"VA Technology Assessment Program Project Report – Patient Summary on Computerized Lower Limb Prosthesis." March 2000. http://www.va.gov/vatap/patientinfo/prosteticlimb.htm (accessed December 27, 2007).

Weingarten, Marc. "For an Irregular Lens, an Optical Blueprint." nyt.com, September 12, 2002. http://query.nytimes.com/gst/fullpage.html?res=9D02E2D81531F931A2575AC0A9649C8B63 (accessed December 27, 2007).

Wiener, Jon. "USC Ophthalmologists Announce Launch of Permanent Retinal Implant Study." April 30, 2002. http://www.eurekalert.org/pub_releases/2002-04/uosc-uoa_1043002.php (accessed January 18, 2008).

RELATED WEB SITES

http://www.alsinfo.org
http://www.fda.gov
http://www.nih.gov
http://www.patientcareonline.com
http://www.telemedicineinsider.com
http://www.va.gov

Security and Privacy in an Electronic Age

LEARNING OBJECTIVES

After reading this chapter, you will be able to

- Define security and privacy.
- Discuss threats to information technology, including crimes, viruses, and the unauthorized use of data.
- Discuss security measures including laws, voluntary codes of conduct, restriction of access to computer systems, and the protection of information on networks.
- Describe the Real ID Act of 2005.
- Describe the impact of information technology on privacy, including the existence of large computerized databases of information kept by both government and private organizations, some of which are on networks linked to the Internet.
- Describe the relationship of privacy and security to health care and appreciate the importance of the privacy of electronic medical records.
- Discuss the Health Insurance Portability and Accountability Act of 1996 (HIPAA) and the USA Patriot Act (2001), specifically their effects on privacy protections.
- Discuss the lack of enforcement of HIPAA.

◼◼ SECURITY AND PRIVACY—AN OVERVIEW

Information technology and the expansion of the Internet have changed the way we live. Almost all of our institutions—schools, businesses, hospitals, and government agencies—depend on computers. By 2014, hospitals are supposed to have installed computerized hospital information systems; eventually, all health care institutions will be linked electronically. Computers enable the collection, storage, and processing of enormous amounts of information quickly and efficiently. At the same time, any harm to computer systems is more threatening to the normal conduct of business. Safeguarding computer systems becomes critical. Guaranteeing the accuracy and **security** and protecting the **privacy** of electronic records, including medical records, are crucial. Our initial discussion of security and privacy, although general, also applies to medical issues of security and privacy. It is an ongoing challenge. In March 2003, the following appeared in *The Centre Daily Times* (Texas): "In Kentucky, state computers put up for sale as surplus . . . contained confidential files naming thousands of people with AIDS and sexually transmitted diseases. The oversight was discovered when the state auditor's office purchased eight of the computers. Thousands of state-owned computers may still be out there."[1]

In 2005, ChoicePoint, a company that collects and sells data to clients with a legitimate interest in the data—including corporations, insurance companies, private investigators, and law enforcement among others—gave away private information. ChoicePoint said "that last year it had unwittingly provided records to some 50 phony businesses posing as legitimate . . . [businesses]." The private information of 145,000–500,000 people was compromised.[2] Less than two weeks later, the Bank of America announced that it had lost tapes containing 1.2 million records.[3]

In August 2006, a Department of Veterans Affairs computer containing data on 38,000 patients at Pennsylvania VA hospitals disappeared.[4] Data on computers are not secure.

Privacy has many aspects. Among them is the ability to control personal information and the right to keep it from misuse. Computer technology makes this much more difficult. Security measures attempt to protect computer systems, including information, from harm and abuse; the threats may stem from many sources including natural disaster, human error, or crime including the spreading of **viruses**. Protection may take the form of anything from professional and business codes of conduct, to laws, to restricting access to the computer.

This chapter deals with threats to information technology, stressing dangers to the privacy of information in electronic databases as well as measures to protect the security of computer systems. Massive government and private databases on the Internet pose dangers to personal privacy. The chapter also deals with computers and trends in health care delivery, including the growth of health maintenance organizations and medical insurance companies, the relationship of telemedicine to issues of privacy and security, the use of electronic medical records and e-mail. The electronic sharing of medical records can help save lives by assuring continuity of care. However, the lack of security in computer systems in health care organizations and on networks in general endangers doctor–patient confidentiality and the privacy of medical information. Even under HIPAA, medical records are accessible not only to your physicians, but also to insurance companies, laboratories, pharmacies, and hospital clerical staffs. Included in this chapter is a discussion of attempts to make electronic medical records secure, including the first federal legislation protecting the privacy of medical records—the Health Insurance Portability and Accountability Act of 1996 (HIPAA).

THREATS TO INFORMATION TECHNOLOGY

Threats to information technology include hazards to hardware, software, networks, and data including information stored in electronic databases. **Data accuracy** and security are what is most relevant to the use of computerized medical records. However, computer hardware, software, and data can be damaged by anything from simple carelessness to power surges, crime, and computer viruses. Computer systems, like any other property, can be hurt or destroyed by disasters such as floods and fires.

Computer Technology and Crime

Computer technology has led to new forms of crime. Crimes involving computers can be crimes using computers or crimes against computer systems. Many times they are both—using computers to harm computer systems. Computer crime includes committing fraud and scams over the Internet, unauthorized copying of software protected by copyright (called **software piracy**), and **theft of services** such as cable TV. Software piracy costs the software industry billions of dollars a year.

According to the Business Software Alliance, over 30 percent of software is pirated.[5] **Theft of information**, including breaking into a medical database and gaining access to medical records, is also considered a crime.

One common computer crime is **fraud**—such as using a computer program to illegally transfer money from one bank account to another or printing payroll checks to oneself. Fraudulent purchases over the Internet are common. Purchases over the Internet are increasing. A favorite target of Internet thieves is software. Because software is delivered instantly—electronically—it is received before credit card numbers are checked.

Viruses can also damage hardware, software, and data. A virus is a program that attaches itself to another program and replicates itself. A virus may do damage to your hardware or destroy your data, or it may simply flash an annoying message. Most states and the federal government make it a crime to intentionally spread a computer virus. Federal law makes it a felony to do $1000 or more worth of damage to any computer involved in interstate commerce; this includes any personal computer connected to the Internet. The penalties for damaging computer systems have been severely increased by the USA Patriot Act and the Homeland Security Act. Spreading viruses is a kind of high-tech vandalism. Virus detection software can find and get rid of many but not all viruses.

One of the most valuable resources of any organization is data or information. An accurate list of a business's customers with their purchases and credit records, or of a doctor's patients with their confidential medical histories, is a vital asset that cannot be replaced. It is crucial that this information be correct and secure. However, this is not always the case. Data may be incorrect simply because of carelessness in data entry; that is, information in a database is erroneous because of faulty entry or an inaccurate source. However, data may be correct and still vulnerable to misuse. Some information, including medical records, is highly personal and subject to abuse. Protecting the privacy of records kept on electronic databases and on networks is extremely difficult, if not impossible.

Identity theft involves someone using your private information to assume your identity. Identity theft rose between 2000 and 2003; however, it has now stabilized: "Identity fraud victims as a percent of the United States adult population . . . declined slightly from 4.7% to 4.0% between 2003 and 2006." Although identity theft predates computers, the existence of computer networks, the centralization of information in databases, and the posting of public information on the Internet could make information much easier to steal. However, currently 68 percent of victims do not experience any financial loss.[6] Many identity thieves start at home; according to a study by the Federal Trade Commission, among those who find out who stole their identity, half are members of the family or household (partners, roommates, children, and parents).[7] An identity thief needs only a few pieces of information (such as Social Security number and mother's maiden name) to steal your identity. Under this false identity—your identity—the thief can take out credit cards, loans, buy houses, and even commit crimes. Identity theft is extremely difficult to prosecute. It is also not easy for the victim to correct all the negative information that the thief has created. False negative information may keep appearing in response to every routine computer check. Currently, some cities are putting all public records including property and court records on the Internet, making identity theft even easier to commit. Think of the information (including your signature) on the ticket you were issued last month.

Biometric methods are going to be used in a new identification system to safeguard your identity. It would include fingerprint sensors within your credit card and would prevent identity thieves from stealing information.[8]

As of 2006, some threats to computer systems include the following. **Spyware** is software that can be installed without the user's knowledge to track their actions on a computer. **Adware** may display unwanted pop-up advertisements on your monitor; the advertisements may be related to the sites you search on the Web or even the content of your e-mail. A **fraudulent dialer** can connect the user with numbers without the user's knowledge; the dialer may connect the user's computer to an expensive 900 number. The user will be totally unaware until he or she receives the telephone bill. A dialer is usually installed with free software. **Keylogging** can be used by anyone to track anyone else's keystrokes. **Malware** includes different forms of malicious hardware, software, and firmware. **Spybot Search and Destroy software** can remove malware, adware, spyware, dialers, and keyloggers from your computer.

Security

Security measures attempt to protect computer systems and the privacy of computerized data. They can include anything from laws and **codes of conduct**, to training employees, to audit trails, to restricting access to computers, to **encryption**—scrambling of data so that it does not make sense. There are federal laws that attempt to protect computer systems and aspects of privacy (Figure 12.1■).

However, in 2006, a GAO (Government Accountability Office) report concluded that "privacy laws do not fully protect personal data when sold by information resellers" like ChoicePoint. In the last thirty-four years, the Federal Trade Commission "initiated more than 20 . . . enforcement actions . . . " but it does not have the authority to penalize companies.[9]

There are also codes of conduct within some businesses and organizations that attempt to safeguard information. Protecting privacy on the Internet is a much more difficult problem. An early attempt at self-regulation occurred in December 1997. To forestall government regulation, several computer companies and look-up services reached an agreement on a code of conduct to limit public access to personal data on the Internet. The code would allow people to have their names removed from databases; but it includes no way of informing people what is online about them or giving them a way to correct it. A person would have to contact all fourteen companies and ask to have his or her name removed from each database. The agreement also would ask marketers to "voluntarily limit the collection of personal data." Encryption would be used to protect private information. Social Security numbers, mother's maiden name, birth date, credit and financial records, and medical records would no longer be available to the general public; private investigators and law enforcement agencies would have access to this information.

Federal Legislation on Computers and Privacy

- **1970—The Fair Credit Reporting Act** regulates credit agencies. It allows you to see your credit reports to check the accuracy of information and challenge inaccuracies. Amended several times, Fair and Accurate Credit Transaction Act of 2003 preempts some state privacy protections, but mandates that you can have a free credit report each year.[10]

- **1974—Privacy Act** prohibits disclosure of government records to anyone except the individual concerned, except for law enforcement purposes. It also prohibits the use of information except for the purpose for which it was gathered. It deals with the use and disclosure of Social Security numbers.[11]

- **1978—Right to Financial Privacy Act** (RFPA) establishes procedures for the federal government to follow when looking at bank records. RFPA amended due to the USA Patriot Act of 2001: to permit the disclosure of financial information to any intelligence or counterintelligence agency in any investigation related to international terrorism (October, 2001).[12]

- **1984 (amended in 1994)—Computer Fraud and Abuse Act** prohibits unauthorized access to federal computers.[13]

- **1986—Electronic Communications Privacy Act** prohibits government agencies from intercepting electronic communications without a search warrant. It also prohibits individuals from intercepting e-mail. However, there are numerous exceptions, and the courts have interpreted this to allow employers to access employees' e-mail. This law does not apply to communications within an organization.[14]

- **1988—Video Privacy Protection Act** prohibits video rental stores from revealing what tapes you rent.[15]

- **1988 (amended in 1990)—Computer Matching and Privacy Protection Act** limits the use of computer matching.[16]

- **1994—Computer Abuse Amendments Act** makes it a crime to "gain unauthorized access to a computer system [used in interstate commerce] with the intent to obtain anything of value, to defraud the system, or to cause more than $1000 worth of damage." This applies to any computer linked to the Internet. It specifically prohibits the transmission of viruses. (Note: Section 1030 was amended on October 26, 2001, by the USA Patriot antiterrorism legislation.)[17]

■ **FIGURE 12.1**   Federal laws intended to protect computer systems and privacy of individuals.

- **1996—National Information Infrastructure Protection Act** establishes penalties for interstate theft of information and for threats against networks and computer system trespassing.[18]

- **1996—Health Insurance Portability and Accountability Act (HIPAA)** puts a national floor under privacy protections for medical information.

- **1997—Driver Privacy Protection Act** limits disclosure of personal information in Motor Vehicles records.[19]

- **1999—The Financial Modernization Act** governs collection and disclosure of customers' personal financial information by financial institutions.[20]

- **2000—Children's Online Privacy Protection Act** requires Web sites targeting children aged thirteen or under to get parental consent to gather information on the children.[21]

- **2001—The USA Patriot Act** gives law enforcement agencies greater power to monitor electronic and other communications, with fewer checks.[22]

- **2002—The Homeland Security Act** expands and centralizes the data gathering allowed under the Patriot Act.[23]

- **2004—Social Security Protection Act**: to amend the Social Security Act and the Internal Revenue Code of 1986 to provide additional safeguards for Social Security and Supplemental Security Income beneficiaries with representative payees, to enhance program protections, and for other purposes.[24]

- **2004—Video Voyeurism Act** would prohibit video voyeurism in the maritime and territorial jurisdiction of the United States.[25]

- **2005—Combat Methamphetamine Epidemic Act**: A new part of the USA Patriot Act that requires anyone who buys cough medicine containing pseudoephedrine to present photo ID.[26]

- **2005—Online Privacy Protection Act** requires the Federal Trade Commission to prescribe regulations to protect the privacy of personal information collected from and about individuals who are not covered by the Children's Online Privacy Protection Act of 1998 on the Internet, to provide greater individual control over the collection and use of that information, and for other purposes.[27]

■ **FIGURE 12.1** *(continued).*

Many organizations restrict access to their computers. This can be done by requiring authorized users to have **personal identification numbers (PINs)** or use **passwords**. Locking computer rooms and requiring employees to carry ID cards and keys are also used to restrict access. **Biometric methods** including **fingerprints, hand prints, retina** or **iris scans, lip prints, facial thermography, body odor sensors, voice recognition,** and **DNA** also help make sure only authorized people have access to computer systems. Biometric technology can use facial structure to identify individuals. **Biometric keyboards** can identify a person by behavior, for example, a typist by fingerprints, a person by fingerprint, voice, and gait. None of these methods is foolproof. Even biometric methods, which for a time were seen as more reliable, are far from perfect. PINs and passwords can be forgotten or shared, and ID cards and keys can be lost or stolen. Biometric methods also pose a threat to privacy, because anyone who can gain access to the database of physical characteristics gains access to other, possibly private information about you. Some biometric measures are inherently different than other security measures. In more traditional methods, such as fingerprinting, you are aware that your identity is being checked. However, iris and retina scans, facial thermographs, **facial structure scans**, and body odor sensors allow your identity to be checked without your knowledge, cooperation, or consent. This can be seen as an invasion of privacy. Now there is the possibility of implanted radio frequency identification (RFID) tags as a security measure.

Since September 11, the federal government has attempted to increase airport security using various measures to screen passengers and baggage. A controversial plan to "deploy 'backscatter' X-ray machines to search air travelers" has been announced by the Transportation Security Administration. It has been referred to as a virtual strip search, because "The level of detail uncovered [is] akin to . . . disrobing in public: the images seen by the screeners reveal the outlines of nipples and genitalia."[28]

Protecting information which is kept on a network is much more difficult because no one knows who can access a network. Even top-secret defense systems have been broken into. One way of protecting data is through encryption. Only authorized persons can see the decrypted data. Electronic blocks (called **firewalls**) can be used to limit access to networks. None of these measures guarantees security; therefore, a protection plan that includes backing up data is always necessary. This guarantees that you have an accurate copy of the data you need, but does nothing to protect data from misuse.

PRIVACY

Computer technology has transformed the way we assemble, store, and protect data—including highly confidential material. It has also changed the way we work at jobs. Almost every white-collar worker has a microcomputer on his or her desk. The personal computer has replaced the typewriter. E-mail is replacing the memo and telephone call. This makes both our words and our work more subject to scrutiny and less private. People think of e-mail as private; it is not. According to Barry Lawrence of the Society of Human Resource Management, ". . . e-mail [is] like a postcard. Anyone can read it along the way." Employees are fired for using e-mail for private communications or to send messages critical of their bosses. The **Electronic Communications Privacy Act of 1986** has been interpreted to allow employers access to employees' e-mail. Not only are your words subject to scrutiny; so is your work. When you are working on your office PC, every keystroke may be monitored and counted by your employer.

As an employee, you have a very restricted right to privacy. In 1977, the Federal Privacy Protection Commission, under pressure from business groups, did not ask Congress to make it a crime for employers to gather information "unrelated to job performance" about employees. As a consumer, when you make a purchase with a credit card, your name, address, and credit card number, along with your purchases, are recorded. The information becomes part of your credit history, and a profile of your buying habits can be put together and sold to direct marketers. Records that used to be kept in physically separate places—your credit history in one store's credit file, or your health records in your doctor's office, or a city's records of births, marriages, and vehicle ownership in a county courthouse—are now organized in databases, stored on computers, linked to networks, and available to anyone with a computer and a modem.

Smart cards are currently being used in many states as driver's licenses. These cards can contain information about the driver and links to government and private databases. However, in May 2005, as part of the military spending bill, President Bush signed the **Real ID Act of 2005** into law. Prior to this, the states were cooperating with the federal government to establish acceptable federal standards. However, the Real ID Act "directly imposes prescriptive federal driver's license standards" by the federal government on the states.[29] This law requires every American to have an electronic identification card. By 2008, states are supposed to start providing ID cards that meet the standards set up by the Real ID Act. "You'll need a federally approved ID card to travel on an airplane, open a bank account, collect Social Security payments . . ." And practically speaking, your driver's license likely will have to be reissued to meet federal standards. To be issued a card, you will need to appear (in person) at a state motor vehicle agency with photo identity, "document your birth date and address, and show that your Social Security number is what you had claimed it to be." This information must be verified, digitized, and stored by the Department of Motor Vehicles (DMV). Your prior licenses and immigration status must also be verified. For the states to be able to check the information an applicant provides, databases containing this information must be put online and standardized so that each state can access the information. The cards will contain (in machine readable form) at least the following information: name, date of birth, sex, ID number, a digital photo, and address. The Department of Homeland Security may unilaterally add other items like a fingerprint or an iris scan.[30] The Department of Homeland Security, the states, and Motor Vehicles Departments are working to set up guidelines; they have not as yet determined what technology or technologies to use: RFID, barcode, or magnetic stripe. The cards must contain features that make them secure against tampering or copying. Data must be encrypted.

Cardholders will be able to block transmission of the information and "ha[ve] to be informed about how the agency issuing the card intended to use it, what information was being collected . . ., the basic risks of the technology . . ., and which precautions were available."[31] State DMVs must share all of the information in their databases with all other state DMVs' databases. This creates a huge database. Police can demand ID from anyone. The law also sets up a "requirement for background checks on employees."

A new threat to personal privacy may come from implanted RFID tags (**Verichips**), according to privacy advocates. The tags are radio transmitters that give off a unique signal, which can be read by a receiver. The person with the tag implanted does not need to know it is being read. Tags have been used in pets and products. The FDA has approved the tags for medical use.[32] In 2006, two employees of an Ohio company had RFID tags embedded in their arms. The company said "it was testing the technology as a way of controlling access to a room."[33]

However, Verichips are very easily counterfeited—". . . you could have a chip implanted, and then your front door would unlock when your shoulder got close to the reader. Let us imagine that you did this; then, I could sit next to you on the subway, and read your chip's ID. This takes less than a second. At this point I can let myself in to your house, by replaying that ID. So now you have to change your ID; but as far as I know, you cannot do this without surgery."[34]

Computer technology and the Internet allow for the inexpensive and easy gathering and distribution of personal information—from the most mundane to the most intimate details of our lives—which may be collected without our consent or knowledge. Laws have been proposed to create some minimal privacy rights on the Internet; for example, sites now have to get parental consent before collecting information from children. The computer may gather information about you without your knowledge as you browse the Net. Cookies are small files that a Web site may put on your hard drive when you visit. Cookies can be programmed to track your movements, collecting information that helps advertisers target you. This information may be sold and shared; the fact is that you do not control your information once it is in cyberspace.

Databases

An electronic **database** is an organized collection of data that is easy to access, manipulate, search, and sort. Gathering facts is not new. A decennial census is mandated by the U.S. Constitution, so that representation in Congress can be determined. Records of birth, marriage, death, divorce, property ownership, taxes, driving, and bankruptcy are all on file. The local library even keeps records of the books you check out until they are returned. These records have always been kept. However, they used to be kept in the local courthouse or motor vehicles department—every file physically and logically separate from every other file. To access the records, you had to travel to where the file was kept. Today, with the use of computerized databases on networked computers, this is not the case. Through the use of Social Security numbers as identifiers, the information in one database can be linked to information in other databases, and a complete and detailed portrait of any individual can be painted.

Government Databases

Large databases of information are kept by the federal and local governments as well as by private businesses. Agencies of the federal government maintain more than two thousand databases. The FBI's National Crime Information Center includes millions of records. The Internal Revenue Service (IRS) keeps a database on the sources and amounts of income we earn and the taxes we pay. The Social Security Administration has records used to determine your eligibility for benefits. The Department of Defense has a database, which includes your draft status. The National Directory of New Hires is a database that the federal government was required to start on October 1, 1997, by the 1996 welfare law. Every time a person is hired, his or her name must be reported along with address, Social Security number, and wages. Wage reports are required every three months. The data collected by the Census Bureau are now computerized, although by law, they cannot be used against a respondent.

Agencies of the government may use computer matching to link data in several databases. For example, the IRS uses computer matching to match tax records with vehicle registration and other records kept by state governments and with private records of large transactions kept by banks. The IRS looks for expensive purchases such as cars and boats, and for large cash transactions. The National Directory of New Hires will be matched against the Department of Health and Human Services' list of everyone owing or owed child support, and the lists will be checked against each other. Some federal agencies (including the IRS, Social Security Administration, and Secret Service) use computer profiling—a technique that puts together a portrait of a person "likely" to commit a crime. Computer profiling is also being used by the Government's Computer-Assisted Passenger Screening program, which "uses several dozen criteria, all but a few secret, to screen for the air travelers most likely to be drug lords or terrorists." Although data gathered by the government are subject to some regulation, data gathered by private companies are not. Government and private companies do cooperate in the gathering of data. Currently, certain jurisdictions are putting all their records online. This means your signature is available on a traffic ticket, and the details of your divorce can be read like a novel.

Since September 11, Congress, concerned with security, passed two bills that affect privacy: the USA Patriot Act (2001) and The Homeland Security Act (2002). The **USA Patriot Act** gives law enforcement agencies greater power to monitor electronic and other communications, with fewer checks. It allows increased sharing of information between the states, the FBI, and the CIA. The law expands the authority of the government to allow roving wiretaps, which intercept communications, wherever the person is. Both e-mail and voice mail may be seized under a search warrant.[35] The government may track web surfing and request information from Internet Service Providers (ISPs) about their subscribers. The law establishes a DNA database that will include anyone convicted of a violent crime. Some of these provisions were originally scheduled to sunset or expire in 2005. However, on March 9, 2006,

President Bush signed an extension of the USA Patriot Act. The sixteen provisions will not expire. The Homeland Security Act expands and centralizes the data gathering allowed under The Patriot Act. A new federal department of Homeland Security is established to analyze data collected by other agencies. The law includes expanded provision for the government to monitor electronic communications and authority for the government to mine databases of personal information, at the same time that it limits Congressional oversight. Any government body at any level can now request information from your ISP without a warrant or probable cause, as long as there is a "good faith" belief that national security is involved. Your local library is required to turn over any record to the FBI, if asked. The act limits an individual's access to information under the Freedom of Information Act. If a business states that its activities are related to security, that information will be kept secret.[36] The law gives government committees more freedom to meet in secret. It limits liability for companies producing antiterrorism products including vaccinations, at the same time that the government would gain wider power to declare national health emergencies, quarantines, and order forced vaccinations.

Since September 11, "new mechanisms . . . for data sharing and mining" have been developed.[37] Many private businesses have been pressed to give customer information to the federal government. One instance of this, which was revealed in 2006, involved large telecommunications companies giving the telephone records of millions of Americans to the National Security Administration without warrants.[38]

In an action that defies classification, "the text of a secret agreement that the Department of Homeland Security executed with the Centers for Disease Control to share airline data" has been revealed. This violates an agreement that the United States reached with the European Union that the latter would share data despite "the lack of privacy laws in the United States. . . . DHS agreed that the passenger data would not be used for any purpose other than the prevention of serious crime." However, DHS has broken the agreement.[39]

Private Databases

Private organizations keep computerized databases of employees and potential customers. Hospitals keep records of patients. You may not be aware that data are being gathered, or that the data gathered may be entered in a database. The information in the databases may be available to the general public over the Internet. Unaware of the existence of the information, you have no opportunity to check its accuracy. When you buy something using a credit card at the supermarket, fill out a warranty card, subscribe to a magazine, fill out a survey questionnaire, or rent a movie, data are collected about your purchasing habits. When you make a telephone call, a record is kept of the telephone number, time, and length of the call. All of this information is collected for commercial purposes; businesses can buy your profile and analyze it, looking for likely customers. However, you do not control what happens to information about you or who will become aware of the brand of soap you use in the shower.

The **Medical Information Bureau** is of particular interest. It is comprised of 650 insurance companies. Its database contains health information on fifteen million people. The information in this huge database is used by medical insurers to help determine insurance rates and whether to grant or deny someone medical coverage. The medical histories in this database are not protected by doctor–patient privilege and are specifically exempt from HIPAA.[40]

Credit bureaus receive information from businesses and banks. From this, they compile a credit history and credit report. Your credit report is used as a basis for granting or denying you a credit card, mortgage, or student loan. It may also be requested by a potential employer and may be used to deny you a job. Although the use and content of credit reports is regulated by the **Fair Credit Reporting Act of 1970**, it is extremely difficult to remove inaccurate negative information.

Some private companies (data warehouses) exist for the sole purpose of collecting and selling personal information. They sell information to credit bureaus and to employers for background checks. Since September 11, the demand for background checks on prospective (or even current) employees has increased. One company experienced a 33 percent increase in the demand for background checks. The linking of information is making these background checks more thorough. Electronic databases are now being linked into larger and more comprehensive super databases. For example, in November 2001, one company linked together criminal records from all U.S. jurisdictions (a database of twenty million convictions). Before that, each jurisdiction had to be searched separately.

Databases and the Internet

When files were first computerized, they were kept in separate computer systems; security could be as easy as locking the door to the computer room and requiring each authorized user to have valid identification. Today, computerized files are kept on networks, many of which linked to the Internet. The information includes highly personal data such as Social Security numbers, dates of birth, mother's maiden name, and unlisted phone numbers. Companies such as Lexis-Nexis and Equifax sell credit and financial information and medical records to banks, insurance companies, and direct marketers. You are not aware of the information that is available about you, or where it is stored, or its accuracy. The impact of this is serious. Anyone with access to your Social Security number can gain access to information about you and even assume your identity.

PRIVACY, SECURITY, AND HEALTH CARE

The privacy of medical records is something people are very concerned about. Several trends combine to threaten the security and privacy of health care information. First, health care information has traditionally been protected by state law. Now, however, this information routinely crosses state lines, which means it needs federal protection. It is very difficult to protect information on computer networks, especially the Internet. The privacy protections of the Health Information Portability and Accountability Act of 1996 began going into effect on April 14, 2003. HIPAA provides the first federal protection for the privacy of medical records.

Health Insurance Portability and Accountability Act of 1996

Given the facts of current medical practice—the use of the electronic medical record stored on networks, telemedicine, and information that routinely crosses state lines—federal protection has become a necessity.

In 1996, Congress passed the **Health Insurance Portability and Accountability Act (HIPAA)**. Guidelines to protect electronic medical records were developed by the Department of Health and Human Services. By encouraging the use of the electronic medical record and facilitating the sharing of medical records among health care providers, it can assure continuity of care and thus save lives. If you are in an accident far from home, the availability of your medical history can prevent medical catastrophes such as allergic reactions to medications. However, the more easily your records are available, the less secure they are. Medical information can be used against you. According to a report by the U.S. Congress cited in the *Telemedicine Newsletter*, it is crucial to safeguard the privacy of health information because, "Inaccuracies in the information or its improper disclosure, can deny an individual access to . . . basic necessities of life, and can threaten an individual's personal and financial well-being."

HIPAA "encourag[es] electronic transactions, but it also requires new safeguards to protect the security and confidentiality" of health information.[41] The new safeguards do not override stronger state protections.

For the first time, all patients have the right to see their medical records and *request* changes; patients will have some knowledge of the use of their medical records and must be notified in writing of their providers' privacy policy. HIPAA gives patients more control over their medical information. Under the rule, medical records must be supplied within thirty days of the patient's request, and the patients are allowed to review and copy their own records as they wish. Prior to HIPAA, many states did not give patients the legal right to see their records. Additionally, the patient can request amendments be made to their records if their appeal is justifiable.

HIPAA regulations began going into effect on April 14, 2001; health plans, clearinghouses, and providers who use electronic billing and funds transfer had until April 14, 2003, to comply. Other entities had until April 2006 to comply. In 2006, the enforcement portion of the law went into effect; that is, health care institutions can be fined for disobeying the law. The regulations cover "all medical records and other individually identifiable health information used or disclosed by a covered entity in any form, whether electronically, on paper, or orally." Higher standards apply to psychotherapy notes, which are not considered part of a medical record under this law and "are never intended to be shared with anyone else." The law applies to both public and private providers and institutions. Providers must give patients a written explanation of how their health information may be used; patients may see, copy, and *request* changes in their medical records. Providers need to make a good faith effort to get a patient's consent before using his or her information. Health information may no longer be used by employers or banks to make decisions regarding employment or loans. Except for the sharing of information for the purpose of treatment, payment, or business operations, "disclosures . . . will be limited to the minimum necessary."[42] In practice, this may mean that any health care business can see personal health information with little regard for treatment.

Health care providers and institutions may design their own procedures to meet the new standards; however, they must be written and must include the following information: who has access to patient information, how this information will be used, and the conditions under which it may be shared. Health care providers are responsible for seeing that those with whom they do business also protect patient privacy. Employees must be trained to respect patient privacy and follow privacy procedures, and one person must be chosen to ensure that the privacy procedures are followed. Under specific conditions, health information may be shared without the patient's consent (e.g., for public health needs, research, and some law enforcement activities, and when the interests of national defense and security are involved). Under HIPAA, violations of the law can be punished by both civil and criminal penalties.[43]

Some of the original privacy protections have been weakened, for example, the requirement of a patient's written consent for disclosure of health information.[44] Because of this, some privacy advocates stress the weaknesses of the privacy protection. According to James Pyles, a lawyer from Washington, DC, "Almost any health care business can now have access to personal health information if it can show that the information is needed for treatment, payment or business operations".[45] However, with all its weaknesses, HIPAA will provide the first national minimum privacy protections for health information.[46]

HIPAA requires health care facilities (protected entities) to conduct a risk analysis to "evaluate risks . . . and to implement policies and procedures to address those risks."[47] Risk management requires the entity to put into place security measures. The use of virus protection software, specifically Spybot Search and Destroy, would be advisable. One of the security measures that health care organizations can use is Single Sign On—Password Management. Single Sign On makes use of smart cards and biometrics. It makes it possible for multiple users to share a workstation without compromising security. It keeps track of users.

Law enforcement responsible for HIPAA (the Department of Health and Human Services Office of Civil Rights) tends to simply respond to complaints. It has only completed a few compliance reviews. Nor has the Department of Health and Human Services Office of Civil Rights chosen to prosecute high-profile cases including "the theft of millions of veterans' records. . . . A California health plan that left personal information about patients on a public Web site for years, and a Florida hospice that sold . . . personal patient information to other hospices."[48]

Between 2003 and 2006, there were 19,420 grievances, most of them alleging privacy violations or difficulty in getting records. There were two criminal prosecutions. "One man was sentenced to 16 months . . . in prison for stealing credit card information from a cancer patient; a woman was convicted of selling an FBI agent's medical records." The government responded to 73 percent of the complaints by saying there was no violation or allowing the violating entity to fix the problem. The

Department of Health and Human Services prefers to work for voluntary compliance. This has been criticized by privacy advocates who state that "the administration's decision not to enforce the law more aggressively has not safeguarded . . . medical records." According to a health care privacy expert at Columbia University, "The law was put in place to give people some confidence when they talk to their doctor or file a claim with their insurance company, that information isn't going to be used against them. [Because] they have done almost nothing to enforce the law . . . we're dangerously close to having a law that is essentially meaningless." HIPAA compliance is falling. Five hundred cases are still open; 309 may involve criminal acts.[49]

Privacy of Medical Records Under HIPAA and the USA Patriot Act

Under both HIPAA and the USA Patriot Act, there are many circumstances that allow police access to your medical records without a warrant. HIPAA allows the release of private medical information in some situations including the assertion that you are a suspect or witness to a crime, or a missing person. Your information may also be released if national security or intelligence is involved or for the protection of VIPs including the president and foreign dignitaries. The government may also access your medical records under the USA Patriot Act "for an investigation to protect against international terrorism or clandestine intelligence activities" (Section 215). Because HIPAA and the USA Patriot Act are so new, the constitutionality of the provisions that allow warrantless access has not been tested.

Telemedicine and Privacy

Telemedicine refers to any kind of health care administered over telecommunications lines. This would include the use of e-mail by physicians to communicate with patients and colleagues, distance exams and consultations, teleradiology, and telepsychiatry, among other specialties. Health care information, comprised of medical records, live videos, psychiatric consultations, and radiologic images, has traditionally been protected by state regulations. But now, this information routinely crosses state lines. Therefore, HIPAA protection is of special importance to this information. HIPAA requires that e-mail be secured either by using encryption or by controlling access. HIPAA specifically discusses privacy issues of telemedicine, including the presence of nonmedical personnel (e.g., camera people and other technicians) and the fact that the more stringent privacy protection (federal or state) has precedence.[50]

E-Mail and Privacy

For some doctors and their patients, e-mail is becoming a common form of communication. It is used as a practical, easy, inexpensive way of confirming or changing appointments, asking and answering questions, and maintaining communication over long distances. Some physicians also see it as a way to rebuild the traditional personal doctor–patient relationship which existed prior to managed care. Some doctors see e-mail as an intimate form of communication. However, e-mail has not been private. It is not like a telephone conversation; a permanent record of e-mail communications exists. Although e-mail is private in transit, it is not protected while stored. As mentioned, courts have ruled that employers have the legal right to read employees' e-mail, and today many doctors are employees of health maintenance organizations. E-mail may be read on any of the computer systems it passes through on its way between doctor and patient. Because of the threats to the privacy of medical information, many doctors are now refusing to use e-mail. The requirements of HIPAA that e-mail be encrypted may help with these issues.

Privacy and Genetic Information

Information-based medicine depends on genetic information. As research focuses on genetics and an individual's genetic predisposition to develop certain diseases, privacy issues arise. Although this research could eventually lead to treatments and cures tailored to each person, it also raises darker possibilities. Employers and insurance companies could use it against employees and consumers.[51] Polls have consistently shown that Americans fear that genetic information would be used against them; one poll found that "63 percent of workers would not take genetic tests if employers could get access to the results." Some individuals become so desperate about negative genetic information that they resort to stealing pages of their medical records.[52] There have been some instances where employers did genetic tests on workers without their knowledge. The government sued and a $2.2 million settlement was reached.[53] In 2005, IBM stated it would not "use genetic information in hiring or in determining eligibility for its health care benefits."

Privacy and Electronic Medical Records

Your medical records include information about your total physical and mental make-up. They may discuss your relationships with family members, sexual behavior, and drug- or alcohol-related problems. One particularly sensitive piece of information is one's human immunodeficiency virus (HIV) status. On a personal level, knowing that anyone has access to intimate details of your life may be humiliating.

Computerizing medical records and making them easily available over networks is, of course, essential to good medical care and can save lives. However, access to networked medical records is not limited to medical personnel. The issues of privacy and the easy availability of records kept on networked databases have special impact on health care and medical ethics. Most people assume the confidentiality of the doctor–patient relationship. This confidentiality is challenged by several trends. The movement to computerize medical records and possibly put them on the Internet, the expanding use of telemedicine, the increasing use of e-mail by health care workers, the increased use of health maintenance organizations, and reliance on third parties to pay for medical care, all raise serious questions of patient confidentiality and medical ethics. Under HIPAA, however, health care providers and their business associates have put some privacy protections in place.

A National Research Council report issued in March 1997 found that although electronic medical records are becoming more and more common, they were not secure, and little was being done to protect them. The report stated that certain precautions can be taken to limit access to medical records. However, six years later, medical records were still not secure. In March 2003, less than one month before HIPAA required privacy protection of medical records, Texas reported that the computer network shared by sixteen state agencies and 225 private and public organizations lacked protection for medical records. Some proposed protections include requiring the use of passwords by authorized users, biometrics, using electronic blocks (called firewalls) to limit the access to networks, and keeping track of who actually sees a record through audit trails. The most obvious precaution is to train personnel not to leave patient information displayed on a computer screen.

Many people now receive health care through health maintenance organizations. Under managed care, people are seen by several health care providers, and records are shared. For example, a patient seen by a general practitioner can be referred to a gastroenterologist for a magnetic resonance imaging (MRI) and blood work. The patient's records are seen by primary care physicians, hospital and laboratory personnel, radiologists, pharmacists, consultants, and office staffs. Patients' records are also available to state health organizations and researchers. This electronic paper trail is then monitored by the health insurance provider and may be seen by an employer seeking to cut medical insurance costs. "Most patients would be surprised at the number of organizations that receive information about their health record," according to Dr. Paul D. Clayton of Columbia Presbyterian Medical Center in New York and Chair of the National Research Council Panel. Dr. Clayton is only referring to authorized users. Incidents have occurred in which unauthorized users (**hackers**) have gained access to hospital computer systems and changed patient information. The possibility of theft of patient information also exists.

The problems of protecting private medical information may multiply if all medical and health records are digitized and put online under a national system proposed by the Health Information Technology Decade. Of course, having a national database of health records could improve health care by making all your medical information (including allergies, medications, and most recent test results) available in any hospital, doctor's office, and emergency room. The challenge of making medical information secure is daunting. However, if data were not secure (and as yet it seems no data are secure), marketers could tailor advertising to people with a particular disease, lenders could disqualify people on the basis of an estimate of how long they would live, and employers could deny employment or promotions.[54]

SECURITY BREACHES

Instituting security measures (passwords, encryption, biometrics, audit trails, and so on) is of course crucial. Still, it should be recognized that breaches of security are common. Just during the past several months:

- Between February 15, 2005, and August 8, 2006, there were 90,000,000 breaches of medical security.[55]

- On August 8, 2006, a computer containing personal information of 38,000 patients at Veterans Administration (VA) hospitals was missing. Another computer disappeared the week before from a VA subcontractor that helped in insurance collections for VA medical centers.
- In July 2006, "Georgetown University suspended an electronic prescription-writing program firm . . . after a computer consultant stumbled upon an online cache of data belonging to thousands of patients."[56] The information was personal (names and Social Security numbers) not medical.
- Breaches of security are common; to see a more complete list go to http://www.privacyrights.org/ar/ChronDataBreaches.htm.

IN THE NEWS

Excerpt from, "THE CONSUMER; How Patients Can Use the New Access to Their Medical Records"

by Mary Duenwald

At one time, polite people never asked to look at their own medical records. To do so would indicate a lack of trust in your physician. Besides, doctors were so resistant to the practice that getting hold of your records could require a subpoena. . . .

Since last April, federal law has required that doctors, clinics and hospitals provide patients with access to their records on demand. As it turns out, many people want to see them, and if you know what you are looking for, medical records can be easy to decipher. . . .

Doctors once suspected that patients who wanted to see their own charts were distrustful or, worse, planning to sue, said George J. Annas, chairman of the health law, bioethics and human rights department at Boston University School of Public Health. And some doctors argued that patients lacked the expertise to understand their own charts.

"'They'd say, you can't possibly understand because it's written in medical language," Mr. Annas said. "You won't know that S.O.B. stands for shortness of breath."

The new federal rules, part of the Health Insurance Portability and Accountability Act, or HIPAA, give patients the right to inspect and copy all their records. Parents are also entitled to their children's medical records.

Access to medical records will soon be very easy for anyone with a personal computer, as hospitals and clinics switch to electronic record-keeping. But even with paper records, obtaining access is easy. Patients need merely telephone their doctor's office or a hospital's records office and ask. . . .

(continued)

Excerpt from, "THE CONSUMER; How Patients Can Use the New Access to Their Medical Records" *(continued)*

Ideally, when looking through the file, the patient should be able to ask a doctor or other informed medical professional questions about anything that seems confusing or hard to understand. . . .

What pieces of the record are most interesting and important?

The ones that a patient might need to provide to future physicians, said Dr. Jinnet B. Fowles, vice president of research for the Park Nicollet Institute, a health research center in Minneapolis. Those might include the dates of immunizations and regular screenings like mammograms, P.S.A. tests and cholesterol checks; the dates of any surgeries and the hospitals where they were performed; a record of all allergies; accounts of any serious medical illnesses; and descriptions of current medical problems and medications. . . .

Patients may want to photocopy the pertinent pages and save them in a file, said Ms. Quinsey of the information management association. Or they may want to transfer the key details to a health history record form. . . .

"I'm allergic to penicillin, sulfa and tetracycline," Ms. Quinsey said. "All those drugs are essentially deadly to me, so I keep that information on a piece of paper that stays in my billfold."

People who suffer from chronic conditions like diabetes or high blood pressure are advised to keep that information with them also, Ms. Quinsey said.

It is important to check for inaccuracies: misfiled pages from another patient's chart, for example, or incorrect notations about allergies or medications.

Contrary to patients' expectations, the doctors' notations are typically not all that interesting, Ms. Quinsey said. "If they think there's gossip in their chart, they are usually disappointed."

Naturally, the trend toward greater openness with patients has discouraged doctors from jotting down ill-considered comments. "They are encouraged to stick to the facts and not characterize patients as 'fat' or 'shabbily dressed,'" Mr. Annas said.

CHAPTER SUMMARY

Chapter 12 introduces the reader to the issue of security for computer systems and the importance of the privacy of the information on those systems—specifically medical records. Although guaranteeing the privacy of medical records was always important, keeping these records on databases on networks raises new problems.

- Threats to information technology may stem from many sources, including crime, viruses, human error, and natural disaster.

- Security measures that attempt to protect computer systems including information may include laws, codes of conduct, encryption, and restricting access. Restricting access may be done by assigning PINs or passwords, requiring ID cards and keys, or through biometric methods. Firewalls (electronic blocks to access) may be used to protect information on networks.
- Computer technology changes the nature of the way we work and makes work more subject to scrutiny.
- The Internet makes gathering personal information easy and inexpensive.
- The existence of networked databases of personal information, especially if they are connected to the Internet, endangers privacy, by making that information accessible to anyone.
- HIPAA provides the first national standards for the privacy and security of health information. However, enforcement has been lax.
- Breaches of security continue to occur.

KEY TERMS

adware
biometric keyboards
biometric methods
body odor sensors
codes of conduct
data accuracy
database
DNA
Electronic
    Communications
    Privacy Act of 1986
encryption
facial structure scans
facial thermography
Fair Credit Reporting
    Act of 1970
fingerprints

firewalls
fraud
fraudulent dialer
hackers
hand prints
Health Insurance Porta-
    bility and Account-
    ability Act (HIPAA)
Homeland Security Act
identity theft
iris scans
keylogging
lip prints
malware
Medical Information
    Bureau
passwords

personal identification
    numbers (PINs)
privacy
Real ID Act of 2005
retina scans
security
software piracy
Spybot Search and
    Destroy software
spyware
theft of information
theft of services
USA Patriot Act
Verichips
viruses
voice recognition

REVIEW EXERCISES

Multiple Choice

1. Threats to information technology include threats to _____.
   A. hardware
   B. software
   C. data
   D. All of the above

2. The unauthorized copying of software protected by copyright is called _____.
   A. theft of services
   B. software piracy
   C. A and B
   D. None of the above

3. Breaking into a medical database and gaining access to medical records is an example of a crime called _____.
   A. theft of services
   B. theft of information
   C. software piracy
   D. network piracy

4. Which of the following is a way of attempting to protect computer systems and data from unauthorized use?
   A. Encryption
   B. Codes of conduct
   C. Restricting access through the use of PINs
   D. All of the above

5. Biometric security methods include _____.
   A. use of passwords
   B. locking the computer room
   C. iris scans, lip prints, and body odor sensors
   D. carrying ID cards

6. Using a computer to create a description of someone who, you believe, is "likely" to commit a crime is called _____.
   A. computer matching
   B. computer profiling
   C. computer graphics
   D. None of the above

7. Privacy means _____.
   A. the ability to control personal information and keep it from misuse
   B. the attempt to protect a computer hardware from criminals
   C. the attempt to protect computer hardware from natural disaster
   D. None of the above

8. Threats to information technology may stem from _____.
   A. crime
   B. human error
   C. natural disaster
   D. All of the above

9. A program that attaches itself to another program, replicates itself, and may do damage to your computer is called a _____.
   A. network
   B. database
   C. virus
   D. None of the above

10. The first federal protection for the privacy of medical information is provided by the _____.
    A. Homeland Security Act
    B. Health Insurance Portability and Accountability Act
    C. USA Patriot Act
    D. All of the above

11. The _____ gives law enforcement agencies greater power to monitor electronic and other communications, with fewer checks.
    A. Health Insurance Portability and Accountability Act
    B. Privacy Act
    C. USA Patriot Act
    D. All of the above

12. _____ are small files that a Web site may put on your hard drive when you visit. They can be programmed to track your movements, collecting information that helps advertisers target you.
    A. Cookies
    B. Tracers
    C. A and B
    D. None of the above

13. _____ limits disclosure of personal information in Motor Vehicles records.
    A. Driver Privacy Protection Act
    B. Motor Vehicle Act
    C. Federal Privacy Act
    D. None of the Above

14. The _____ has a database that contains health histories of fifteen million people.
    A. Immigration and Naturalization Service (INS)
    B. Medical Information Bureau (MIB)
    C. National Crime Information Center (NCIC)
    D. None of the above

15. The RFID tags (radio transmitters that give off a unique signal, which can be read by a receiver) are called _____.
    A. identichips
    B. verichips
    C. solochips
    D. multichips

True/False Questions

1. Most computer frauds are committed by employees of the organization being defrauded. _____
2. E-mail is a private communication. _____
3. According to the Electronic Privacy Information Center, most Web sites have privacy policies. _____

4. Computer matching links the information in one database to the information in other databases. _____
5. The Medical Information Bureau contains medical information on millions of people and it guards the privacy of these records. _____
6. Traditionally, health care information has been protected by state law. _____
7. Computerizing medical records and making them available over networks helps facilitate sharing of medical records among health care providers and, therefore, can help assure continuity of care. _____
8. Medical records on the Internet are guaranteed to be secure. _____
9. Hackers have never gained access to hospital computer systems. _____
10. It is a crime for employers to gather information about their employees. _____
11. Under HIPAA, medical records get some federal privacy protection. _____
12. Under some circumstances, government agencies have access to your medical information without a warrant. _____
13. The Real ID Act requires a national identity card. _____
14. Your rights under HIPAA are affected by the USA Patriot Act. _____
15. Under HIPAA, you have the right to examine your medical records. _____

Critical Thinking

1. Assume that the information you provide when you register as a college student is kept in a networked database. This includes personal details such as your name, Social Security number, birth date, address, financial and marital status, and prior educational records. How would you safeguard the privacy of this information?
2. Numerous medical organizations are keeping records online. Some are linking their hospital networks to the Internet. How would you propose protecting the confidentiality of the doctor–patient relationship in this situation?
3. Critically examine the Real ID Act and its implications for privacy and security.
4. Computer profiling is being used to identify people "likely" to commit a crime. Although these people are not automatically arrested, they may be stopped and questioned for no reason other than their profile "fits." In a democracy, people are supposed to be arrested only after a crime is committed, and even then they are presumed innocent. Does computer profiling violate these tenets of democracy?
5. Where would you draw the line on how much private information (name, Social Security number, mother's maiden name, unlisted phone number and address, financial and medical information, for example) should be available on the Internet? What are the pros and cons of government regulation?
6. Discuss why privacy and security are especially important issues in the new millennium.
7. How do HIPAA and the USA Patriot Act affect the privacy of medical information? Does the possible loss of privacy guarantee greater national security?
8. Discuss how the apparent lack of enforcement of HIPAA could impact on the privacy and security of medical information.

NOTES

1. Mitch Mitchell, "Medical Privacy Law Stirs Controversy," *Star Telegram,* February 23, 2003, http://www.gardere.com/Content/hubbard/tbl_s31Publications/FileUpload137/498/Star-Tel.Hoffman-02-23-03.pdf (accessed December 1, 2006).
2. Tom Zeller Jr., "Breach Points Up Flaws in Privacy Laws," nyt.com, February 24, 2005, http://www.nytimes.com/2005/02/24/business/24datas.html (accessed December 28, 2007).
3. Declan McCullagh and Robert Lemos, " 'Perfect Storm' for New Privacy Laws?" CNET News.com, March 1, 2005, http://www.news.com/Perfect-storm-for-new-privacy-laws/2100-1029_3-5593225.html (accessed December 28, 2007).
4. "Another Veterans Affairs Computer with Sensitive Data Is Missing," privacy.org, August 8, 2006, http://www.privacy.org/archives/2006_08.html (accessed December 28, 2007).
5. George Beekman, *Computer Confluence: Exploring Tomorrow's Technology,* 5th ed. (Upper Saddle River, NJ: Prentice Hall, 2003).
6. "New Research Shows Identity Fraud Contained and Consumers Have More Control Than They Think," bbbonline.com, January 2006, http://www.bbbonline.org/IDTheft/safetyQuiz.asp (accessed December 28, 2007).
7. John Leland, "Identity Thief Is Often Found in Family Photo," nyt.com, November 13, 2006, http://www.nytimes.com/2006/11/13/us/13identity.html (accessed December 28, 2007).
8. A. K. Jain and S. Pankanti, "A Touch of Money," *IEEE Spectrum* 43, no. 7 (July 2006): 22–27 [abstract] (accessed January 23, 2008).
9. David Hubler, "GAO Finds Holes in Privacy Laws," FCW.com, July 26, 2006, http://www.fcw.com/online/news/95427-1.html (accessed December 28, 2007).
10. "Fair Credit Reporting Act and the Privacy of Your Credit Report," October 7, 2005, http://epic.org/privacy/fcra/ (accessed December 28, 2007).
11. "What Is the Privacy Act?" http://www.fs.fed.us/im/foia/pa.htm (accessed November 29, 2006).
12. "The Right to Financial Privacy Act," 2003, http://epic.org/privacy/rfpa/ (accessed December 28, 2007).
13. "Computer Fraud and Abuse Act," 2003, http://legal.web.aol.com/resources/legislation/comfraud.html (accessed November 29, 2006).
14. "Electronic Communications Privacy Act," http://www.usiia.org/legis/ecpa.html (accessed November 29, 2006).
15. "The Video Privacy Protection Act (VPPA)," 2002, http://epic.org/privacy/vppa/ (accessed December 28, 2007).
16. "Overview of the Privacy Act of 1974, 2004 Edition Computer Matching," http://www.usdoj.gov/oip/1974compmatch.htm (accessed November 29, 2006).
17. "The Computer Fraud and Abuse Act (as Amended 1994 and 1996)," http://www.panix.com/~eck/computer-fraud-act.html (accessed November 29, 2006).
18. "National Information Infrastructure Protection Act of 1996," http://epic.org/security/1996_computer_law.html (accessed December 28, 2007).
19. "Driver Privacy Protection Act (DPPA)," 2005, http://www.maine.gov/informe/subscriber/dppa.htm (accessed December 28, 2007).
20. "Gramm-Leach Billey," 2005, http://www.cleo.com/about/glb.asp (accessed December 28, 2007).
21. "How to Comply with the Children's Online Privacy Protection Rule," 1999, http://www.ftc.gov/bcp/conline/pubs/buspubs/coppa.htm (accessed November 29, 2006).
22. "The USA Patriot Act," November 17, 2005, http://epic.org/privacy/terrorism/usapatriot/ (accessed December 28, 2007).
23. "A BILL: To Establish a Department of Homeland Security, and for Other Purposes," 2002, http://www.whitehouse.gov/deptofhomeland/bill/ (accessed December 28, 2007).

24. 108th U.S. Congress (2003–2004), "H.R. 743 [108th]: Social Security Protection Act of 2004," http://www.govtrack.us/congress/bill.xpd?bill=h108-743 (accessed December 3, 2007).

25. 109th U.S. Congress (2005–2006), "H.R. 84 [109th]: Online Privacy Protection Act of 2005," http://www.govtrack.us/congress/bill.xpd?bill=h109-84 (accessed December 28, 2007).

26. "Combat Methamphetamine Epidemic Act 2005 (Title VII of Public Law 109-177)," http://www.deadiversion.usdoj.gov/meth/index.html (accessed December 3, 2007).

27. "Cegavske Targets 'Video Voyeurism,'" February 17, 2005, http://www.reviewjournal.com/lvrj_home/2005/Feb-17-Thu-2005/news/25883310.html (accessed November 29, 2006).

28. "Spotlight on Surveillance," 2005, http://epic.org/privacy/surveillance/spotlight/ (accessed December 28, 2007).

29. "Real ID Act of 2005 Driver's License Title Summary," 2006, http://www.ncsl.org/standcomm/sctran/realidsummary05.htm (accessed January 18, 2008).

30. Declan McCullagh, "FAQ: How Real ID Will Affect You," CNET News.com, May 6, 2005, http://www.news.com/FAQ-How-Real-ID-will-affect-you/2100-1028_3-5697111.html (accessed December 28, 2007).

31. Anush Yegyazarian, "Tech.gov: Real ID's Real Problems," washingtonpost.com, October 11, 2006, http://www.pcworld.com/article/id,127419-c,techrelatedlegislation/article.html (accessed December 28, 2007).

32. Barnaby J. Feder and Tom Zeller Jr., "Identity Chip Under Skin Approved for Use in Health Care," nyt.com, October 14, 2004, http://www.nytimes.com/2004/10/14/technology/14implant.html (accessed December 28, 2007).

33. Richard Waters, "US Group Implants Electronic Tags in Workers," FT.com, February 12, 2006, http://www.ft.com/cms/s/2/ec414700-9bf4-11da-8baa-0000779e2340.html (accessed December 28, 2007).

34. "Demo: Cloning a Verichip," July 2006, http://cq.cx/verichip.pl (accessed December 1, 2006).

35. Ronald Plesser, James J. Halpert, and Milo Cividanes, "Summary and Analysis of Key Sections of USA PATRIOT ACT of 2001," http://www.cdt.org/security/011031summary.shtml (accessed December 3, 2007).

36. Lauren Weinstein, "Taking Liberties with Our Freedom," Wired News, December 2, 2002, http://www.wired.com/politics/law/news/2002/12/56600 (accessed December 28, 2007).

37. Jacqueline Klosek, *The War on Privacy* (Westport, CT: Praeger, 2007).

38. Ibid.

39. "Statement of Barry Steinhardt, Director of the ACLU Technology and Liberty Program, on RFID Tags Before the Commerce, Trade and Consumer Protection Subcommittee of the House Committee on Energy and Commerce," July 14, 2004, http://www.aclu.org/privacy/spying/15744leg20040714.html (accessed January 7, 2008).

40. Sunshine Red, "Medical Records: About the Medical Information Bureau," June 22, 2007, http://www.associatedcontent.com/article/286156/medical_records_about_the_medical_information.html (accessed November 23, 2007).

41. "Protecting the Privacy of Patients' Health Information," July 6, 2001, http://www.nchica.org/HIPAAResources/Samples/privacylessons/P-110%20Article%20-%20HHS%20Fact%20Sheet%20-%20July%206%202001.doc (accessed December 3, 2007).

42. Ibid.

43. Ibid.

44. Office for Civil Rights—HIPAA, "Medical Privacy—National Standards to Protect the Privacy of Personal Health Information," http://www.hhs.gov/ocr/hipaa/finalreg.html (accessed December 3, 2007).

45. Mitchell, "Medical Privacy Law Stirs Controversy."

46. "Protecting the Privacy of Patients' Health Information."

47. "HIPAA Security Series," June 6, 2005, http://64.233.169.104/search?q=cache:BK34bm5c668J:www.cms.hhs.gov/EducationMaterials/Downloads/SecurityStandardsAdministrativeSafeguards.pdf+HIPAA+Security+Series&hl=en&ct=clnk&cd=1&gl=us (accessed January 18, 2008).

48. Rob Stein, "Medical Privacy Law Nets No Fines: Lax Enforcement Puts Patients' Files At Risk, Critics Say," Monday June 5, 2006; AO1, http://www.washingtonpost.com/wp-dyn/content/article/2006/06/04/AR2006060400672_pf.html (accessed February 2, 2008).

49. Rob Stein, "Medical Privacy Law Nets No Fines," washingtonpost.com, June 5, 2006, http://www.washingtonpost.com/wp-dyn/content/article/2006/06/04/AR2006060400672.html (accessed December 28, 2007).

50. HIPAA Privacy Update, "Issue: Privacy and Telemedicine," 2000, http://www.hrsa.gov/telehealth/pubs/privac.htm (accessed December 3, 2007).

51. "Medicine and the New Genetics," 2006, http://genome.gsc.riken.jp/hgmis/medicine/medicine.html (accessed December 28, 2007).

52. Robert Klitzman, "The Quest for Privacy Can Make Us Thieves," nyt.com, May 9, 2006, http://www.nytimes.com/2006/05/09/health/09essa.html?_r=1&oref=slogin (accessed December 28, 2007).

53. Steve Lohr, "I.B.M. to Put Genetic Data of Workers Off Limits," nyt.com, October 10, 2005, http://www.nytimes.com/2005/10/10/business/10gene.html (accessed December 28, 2007).

54. "The New Threat to Your Medical Privacy," ConsumerReports.org, 2006, http://www.consumerreports.org/cro/health-fitness/health-care/electronic-medical-records-306/overview/index.htm (accessed December 28, 2007).

55. "A Chronology of Data Breaches," Privacy Rights Clearinghouse, August 5, 2006, http://www.privacyrights.org/ar/ChronDataBreaches.htm (accessed August 9, 2006).

56. *HIPAA Advisory,* July 2006 News Archives, Phoenix Health Systems, http://www.hipaadvisory.com/News/NewsArchives/2006/jul06.htm (accessed February 2, 2008).

ADDITIONAL RESOURCES

109th U.S. Congress (2005–2006). "H.R. 82 [109th]: Social Security On-line Privacy Protection Act." http://www.govtrack.us/congress/bill.xpd?bill=h109-82 (accessed December 28, 2007).

"Answers to Frequently Asked Questions About Government Access to Personal Medical Information (Under the USA Patriot Act and the HIPAA Regulations)." American Civil Liberties Union, May 30, 2003. http://www.aclu.org/privacy/medical/15222res20030530.html (accessed December 28, 2007).

Austen, Ian. "A Scanner Skips the ID Card and Zooms In on the Eyes." nyt.com, May 15, 2003. http://query.nytimes.com/gst/fullpage.html?res=9907E0D71F3FF936A25756C0A9659C8B63 (accessed December 28, 2007).

Baase, Sara. *A Gift of Fire: Social, Legal, and Ethical Issues in Computing.* Upper Saddle River, NJ: Prentice Hall, 1996.

Bernstein, Nina. "Personal Files Via Computer Offer Money and Pose Threat." *New York Times,* June 12, 1997, A1, B14.

Burton, Brenda K. and Erik Kangas. "HIPAA Email Security Management in Email Communications, Secure Email White Paper." 2006. http://luxsci.com/info/hipaa-email.html (accessed December 2, 2006).

Chaddock, Gail Russell. "Security Act to Pervade Daily Lives." *Christian Science Monitor,* November 21, 2002. http://www.csmonitor.com/2002/1121/p01s03-usju.html (accessed November 30, 2006).

Clymer, Adam. "Conferees in Congress Bar Using a Pentagon Project on Americans." February 12, 2003. http://foi.missouri.edu/totalinfoaware/conference.html (accessed December 1, 2006).

Cronin, Anne. "Census Bureau Tells Something About Everything." *New York Times,* December 1, 1997, D10.

Donovan, Larry. "Privacy Law Update." 2001. http://library.findlaw.com/2001/Feb/1/129062.html (accessed December 28, 2007).

"EFF Analysis of the Provisions of the USA Patriot Act That Relate to Online Activities (October 31, 2001)." October 27, 2003. http://w2.eff.org/Privacy/Surveillance/Terrorism/20011031_eff_usa_patriot_analysis.php (accessed December 1, 2006).

Electronic Privacy Information Center. "Latest News." epic.org, December 2, 2006 (accessed December 2, 2006).

Electronic Privacy Information Center. "Medical Privacy." April 3, 2006. http://www.epic.org/privacy/medical (accessed December 1, 2006).

"Face Recognition." January 19, 2006. http://epic.org/privacy/facerecognition/ (accessed December 28, 2007).

Fein, Esther B. "For Many Physicians, E-Mail Is the High-Tech House Call." *New York Times,* November 20, 1997, A1, B8.

Fitzgerald, Thomas J. "A Trail of Cookies? Cover Your Tracks." nyt.com, March 27, 2003. http://query.nytimes.com/gst/fullpage.html?res=9407E6DC1E30F934A15750C0A9659C8B63 (accessed December 28, 2007).

Glass, Andrew. "Computer Industry Adopts Internet Privacy Code." Accessmylibrary.com, 1997, 1–2. http://www.accessmylibrary.com/coms2/summary_0286-5567738_ITM (accessed December 28, 2007).

Guernsey, Lisa. "What Did You Do Before the War," nyt.com, November 22, 2001, http://query.nytimes.com/gst/fullpage.html?res=9B0CE6DE173AF931A15752C1A9679C8B63 (accessed December 2, 2006).

Hafner, Katie. "'Dear Doctor' Meets 'Return to Sender.'" nyt.com, June 6, 2002. http://query.nytimes.com/gst/fullpage.html?res=9C0CE1DC1F3AF935A35755C0A9649C8B63 (accessed December 28, 2007).

Holtzman, David. "Homeland Security and You." CNET News.com, January 21, 2003. http://www.news.com/2010-1071-981262.html (accessed December 28, 2007).

Leary, Warren E. "Panel Cites Lack of Security on Medical Records." *New York Times,* March 6, 1997, A1, B11.

Lee, Jennifer. "Dirty Laundry, Online for All to See." nyt.com, September 5, 2002. http://query.nytimes.com/gst/fullpage.html?res=9A04E4D9173EF936A3575AC0A9649C8B63 (accessed December 28, 2007).

Lee, Jennifer. "Identity Theft Complaints Double in '02, Continuing Rise." nyt.com, January 23, 2003. http://query.nytimes.com/gst/fullpage.html?res=9F04EFD61130F930A15752C0A9659C8B63 (accessed December 28, 2007).

Lee, Jennifer. "Dirty Laundry, Online for All to See." nyt.com, September 5, 2002. http://query.nytimes.com/gst/fullpage.html?res=9A04E4D9173EF936A3575AC0A9649C8B63 (accessed December 28, 2007).

Lewis, Peter H. "Forget Big Brother." *New York Times,* March 19, 1998, G1, G6.

Lichtblau, Eric. "Republicans Want Terror Law Made Permanent." CommonDreams.org, April 2003. http://www.commondreams.org/headlines03/0409-01.htm (accessed December 28, 2007).

Markoff, John. "Guidelines Don't End Debate on Internet Privacy." *New York Times,* December 18, 1997.

McCullagh, Declan. "Bush Signs Homeland Security Bill." CNET News.com, November 25, 2002. http://www.news.com/Bush-signs-Homeland-Security-bill/2100-1023_3-975305.html (accessed December 28, 2007).

Murphy, Dean E. "Librarians Use Shredder to Show Opposition to New F.B.I. Powers." Originally in the nyt.com, April 7, 2003. http://www.commondreams.org/headlines03/0407-03.htm (accessed December 1, 2006).

"National ID Cards and REAL ID Act." November 29, 2006. http://www.epic.org/privacy/id_cards/default.html (accessed December 1, 2006).

Newman, Andy. "Those Dimples May Be Digits." nyt.com, May 3, 2001. http://query.nytimes.com/gst/fullpage.html?res=9E04E2DE1538F930A35756C0A9679C8B63 (accessed December 28, 2007).

Parsons, June, Dan Oja, and Stephanie Low. *Computers, Technology, and Society.* Cambridge, MA: ITP, 1997.

Pear, Robert. "Bush Acts to Drop Core Privacy Rule on Medical Data." nyt.com, March 22, 2002. http://query.nytimes.com/gst/fullpage.html?res=9C0DEFD61E38F931A15750 C0A9649C8B63 (accessed December 28, 2007).

Pear, Robert. "Health System Warily Prepares for Privacy Rules." nyt.com, April 6, 2003. http://query.nytimes.com/gst/fullpage.html?res=9B06E2DC1238F935A35757C0A9659 C8B63 (accessed December 28, 2007).

———. "Vast Worker Database to Track Deadbeat Parents." *New York Times,* September 22, 1997.

Reuters. "Senate Rebuffs Domestic Spy Plan." *Wired News,* January 23, 2003. http://www. wired.com/politics/law/news/2003/01/57386 (accessed December 28, 2007).

Safire, William. "You Are a Suspect." nyt.com, November 14, 2002. http://query. nytimes.com/gst/fullpage.html?res=9F0CE6D71630F937A25752C1A9649C8B63 (accessed December 28, 2007).

Schwaneberg, Robert. "Questions Leave 'Smart Card' in Limbo for Now." *Star-Ledger,* June 30, 1998, 11, 14.

———. "Smart Cards Take a Step in Legislature." *Star-Ledger,* June 23, 1998, 11, 15.

Schwartz, John. "Threats and Responses: Surveillance; Planned Databank on Citizens Spurs Opposition in Congress." nyt.com, January 16, 2003. http://query.nytimes.com/gst/ fullpage.html?res=940CE4D61131F935A25752C0A9659C8B63 (accessed December 28, 2007).

Seelye, Katharine Q. "A Plan for Database Privacy, but Public Has to Ask for It." *New York Times,* December 18, 1997, A1, A24.

Shelley, Gary and Thomas Cashman. *Discovering Computers a Link to the Future.* Cambridge, MA: ITP, 1997.

"Surfer Beware: Personal Privacy and the Internet." Report of the Electronic Privacy Information Center, Washington, DC, June 1997. http://www.epic.org/Reports/ surfer-beware.html (accessed December 1, 2006).

"Telehealth Update: Final HIPAA Privacy Rules." February 20, 2001. http://www.hrsa.gov/ telehealth/pubs/hippa.htm (accessed December 28, 2007).

Wayner, Peter. "Code Breaker Cracks Smart Cards' Digital Safe." *New York Times,* June 22, 1998, D1–D2.

Zuzek, Ashley. "Changes to Patriot Act Limit Medicinal Purchases," April 18, 2006, http:// thedartmouth.com/2006/04/18/news/changes/ (accessed November 24, 2007).

RELATED WEB SITES

http://www.biometrics.dod.mil/

http://www.dol.gov

http://www.eff.org

Electronic Privacy Information Center (http://www.epic.org) is a research organization concerned with privacy issues. It keeps a Privacy Archive with "an extensive collection of documents, reports, news items, policy analysis and laws relating to privacy issues."

http://www.ftc.gov

http://www.govtrack.us/congress/billsearch.xpd lists 202 bills under the USA Patriot Act (2007–2008).

http://www.hhs.gov

http://www.hipaaadvisory.com/news

http://www.mib.com

http://www.patientprivacyrights.org

http://www.privacyrights.org

Glossary

accounts receivable (A/R)—include any invoice or any payment from the patient or insurance carriers to the medical practice

ADAM—simulation software that teaches anatomy and physiology, using two- and three-dimensional images (some of them created from the Visible Human data); versions available for both patients and professionals; interactive, allowing the user to click away over one hundred layers of the body and see more than four thousand structures

adaptive technology—(assistive technology) makes it possible for people with disabilities to exercise control over their home and work environments

adjustment—a positive or negative change to a patient account

administrative applications—use of information technology for tasks such as office management, finance and accounting, and materials management

adware—may display unwanted pop-up advertisements on your monitor; it may be related to the sites you search on the Web or even the content of your e-mail

AESOP (automated endoscopic system for optimal positioning)—introduced in 1994 by Computer Motion Inc. is the first FDA-cleared surgical robot; originally developed for the space program, AESOP is now used as an assistant in endoscopic procedures

AIDS (acquired immune deficiency syndrome)—AIDS attacks the immune system leading to susceptibility to opportunistic infection

Americans with Disabilities Act of 1990—federal law that prohibits discrimination against people with disabilities and requires that businesses with more than fifteen employees provide "reasonable accommodation" to allow the disabled to perform their jobs

antisense technology—one experimental technology used to develop drugs to shut off disease-causing genes

application software—programs that perform specific tasks for the user, also called productivity software; include word processing, spreadsheet, database management, graphics, and communications programs

Aquarius—the only undersea laboratory in the world used by Neemo

arithmetic-logic unit—the part of the central processing unit that performs arithmetic and logical operations

ARPAnet—a project of the Advanced Research Projects Agency of the U.S. Department of Defense (1969); an attempt to create both a national network of scientists and a communications system that could withstand nuclear attack; later became the Internet

arrhythmia monitor—a device that monitors heart rate

ARTEMIS—a robotic system that works with the simulation software KISMET; allows a surgeon to perform minimally invasive surgery while viewing three screens that show the view presented by the endoscope and simulations

artificial intelligence (AI)—the branch of computer science that seeks to make computers simulate human intelligence

assignment—the amount the insurance company pays

assistive technology—see adaptive technology

augmentative communication device—a device that helps those who cannot speak or whose speech is incomprehensible to communicate

augmented reality surgery—(enhanced reality surgery) makes use of computer-generated imagery to provide the surgeon with information that would otherwise be unavailable; these images may be either fused with the image on the monitor or projected directly onto the patient's body during the operation allowing the doctor to virtually see inside the patient

authorization—permission by the insurance carrier for the provider to perform a medical procedure

automatic recalculation—refers to the fact that when one value in a spreadsheet is changed, any cell that refers to it is automatically changed

Baby CareLink—originated in Massachusetts. Its purpose was to compare high-risk, premature infants receiving traditional care with an experimental group, which in addition to traditional care received a telemedicine link to the hospital while the babies were hospitalized and for six months after. The addition of telemedicine to the care of premature babies has been so successful that Baby CareLink is now used throughout the United States

balance billing—bucket billing (or balance billing) is specific to health care office environments, where each insurer must be billed and payment received before the patient is billed

bandwidth—a measure of the capacity of transmission media to carry data; the broader the bandwidth, the faster the medium

bar-code scanner—direct-entry scanning input device; reads the universal product code (UPC)

binary digit—(bit) a one or a zero; binary digits are used to represent data and information in the computer

bioinformatics—the application of information technology to biology

biometric keyboard—a keyboard that can identify a typist by fingerprints

biometric methods—ways of identifying a user by some physical characteristic; include fingerprints, hand prints, retina or iris scans, lip prints, facial thermography, and body odor sensors

biometrics—the science that measures body characteristics; enables security devices to identify a user by these characteristics

biomicroscopes—used for diagnosis of cataracts

Biomove 3000—for stroke patients; helps to stimulate the muscles to avoid atrophy and increase both the range of motion and blood circulation

biotechnology—discipline that sees the human body as a collection of molecules and seeks to understand and treat disease in terms of these molecules

bird flu (avian flu)—the first human cases of avian flu were confirmed in 1997. The virus called H5N1 or A(H5N1) that causes the disease currently presents itself in the animal population. The virus would have to mutate to easily spread to humans

bit (binary digit)—binary digit (1 or 0)

Bluetooth—a wireless technology that can connect digital devices from computers to medical devices to cell phones

body odor sensor—a biometric device enabling the identification of user by odor

bonding—involves the application of a material to the tooth that can be shaped and polished

boot—load the operating system into memory

BrainGate Neural Interface System—for ALS (Lou Gehrig's Disease). The system involves implanting a chip in the brain that will convert brain cell impulses to computer signals

bucket billing—see balance billing

capitated plan—a physician is paid a fixed fee (the capitation), and the physician is paid regardless of the amount of treatment he or she provides

case—the condition for which the patient visits the doctor

CD (compact disk)—optical disks, CDs (compact disks), or DVDs (digital video disks) store data as pits and lands burnt into a plastic disk

CD-ROM (compact disk-read-only memory)—optical disk created at a factory that can be read, but not written to; lasers are used to create pits and lands to store data

cell phone—the most common wireless device in use today; allows text messaging, music, videos, and, of course, telephone calls

Centers for Medicare and Medicaid Services (CMS)—government insurance plans are administered by the federal Centers for Medicare and Medicaid Services (CMS), formerly the Health Care Financing Administration (HCFA)

Centerwatch—maintains a Web site that lists 7,000 (of the 70,000) current clinical trials in the United States, many of which are recruiting participants

central processing unit (CPU)—contains the arithmetic-logic unit and control unit

CHAMPUS—covers medical necessities for those eligible: retired military, dependents of those on active duty, retired, or dead military

CHAMPVA—covers the immediate families of veterans who are totally disabled; surviving spouse and children of a veteran who died from a service-related disability; widow and children of a veteran who was permanently disabled; and the surviving spouse and children of a member of the military who died in the line-of-duty

channel—medium used to connect the nodes on a network

charge—the amount a patient is billed for the provider's service

claim—a request to an insurance company for payment for services

clearinghouse—practices that submit electronic claims use a clearinghouse—a business that collects insurance claims from providers and sends them to the correct insurance carrier

clinical application—the use of information technology for direct patient care; includes patient monitoring, interventional radiology, surgery, and electronic prosthetics

clinical decision-support systems (CDSS)—computer programs (also called expert systems) that help health care professionals in making diagnoses by analyzing patient data

clinical information system (CIS)—uses computers to manage clinical information

clinical pharmacology—a database of the latest drug information

CMS-1500—the most widely accepted claim form (formerly called HCFA-1500)

code of conduct—internal company policy that attempts to safeguard information and guarantee privacy

communications software—application software that allows the connection of one computer to other computers

Composite International Diagnostic Interview (CIDI)—a tool for diagnosing mental disorders

Composite International Diagnostic Interview-Auto—a computerized version of CIDI; can be self-administered

computer—an electronic device that can accept data (raw facts) as input, process or alter them in some way, and produce useful information as output

computer information systems—used in some hospitals and other health care facilities to help manage and organize relevant patient, financial, pharmacy, laboratory, and radiological information

computer literacy—familiarity with and knowledge about computers, the Internet, and the World Wide Web; the ability to use computers to perform tasks in one's own field

computer-assisted surgery—makes use of computers, robotic devices, and/or computer-generated images in the planning and carrying out of surgical procedures

computer-assisted trial design—software that allows the simulation of clinical drug trials before the actual trials begin

computerized functional electrical stimulation (CFES or FES)—a technique involving the use of low-level electrical stimulation; has been used for many years in pacemakers and other implanted devices; now used to strengthen paralyzed muscles with simulated exercise; low-level electrical stimulation is applied directly to muscles that cannot receive these signals from the brain because of spinal cord injury

computerized medical instruments—contain microprocessors and provide direct patient services such as monitoring, administering medication, or treatment

computerized tomography (CT)—an imaging technique that involves taking a series of X-rays at different angles from which the computer constructs a cross-sectional image

connectivity—the fact that computers can be connected to each other

control unit—the part of the central processing unit that controls processing following the instructions of a program; it directs the movement of electronic signals between parts of the computer

cookies—small programs put on a user's hard drive every time a Web site is visited

co-payment—the part of the charge for which the patient is responsible

corneal topography—uses a computer to create an accurate three-dimensional map of the cornea, so the health care professional can see the shape and power of the cornea

cosmetic dentistry—attempts to create a more attractive smile

Cumulative Index to Nursing and Allied Health Literature (CINAHL)—a database specifically geared to the needs of nurses and other professionals in seventeen allied health fields, including dental hygiene, occupational therapy, and radiology; includes an index of 1,000 journals from 1982 to the present, bibliographic citations of books, pamphlets, software, and standards of practice, abstracts or full text of articles where they are available, journals and descriptions of Web sites of interest

current procedural terminology (CPT)—codes laboratory tests, treatments, and other procedures

cyber knife—a device that compensates for patient movement and can be used to treat brain and spinal tumors with radiosurgery

da Vinci®—robot (Intuitive Surgical, Inc.) was first cleared for assisting in surgery in 1997, for performing some surgeries in 2000, and for performing cardiac surgery, such as mitral valve repair in November 2002. It performs minimally invasive surgeries

data accuracy—correctness and currency of information

Databank for Cardiovascular Disease—at Duke University, a highly specialized expert system that combines computer monitoring with extensive collections of information on cardiac patients

database—a large organized collection of information that is easy to maintain, search, and sort

database management system (DBMS)—application software that allows the user to enter organized lists of data and easily edit, sort, and search them

deductible—a certain amount the patient is required to pay each year before the health insurance begins paying

demineralize—deterioration of the enamel of the teeth caused by acids

dental implants—used to replace missing teeth; computers help plan the exact placement of the implant

dental informatics—combines computer technology with dentistry to create a basis for research, education, and the solution of real-world problems in oral health care using computer applications

DentSim—a program that uses virtual reality. Its purpose is to teach technical dexterity to dental students. A small pilot study has been completed

diagnostic-related group (DRG)—code used for diagnosis; hospital reimbursement by insurers is based on a formula using DRGs

DICOM (digital imaging and communications in medicine)—the standard communication protocols of imaging devices are called DICOM

diffusion tensor imaging (DTI)—a new MRI-related imaging technique; it shows the white matter of the brain, the connections between parts of the brain, so that these are not damaged during surgery

DIFOTI® (Digital Imaging Fiber-Optic Transillumination)—involves using a digital camera to obtain images of teeth illuminated with laser light. The images are analyzed using computer algorithms

digitize—to translate into zeroes and ones that the computer can understand

digitizing tablet—a direct-entry input device, pointing device; the user works on a tablet on the desk (instead of directly on the screen) with a stylus

direct access storage device—a secondary storage device that allows reading from or writing to any part of the storage medium (disk)

direct-entry devices—input devices including scanning and pointing devices and sensors

disk drive—storage device in which a medium (disk) is inserted; the drive includes a motor to spin the disk and a read/write head that reads data from or writes it to the disk

distance surgery—(telepresence surgery) surgery performed by robotic devices controlled by surgeons at another site

DNA (deoxyribonucleic acid)—a nucleic acid molecule containing genetic instructions for living things

dual X-ray absorptiometry (DEXA) scan—a special kind of low-radiation X-ray that shows changes in the rays' intensity after passing through bone. Doctors can see small changes in bone density from the amount of change in the X-ray

DVD disk—optical medium with enormous storage capacity (several gigabytes)

Ebola virus—first identified in Zaire in 1976. The same disease appeared in Sudan. It has been seen in the United States in monkeys, but no human cases are known to have occurred here. Very little is known about the disease. It appears only sporadically

electrical conductance—currently used to diagnose cavities. An electric current is passed through a tooth, and the tooth's resistance is measured. A decayed tooth has a different resistance reading than a healthy tooth

Electronic Communications Privacy Act of 1986—prohibits government agencies from intercepting electronic communications without a search warrant. It also prohibits individuals from intercepting e-mail. However, there are numerous exceptions, and the courts have interpreted this to allow employers to access employees' e-mail. This law does not apply to communications within an organization

electronic dental chart—dental chart in an electronic form; standardized, easy to search, and easy to read. It will integrate practice management tasks (administrative applications) with clinical information

electronic health record (EHR)—electronic record of patient health information generated by one or more encounters in any care delivery setting

electronic medical record (EMR)—in a computerized office, the information that was gathered and entered onto a patient information form will then be entered into a computer into electronic medical records. This will form the patient's medical record

electronic remittance advice (ERA)—accompanies the response to an electronic claim to an insurance company

electronic spreadsheet—application software that allows the user to store and manipulate numbers

embedded computer—a single-purpose computer on a chip of silicon, which is embedded in anything from appliances to humans. An embedded computer may help run your car, microwave, pacemaker, or watch

encounter form (superbill)—list of diagnoses and procedures common to a practice

encryption—used to protect information from unauthorized users; involves encoding of messages

endodontics—dental specialty that diagnoses and treats diseases of the pulp

endoluminal surgery—one form of minimally invasive robotic surgery is called endoluminal

surgery. Endoluminal surgery does not require incisions. It is also called natural orifice surgery

endoscope—a thin tube with a light source that either allows a direct view into the body or is connected to a minuscule camera that projects an image of the surgical site onto a monitor

environmental control system (ECS)—hardware and software that help physically challenged people control their environments

EOB (explanation of benefits)—the response of an insurance company to a paper claim includes an explanation of benefits (EOB), which explains why certain services were covered and others not

epidemic—an excess in the number of cases of a given health problem

epidemiology—the study of diseases in populations by collecting and analyzing statistical data

e-prescribing (electronic prescribing)—the use of computers and software to enter prescriptions and send them to pharmacies electronically

expansion boards—circuit boards that are plugged into the expansion slots on the main circuit board; they include the electronic circuitry needed by add-on hardware

expansion slots—slots in the main circuit board that allow expansion boards to be inserted

expert system—a program that attempts to make computers mimic human expertise in limited fields; uses a database of numerous facts and rules about how decisions are made; also called decision support system

EXPERTMD—software that allows the creation of medical and dental expert systems

Explorable Virtual Human—will include authoring tools that engineers can use to build anatomical models that will allow students to experience how real anatomical structures feel, appear, and sound

extranet—a corporate intranet connected to other intranets outside the corporation

EYESI surgical simulator—allows doctors to learn new surgical skills and techniques for eye surgery

facial structure scan—a biometric method that identifies users by facial structure

facial thermography—a biometric method that identifies users by the heat generated by their faces

Fair Credit Reporting Act of 1970—a federal law that regulates credit agencies; it allows you to see your credit reports to check the accuracy of information and to challenge inaccuracies

fax machine—a direct-entry input device, scanning device; scans the text or image and converts it to electronic signals that are sent over telephone lines; the receiving fax machine converts it back into text and images

fee-for-service plans—health insurance plans that are not restricted to a network of providers; they do not need referrals to specialists

fetal monitor—measures fetal heart rate

fiber optic camera—analogous to the endoscope used in surgery. It is used to view an area of the mouth that is normally difficult to see

fiber-optic transillumination—finds early lesions (affecting enamel) but is limited in diagnosing advanced caries

field—each record in a table is made up of related fields. One field holds one piece of information, such as a patient's last name, or Social Security number, or chart number

file—a practice can store all of its data and information in a database file stored on a computer. Within the file, there can be several tables

financial information system (FIS)—is concerned with the financial details of running a hospital

fingerprint—biometric method of identification

firewall—software used to protect LANs from unauthorized access through the Internet

firmware—a computer program that is embedded in a hardware device

focused ultrasound surgery—in the early experimental stages; uses sound waves to raise the temperature of cancerous tissue until it dies; also being examined as a way to stop massive bleeding

Food and Drug Administration (FDA)—federal agency in the Department of Health and Human Services in charge of reviewing, approving, and regulating the purity of food and the safety and effectiveness of drugs

fraud—includes such crimes as using a computer program to illegally transfer money from one bank account to another or printing payroll checks to oneself

fraudulent dialer—can connect the user with numbers without the user's knowledge; the dialer may connect the user's computer to an expensive 900 number. The user will be totally unaware until he or she receives the telephone bill

functional electrical stimulation (FES or CFES)—see computerized functional electrical stimulation

functional MRI (fMRI)—measures small metabolic changes in an active part of the brain. fMRI identifies brain activity by changes in blood oxygen

gamma knife—bloodless surgical device; works by delivering 201 focused beams of radiation directly at a brain tumor, killing the tumor and sparing the surrounding tissue

gamma knife surgery—bloodless surgery using a gamma knife

GDx Access—uses an infrared laser to measure the thickness of the retinal nerve fiber. It is used for the early detection of glaucoma

global warming—our planet is warming, and we are helping to make it happen by adding more heat-trapping gases, primarily carbon dioxide (CO_2), to the atmosphere. Global warming is already having a devastating effect on the earth and on human health: more intense heat waves lead to more heat-related deaths. Asthma and eczema in children and adults have been linked to global warming

graphical user interface (GUI)—an operating environment or interface used by Windows and Macintosh OS that allows users to interact with the computer by clicking on icons with a mouse

guarantor—the person responsible for payment of a medical bill; it may be the patient or a third party

hacker—a proficient computer user without authorized access to systems

hand print—biometric method of identification used to restrict access to computers

hard copy—printed output

hardware—the physical components of a computer

HCFA-1500 (CMS-1500)—the most commonly accepted claim form

head mouse—input device that moves the cursor according to the user's head motions

Health Care Financing Administration (HCFA) (now CMS)—administers government health plans

Health Insurance Portability and Accountability Act (HIPAA)—in 1996, Congress passed the Health Insurance Portability and Accountability Act (HIPAA). Guidelines to protect electronic medical records were developed by the Department of Health and Human Services. By encouraging the use of the electronic medical record and facilitating the sharing of medical records among health care providers, it can assure continuity of care and thus save lives

health maintenance organization (HMO)—a patient who uses a health maintenance organization (HMO) pays a fixed yearly fee and must choose among an approved network of health care providers and hospitals

Healthfinder—a listing of "sites 'hand-picked' . . . by health professionals"

Heidelberg retinal tomograph (HRT)—uses lasers to scan the retina resulting in a three-dimensional description. This technique can detect glaucoma before any loss of vision

HELEN (HELp Neuropsychology)—a computerized program that contains diagnostic analyses that keep track of specific tests and tasks performed by the stroke patient

HERMES—an FDA-cleared computer operating system that controls all the electronic equipment in the operating room, coordinating the endoscope and robotic devices

HIV (human immunodeficiency virus)—the virus that causes AIDS

Homeland Security Act—expands and centralizes the data gathering allowed under the Patriot Act

hospital information system (HIS)—attempts to integrate the administrative and clinical functions in a hospital. Ideally, the HIS includes clinical information systems, financial information systems, laboratory information systems, nursing and pharmacy information systems, and picture archiving and communication systems and radiology information systems

Human Genome Project (HGP)—international project (begun in 1990) seeking to understand the human genetic makeup; to find the location of the 100,000 or so human genes and to read the entire genetic script, all three billion bits of information, by the year 2005

human patient simulators (HPS)—programmable mannequins on which students can practice medical and dental procedures

human-biology input device—uses sensors to interpret body movements and characteristics, allowing the user's body to be used as an input device

identity theft—involves someone using your private information to assume your identity

iHealth Record—a personal medical record that the patient can create and maintain at no cost. It is available at some doctors' offices

ILIAD—a program that provides hypothetical cases for the student to evaluate. The student's diagnostic abilities are then compared to the computer's

image scanner—a direct-entry input device, scanning device; can scan whole pages of graphics and text and digitize them so that the computer can process them

image-guided (or directed) surgery—surgery guided by computer-generated images of the surgical field, not a direct view

indemnity plan—fee-for-service health insurance plan

information technology (IT)—includes computers, communications networks, and computer literacy

Innova—can image fine vessels and cardiovascular anatomy, producing three-dimensional images of the vascular system, bone and soft tissue

input device—a device that translates data into a form the computer can process (bits)

input/output device—a device that contains a monitor for output and a keyboard for input

interactive videoconferencing—(teleconferencing) allows doctors and patients to consult in real time, at a distance

International Classification of Disease (ICD-9-CM)—codes 1,000 diseases

Internet (interconnected network)—a global network of networks, connecting innumerable smaller networks, computers, and users

INTERNIST—medical expert system used as decision-support system to help in diagnosis

interoperability—the connection of people and diverse computer systems

interventional radiology—the use of the tools of radiology to treat conditions that once required surgery

intranet—a private corporate network that uses the same structure as the Internet and the same TCP/IP protocols

intra-oral fiber optic camera—allows both patient and dentist to get a close-up tour of the patient's mouth. A fiber optic device is aimed at an area of the patient's mouth, and the image appears on the screen

iris scan—a biometric method of identification used to restrict access to computers

key field—uniquely identifies each record in a table

keyboard—an input device

keylogging—can be used by anyone to track anyone else's keystrokes

KISMET—simulation software used in surgery

Kurzweil scanner—a direct-entry input device, scanning device, also an output device; scans printed text and reads it aloud to the user

laboratory information systems (LIS)—use computers to manage both laboratory tests and their results

LAN (local area network)—a small private network that spans a room or building

laparoscope—endoscope used for abdominal surgery

laser (light amplification by stimulated emission of radiation)—delivers light energy. There are several uses of lasers in dentistry. Low-level lasers can find pits in tooth enamel that may become cavities. The FDA has approved laser machines for drilling and filling cavities; lasers also reduce the bacteria in the cavity; lasers are also used in surgery

light illumination—several methods use light to help diagnose tooth disease. To find decay, a bright light is used to illuminate the tooth, revealing color differences

light pen—direct-entry input device, pointing device; allows the use of a pen-like device to identify exact points to draw on the screen

line-of-sight system—allows you to use your body as an input device; the user's eyes can point to a part of the screen; a camera and computer can identify the area you are looking at

lip print—biometric method of identification used to restrict access to computers

local area network (LAN)—small private network

LOINC (Logical Observation Identifiers, Names, and Codes)—standardizes laboratory and clinical codes

LUMA Cervical Imaging System—helps detect cervical cancer

mad cow disease—or "[b]ovine spongiform encephalopathy (BSE) is a progressive neurological disorder of cattle that results from infection . . ."

magnetic disk—storage medium that stores data as magnetic spots

magnetic ink character recognition (MICR)—technology used only by banks to read the magnetic ink characters at the bottoms of checks

magnetic resonance imaging (MRI)—an imaging technique that uses computer technology to produce images of soft tissue within the body that could not be pictured by traditional X-rays; can produce images of the insides of bones; uses computers and a very strong magnetic field and radio waves to generate mathematical data from which an image is constructed

Magnetic tape—sequential access storage medium; magnetic tape was widely used as secondary storage in the 1950s and 1960s; now used mainly for backup and archives

main circuit board—motherboard

mainframe—large, fast computer designed for multiple users; used for input/output intensive tasks

malware—includes different forms of malicious hardware, software, and firmware

managed care—a type of health insurance that requires the patient to choose among a network of providers

MEDCIN—provides 250,000 codes for such things as symptoms, patient history, physical examinations, tests, diagnoses, and treatments. MEDCIN codes can be integrated with other coding systems

Medicaid—jointly funded, federal-state health insurance for certain low-income and needy people

medical informatics—the use of computers and computer technology in health care and its delivery

Medical Information Bureau—composed of 650 insurance companies. Its database contains health histories of fifteen million people; used by medical insurers to help determine insurance rates and whether to grant or deny someone medical coverage; not protected by doctor–patient privilege and, at present, not protected by any federal law; may be available to your employer without your consent

Medicare—a government plan that serves people aged 65 years and over and disabled people with chronic renal disorders

MEDI-SPAN—a database of information on drug/drug interactions and drug/food interactions

MEDLARS (Medical Literature Analysis and Retrieval System)—a collection of forty computerized databases containing eighteen million references, available free via the

Internet; can be searched for bibliographical lists or for information

MEDLINE—a comprehensive online database of current medical research including publications from 1966 to the present; it contains 8.5 million articles from 3,700 journals; 31,000 citations are added each month

memory—temporary storage area used during processing; internal storage made up of RAM and ROM

microcomputer—personal computer (PC), designed for use by one person at a time

microdialysis—a technique that attempts to look at the body's response to an implant at the cellular level

microprocessor—a tiny computer on a chip; contains millions of miniaturized transistors

MIDAS (models of infectious disease agent study)—a collaboration of research and informatics groups to develop computational models of the interactions between infectious agents and their hosts, disease spread, prediction systems, and response strategies, according to the NIH

MINERVA—a robot developed to perform stereotactic neurosurgical procedures

minicomputer—a smaller, less expensive version of the mainframe; designed for multiple users

minimally invasive dentistry—emphasizes prevention and the least possible intervention

minimally invasive surgery (MIS)—surgery performed through small incisions

monitor—screen

motherboard—main circuit board of the computer

motion monitor—a real-time computer-based system which objectively measures joint motion in a patient for a therapist

mouse—a direct-entry input device, pointing device; used to select items from a menu and position the insertion point

MYCIN—an expert system used as a decision-support system to help in the diagnosis and treatment of bacterial infections

myoelectric limbs—artificial limbs containing motors and responding to the electrical signals transmitted by the residual limb to electrodes mounted in the socket

nanotechnology—A nanometer is one-billionth of a meter. Nanotechnology works with miniscule materials the size of atoms and molecules. It holds promise for regenerative medicine

national drug codes (NDC)—developed by the FDA, it identifies drugs

National Health Information Network (NHIN)—the infrastructure that would allow communication between RHIOs

NEDSS initiative—the National Electronic Disease Surveillance System (part of the Public Health Information Network) will promote "integrated surveillance systems that can transfer . . . public health, laboratory and clinical data . . . over the Internet." This would be a national electronic surveillance system that would allow epidemics to be identified quickly

NEEMO (NASA Extreme Environment Mission Operation)—a series of NASA missions in which groups of scientists live in Aquarius

neonatal monitor—monitors infant heart and breathing rates

network—computers and other hardware devices linked together via communications media

Neuromove—for stroke patients; helps to stimulate the muscles to avoid atrophy and increases both the range of motion and blood circulation

neuroprosthesis—in 2006, a new implantable device using FES—a neuroprosthesis—was developed. It uses "low levels of electricity in order to activate nerves and muscles in order to restore movement"

New Medicines in Development—a database that provides information on newly approved drugs and drugs awaiting approval

nursing information systems (NIS)—are supposed to improve nursing care by using computers to manage charting, staff scheduling, and the integration of clinical information

open architecture—computer design that allows hardware devices to be added by plugging expansion boards into expansion slots on the main circuit board

operating system—the system software that controls the basic operation of the computer hardware, managing the resources of the computer including input and output, the execution of programs, and processor time; provides the user interface

optical biometry—in cataract surgery, the eye's lens is replaced by an intra-ocular lens (IOL). The measurements used to determine which IOL to use are determined by calculations referred to as optical biometry

optical card—holds about 2,000 pages of data

optical character recognition (OCR)—direct-entry input device, scanning device; reads printed characters

optical disk—secondary storage device on which data are represented by pits and lands burnt in by a laser

optical mark recognition (OMR)—direct-entry input device, scanning device; reads marks on paper

Optomap Panoramic200—can examine the retina without dilation using low-powered red and green lasers

osseointegration—a technology that allows the integration of living bone with titanium implants

output devices—hardware that presents information in a form a human user can comprehend

page scanner—a direct-entry input device that digitizes printed text

pandemic—a global disease outbreak to which everyone is susceptible

password—a secret code assigned to (or chosen by) an authorized user

patient aging report—used to show a patient's outstanding payments

patient day sheet—lists the day's patients, chart numbers, and transactions

payment day sheet—a grouped report organized by providers

payments—made by a patient or an insurance carrier to the practice

PDUFA (Prescription Drug User Fees Act)—requires drug companies to pay fees to support the drug review process

PediaSim—a programmable human patient simulator of a child used for teaching purposes

pen-based system—direct-entry input device, pointing device; allows handwritten input

periodontics—concerned with diagnosing and treating diseases of the gums and other structures supporting the teeth. Periodontal disease is caused by bacteria

personal computer (PC)—microcomputer

personal digital assistant (PDA)—hand-held computer

personal identification number (PIN)—a secret code assigned to (or chosen by) an authorized user

pharmacy information systems (PIS)—monitor drug allergies and interactions and fill and track prescriptions. They also track inventory and create patient drug profiles

physiological monitoring systems—monitor physiological processes; analyze blood and other fluids

Physiome Project—project attempting to develop accurate and complete human physiological models, which may in the future be used as simulated patients in drug trials

picture archiving and communication systems (PACS)—manage digital images. Digital images are immediately available on the monitor and can be shared over a network

PLATO (Programmed Logic for Automatic Teaching Operations)—an early (1960s) simulation program for nurses

plotter—output device that produces hard copy; used for graphics, such as maps and architectural drawings

pointing devices—input devices including the mouse, trackball, light pen, and touch screen

polio—a contagious virus that can cause paralysis and even death. It became very rare in the United States in the second half of the twentieth century

port—socket, usually on the back of the computer

positron emission tomography (PET)—an imaging technique that uses radioisotope technology to create a picture of the body "in action"; uses computers to construct images from the emission of positive electrons (positrons) by radioactive substances administered to the patient

Post Operative Expert Medical System (POEMS)—an expert system that focuses on patients who become sick while recovering from surgery

practice—a group of health care practitioners in business together

practice analysis report—generated on a monthly basis; a summary total of all procedures, charges, and transactions

preferred provider organization (PPO)—a patient with PPO insurance can seek care within an approved network of health care providers who have agreed with the insurance company to lower their charges and accept assignment

printer—output device that produces hard copy

privacy—the ability to control personal information and the right to keep it from misuse

procedure day sheet—a grouped report organized by procedure

processor (system unit)—contains the CPU and memory; does the actual manipulation of data

program—step-by-step instructions; also called software

prosthetic devices—replacement limbs and organs

protocols—technical standards governing communication between computers

public health—is where the largest numbers of lives are saved, usually by understanding the epidemiology of a disease—its patterns, where and how it emerges and spreads—and attacking it at its weak points. This can lead to prevention by means of public health measures like better sanitation or providing cleaner water. It can also lead to the development and widespread distribution of vaccinations

public health informatics—supports public health practice and research with information technology

PubMed—search engine for Medline

puff straw—an input device that allows people to control the mouse with their mouths

pulmonary monitor—measures blood flow through the heart and respiratory rate

radiology information systems (RIS)—manage patients in the radiology department including scheduling appointments, tracking film, and reporting results

random-access memory (RAM)—the part of temporary, volatile internal storage that holds the work you are currently doing while you are doing it, including the program and data you are using; the operating system must be in RAM for other programs to run

rational drug design—a technique that utilizes computers to model molecules and develop chemical compounds that will bind to the target molecule and inhibit or stimulate it; used in the development of drugs that are used for Alzheimer's, hypertension, and AIDS

Raven—a 50-pound, mobile surgical robot used on NEEMO

read-only memory (ROM)—part of internal memory; firmware; permanent instructions that the user normally cannot change

Real ID Act of 2005—"directly imposes prescriptive federal driver's license standards" by the federal government on the states. This law requires every American to have an electronic identification card

record—a table is made up of related records; each record holds all the information on one item in the table

regional health information organizations (RHIOs)—regional cooperation is being fostered through the establishment of regional health information organizations (RHIOs) in which data could be shared within a region

relational database—organized collection of related data

remineralize—repair damage to the tooth's enamel using phosphate and fluoride

remote monitoring device—transmits signals over communications lines, making it possible for patients to be monitored at home or in ambulances

retina scan—a biometric method of identifying users

RFID tag—radio frequency identification tags are becoming more and more common. RFID tags can be incorporated into products; they receive and send a wireless signal

ribonucleic acid (RNA)—made in the nucleus of a cell, but not restricted to the nucleus. It is a long coiled-up molecule whose purpose is to take the blueprint from DNA and build our actual proteins

RNA interference (RNAi)—a new technology aimed at drug development

ROBODOC—a computer-controlled, image-directed robot used in hip-replacement surgery

robot—a programmable machine that can manipulate its environment

SARS—sudden acute respiratory disease appeared in 2002, first in China. The epidemic was caused by the corona virus

SATELLIFE—founded in 1989, its purpose was to deliver journals and other information to health care workers in developing areas

scanning devices—direct-entry input devices; include fax machines, optical character recognition, optical mark recognition, magnetic ink character recognition, image scanners

schedule of benefits—a list of those services that the insurance carrier will cover

scientific visualization—the process of graphically representing the results of numerical calculations

screen reader software—used with page scanners and synthesizers, tells the speech synthesizer what to say, for example, to read the text description of an icon

SDILINE (Selective Dissemination of Information Online)—contains only the latest month's additions to MEDLINE

search engine—software that allows you to search the Web

secondary storage devices—include disk drives and tape drives that, with their media, allow the more permanent storage of data, programs, and information than primary storage

secondary storage media—include disks and tape, which provide more permanent storage than random-access memory

security—measures attempting to protect computer systems (including hardware, software, and information), from harm and abuse; the threats may stem from many sources including natural disaster, human error, or crime

sensor—a direct-entry input device that collects data directly from the environment and sends it to a computer; used to collect patient information for clinical monitoring systems

simulation software—software that attempts to recreate a real situations

simulations—computers can create what-if scenarios or simulations of what would happen to an infectious disease if something else happened

smart card—includes a microprocessor and memory and holds about thirty pages of data; used as a debit card

smart glasses—glasses developed at the University of Arizona that will soon be able to automatically change focus

SNOMED (Systematized Nomenclature of Medicine)—"provides a common language that enables a consistent way of capturing, sharing, and aggregating health data . . ."

SOCRATES—system that allows long-distance mentoring of surgeons in real time

soft copy—output on a monitor or voice output

SoftScanR—is now in clinical trials. It is meant to be a diagnostic tool which will complement mammography

software—(programs), the step-by-step instructions that tell the computer what to do

software piracy—unauthorized copying of copyrighted software

solid state memory devices—include flash memory cards used in notebooks, memory sticks, and very compact key chain devices; they have no moving parts, are very small, and have a high capacity. USB flash drives have a huge capacity for information

special-purpose application—the use of information technology for applications not included in clinical or administrative applications, such as drug design and education

SPECT (single-photon emission computed tomography)—an imaging technique that, like the PET scan, shows movement; less precise and less expensive than PET

speech synthesizer—a device with a processor, memory, and output capability, which turns digital data into speech-like sounds, allowing the computer to talk

Spybot Search and Destroy software—can remove malware, adware, spyware, fraudulent dialers, and keyloggers from your computer

spyware—software that can be installed without the user's knowledge to track their actions on a computer

Starbright World—a network linking seriously ill children in one hundred hospitals in the United States (1998); children in the networked hospitals can play games, chat, send and receive e-mail, and receive medical information

stem cells—cells that can develop into different types of body cells; theoretically, they can repair the body. As a stem cell divides, the new cells can stay a stem cell or become another kind of cell

stereotactic radiosurgery—gamma knife surgery; used to treat brain tumors

store-and-forward technology—technique in which the data to be sent is digitized, stored, and transmitted over a telecommunications network

superbill—encounter form

supercomputer—the fastest, largest, most expensive computer at any time; used for complex processor-intensive, scientific tasks such as weather forecasting and weapons research

syndromic surveillance—uses health-related data that precede diagnosis and signal a sufficient probability of a case or an outbreak

system software—programs that control hardware operations and interact between the applications and the computer; includes the operating system, utility programs, and language translators

system unit—processor, contains the CPU and memory

table—in a relational database, each table holds related information

telecommunications network—network using telephone lines as media

teleconferencing—may involve anything from a conference call to a meeting between people who are not in the same place, but who can see and hear each other via video and audio equipment. It may also involve sharing documents on monitors and being able to work on them cooperatively

teledentistry—programs to help dentists access specialists in order to improve patient care

teledermatology—the practice of dermatology using telecommunications networks

telehealth—includes telemedicine and other health-related activities using telecommunications lines and computers, including education, research, public health, and administration of health services

telehome care—involves the monitoring of vital signs from a distance via telecommunications equipment and the replacement of home nursing visits with videoconferences

telemedicine—the delivery of health care over telecommunications lines

teleneurology—neurology was slower to use telemedicine than other specialties. Now, however, email and videoconferencing are replacing the letter and telephone call. One of the first subspecialties to use telemedicine in neurology is stroke diagnosis

telenurse—telenursing involves teletriage and the telecommunication of health-related

data, the remote house call, and the monitoring of chronic disease

teleoncology—use of telemedicine to treat cancer

telepathology—the transmission of microscopic images over telecommunications lines

telepharmacy—the linking of the prescribing doctor's office with the dispensing pharmacy via telecommunications lines

telepresence surgery—see distance surgery

telepsychiatry—the delivery of therapy using telecommunications lines

teleradiology—the sending of radiological images in digital form over telecommunications lines

telespirometry—monitoring system used by asthmatic patients; it is designed to transmit over the telephone to a remote location

telestroke—a program that connects small local hospitals with stroke experts. When a stroke victim appears at the local hospital, the doctors do CT scans and forward them to stroke specialists

teletriage—telemedicine application in which calls are screened and directed to the proper services

theft of information—unauthorized access to and use of information

theft of services—unauthorized use of services such as cable TV

tonometers—measure eye pressure

touch screen—a direct-entry input device, pointing device; a screen that can receive input through touch; used at ATMs, in airports, in stores, in restaurants, and in kiosks in malls

Tracey visual function analyzer—measures how well you can see by measuring how your eye focuses light. These data help in surgical or laser vision correction. Computers are also used to custom design contact lenses

transactions—charges, payments, and adjustments

transmission control protocol/Internet protocol (TCP/IP)—the protocols that govern the Internet

TRICARE—the U.S. health program for armed service members and their families

ultrafast CT—a variation of the traditional CT scan; may be used in place of a coronary angiogram to examine coronary artery blockages. Compared to a coronary angiogram, the ultrafast CT is painless, less dangerous, noninvasive, and less expensive

ultrasound—an imaging technique that uses no radiation; uses very high-frequency sound waves and the echoes they produce when they hit an object to generate information that is used by a computer to create a two-dimensional moving image on a screen; used to examine a moving fetus, to study blood flow, and to diagnose gallstones and prostate disease

uniform resource locator (URL)—address of a Web page

universal product code (UPC)—or bar code that appears on products for sale

USA Patriot Act (2001)—gives law-enforcement agencies greater power to monitor electronic and other communications, with fewer checks

user interface (operating environment)—defines how the user communicates with the computer

vaccination—protects people against infection

verichip—radio transmitters that give off a unique signal, which can be read by a receiver

Vesalius Project—a project that is creating models of anatomical regions and structures to be used in teaching anatomy

virtual environment—technology used to provide surgeons with realistic accurate models on which to teach surgery and plan and practice operations

Virtual Hospital—a comprehensive and authoritative Web site maintained by the University of Iowa. Its information (available for patients and health care providers) comes from 350 peer-reviewed sources

Virtual Human Embryo—a project that is digitizing some of the 7,000 human embryos lost in miscarriages, which have been kept by the National Museum of Health and Medicine of the Armed Forces Institute of Pathology since the 1880s

virtual reality (VR)—technology that allows the computer to create an environment that seems real, but is not; used in planning and teaching surgical and other procedures

virus—a program, attached to another file, which replicates itself and may do damage to your computer system

Visible Human Project—a computerized library of human anatomy at the National Library of Medicine, seeking to create accurate, three-dimensional representations of the male and female body. The project began in the late 1980s. It now contains images of 1,800 cross-sections of a male cadaver (39 years old) and 5,000 of a female cadaver (59 years old) stored in a computer and accessible over the Internet

vision input—input via a digital camera

vision replacement therapy (VRT)—retrains the brain. Using dots on a computer screen, the aim is to stimulate peripheral vision. This therapy can be effective years after the stroke occurred

Web browser—software needed to browse the Web

Web page—(page) Web site

Web site—files in which information on the Web is stored

West Nile virus—first appeared in the 1930s. It is a form of encephalitis or brain inflammation. It cycles between mosquitoes and birds. Infected birds will infect mosquitoes. Mosquitoes can spread the disease to humans. It can be diagnosed by MRIs

what-if scenarios—computers can create what-if scenarios or simulations of what would happen to an infectious disease if something else happened

WHO (World Health Organization)—the directing and coordinating authority for health within the United Nations system

WHONET—an information system developed to support the World Health Organization's (WHO) goal of global surveillance of bacterial resistance to antimicrobial agents

wide area network (WAN)—a network that may span a state, country, or even the world

Wi-Fi—a wireless technology that allows you to connect a PDA (and other devices), to a network (including the Internet), if you are close enough to a Wi-Fi access point

word processing software—application software that allows the user to create, edit, format, save, retrieve, and print text documents

worker's compensation—a government program, which covers job-related illness or injury

World Wide Web (Web or WWW)—the part of the Internet that is most accessible and easiest to navigate, organized as sites with hyperlinks to one another

X-ray—a traditional imaging technique that uses high-energy electromagnetic waves to produce a two-dimensional picture on film; does not produce good images of all organs and cannot see behind bones

ZEUS—a robotic surgical system that will make possible minimally invasive microsurgery; has three interactive robotic arms, one of which holds the endoscope, whereas the other two manipulate the surgical instruments; the surgeon, sitting at a console, controls them; includes a feedback system so that the surgeon "feels" the tissue

Index